Nature Cures

Also by James C. Whorton

Crusaders for Fitness: A History of American Health Reformers
Inner Hygiene: Constipation and the Pursuit of Health in Modern Society

Nature Cures

The History of Alternative Medicine in America

James C. Whorton

OXFORD
UNIVERSITY PRESS
2002

OXFORD
UNIVERSITY PRESS

Oxford   New York
Auckland   Bangkok   Buenos Aires   Cape Town   Chennai
Dar es Salaam   Delhi   Hong Kong   Istanbul   Karachi   Kolkata
Kuala Lumpur   Madrid   Melbourne   Mexico City   Mumbai   Nairobi
São Paulo   Shanghai   Singapore   Taipei   Tokyo   Toronto

and an associated company in Berlin

Copyright © 2002 by Oxford University Press, Inc.

Published by Oxford University Press, Inc.
198 Madison Avenue, New York, New York 10016

www.oup.com

Library of Congress Cataloging-in-Publication Data

Whorton, James C., 1942–
Nature cures : the history of alternative medicine
in America / James C. Whorton.
p.   cm. Includes bibliographical references and index.
ISBN 0-19-514071-0
1. Alternative medicine—United States—History.   2. Alternative
medicine—United States—History—20th century.
I. Title.

R733.W495   2002   615.5'0973—dc21   2002022023

1 3 5 7 9 8 6 4 2

Printed in the United States of America
on acid-free paper

For Jackie

Contents

Preface

I n the autumn of 1994, a *New Yorker* cartoonist imagined a clinical scene in which a patient who is literally radiant with health, his body throwing off a nearly blinding aura of wellness, is nevertheless being sternly admonished by his physician because he has achieved his health the wrong way: "You've been fooling around with alternative medicines, haven't you?" the doctor scolds.[1]

New Yorker cartoons constitute the most sensitive of barometers to shifting currents in America's cultural atmosphere. And in truth, whatever one chooses to call it—alternative medicine, unconventional medicine, holistic medicine, complementary medicine, integrative medicine (some even like the term vernacular medicine)—a lot of people have been fooling around with unorthodox forms of therapy in recent years. In a now legendary survey published in 1993, Harvard's David Eisenberg reported that one in three Americans had used one or more forms of alternative medicine in 1990, and expressed surprise at the "enormous presence" of healing alternatives in American society. When Eisenberg and colleagues repeated the survey in 1997, furthermore, they found that "alternative medicine use and expenditures have increased dramatically" since the first study: now 40 percent of the population employed such procedures.[2]

That alternative methods were so widespread in the presumably enlightened 1990s was a startling realization for the medical profession. It shouldn't have been, for there's nothing at all new in the current enthusiasm for unconventional therapies. Comparable levels of support have been the norm for most of the last two centuries: Americans, in short, have been fooling around with alternative medicine for a long time.

That such activity has been mere foolishness has been the opinion, of course, of orthodox practitioners. From the start, MDs have scorned alternative systems of treatment as a grab-bag of inert (when not dangerous) therapies foisted upon gullible hypochondriacs by scientifically uncritical quacks. Alternative doctors, Spalding Gray has joked on behalf of physicians, believe that "*everything* gives you cancer," but there's no need to worry, because they also believe that "everything else heals you of it." (The emphasis is Gray's; italicized words in quoted passages throughout this book were italicized in the original.)[3]

Yet in just the few years since the publication of that *New Yorker* cartoon, mainstream medicine's historic disdain for alternative medicine has softened remarkably. The decision by the U.S. Congress in 1991 to establish an Office of Alternative Medicine at the National Institutes of Health was, to be sure, a political act, and one that enraged many MDs. Nevertheless, the founding of the OAM, followed by Eisenberg's study (1993), the opening of the first publicly funded natural medicine clinic in the country (King County, Washington, 1996), and other revelations of public support for non-standard therapies forced physicians to pay closer attention to their alternative counterparts. At first, attention was motivated primarily by the recognition that practitioners needed to know more about unconventional systems of care in order to engage their alternatively inclined patients in open discussion of their habit (in contrast to shaming them in the manner of the cartoon physician). Eisenberg had found in 1990 that 72 percent of patients who received treatment from unconventional practitioners did not inform their medical doctor of that fact, suggesting "a deficiency in current patient-doctor relations" that could be harmful to patients. To remedy the deficiency, Eisenberg urged that physicians begin to ask patients about their use of alternative therapies and that medical schools introduce instruction on alternative medicine into their curricula. Since then, more than half the medical schools in the country have established courses on unconventional medicine, and the remainder seem likely to follow.[4]

In the process, the forced familiarity with alternative systems has bred a lessening of the contempt of past times, as physicians have discovered an unexpected level of professionalism among their alternative counterparts, as well as evidence of effectiveness for several popular alternative therapies. In December 1997 the editorial board of the *Journal of the American Medical Association* announced that unconventional medicine had been ranked third among eighty-six subjects in terms of interest and importance for readers, and that the topic would be the focus of a special issue of the journal. That issue appeared in November 1998. It included reports on clinical trials of seven different alternative therapies (including chiropractic, acupuncture, yoga, and herbs); four of the seven trials found positive benefits from the tested treatment.[5] Now, it would seem, conventional physicians were going to start fooling around with alternative medicine themselves.

Even so, the past will not be left behind without a struggle. Wounds from historic conflicts between mainstream and marginal practitioners have not fully healed and are easily reopened. Since 1986 I have given an elective course on alternative approaches to healing to students at the University of Washington School of Medicine. Initially, the project seemed a bit like teaching druidism in a Christian Sunday school, although my object never was to convert students to unconventional medicine. (Indeed, except for a monthly indulgence in therapeutic massage, I personally have never patronized an alternative practitioner.) Nor have I been interested in using the class as a forum for attacking alternative medicine. My intent, rather, has been simply to alert medical (as well as nursing, pharmacy, and other health profession) students to the prominence of alternative therapies in the American health care environment and to provide them with at least an introduction to the treatments, theories, and claims of the most popular alternative systems. The latter is accomplished primarily through presentations made by prominent local practitioners of naturopathic medicine, homeopathy, chiropractic, and other unorthodox methods. The first year I offered the class, the very first guest speaker was an osteopathic physician (I elected to begin with the most familiar and accepted alternative) who was respectfully asked by a medical student if the generally lower grade point average and medical school admission test scores of osteopathic medical students meant that osteopathic schools placed more emphasis on non-academic qualities in selecting their classes. "Most definitely," was the answer; "for example, we like for our students to be human beings."

So confrontational a beginning to my consciousness-raising project was an unsettling reminder to me, as a medical historian, that the long record of interprofessional warfare continues to strain interactions between the two sides. Time is in the process of relieving the tension, but the change can be quickened by mainstream health professionals acquiring some awareness of the mistreatment that alternative practitioners feel they have suffered over the years at the hands of the medical establishment; similarly, alternative doctors can benefit from a deeper understanding of why the orthodox profession has tried to suppress their activities.

A second way that an appreciation of the history of unconventional medicine might assist in the process of conciliation is to acquaint mainstream doctors with the culture of natural healing. It will not be enough for physicians to learn more about the treatments and theories of alternative practitioners and about what evidence exists for the efficacy of their therapies. They must also learn more about the practitioners themselves. I am thinking here not of the individual relationships that MDs might establish with NDs, DCs, and other unconventional healers as they coordinate the care their patients receive.

I have in mind instead the need to appreciate the philosophical outlook common to alternative doctors of all persuasions. For while the dozens of different alternative systems are quite distinct from one another with respect to therapies and theories, they are united at the level of values. All share a certain perception of themselves, and of conventional medicine, that has been forged over two centuries of effort to define the ways in which they differ from medical orthodoxy. This alternative interpretation of healing will be discussed in Chapter 1.

The importance of this philosophical foundation shared by all systems of alternative medicine can hardly be overstated. When the leaders of naturopathy today aver that their medicine is "more than simply a health care system; it is a way of life," they are stating that they think of human beings, their relation to their environment, and their responses to environment and therapy in fundamentally different ways than mainstream physicians do. It is an orientation that since the 1970s has been called "holistic medicine," but long before the word "holistic" had been coined and glorified as a "new paradigm" for healing, alternative practitioners were advocating a philosophy of healing that was nothing if not "holistic."[6]

"Nature cures" is another term for describing the various medical alternatives. The phrase "nature cure" has long been used by naturopaths to identify their system as one that relies on the body's own natural healing mechanisms to restore the sick to health. But in truth, alternative therapists of every denomination have always claimed to heal by supporting and stimulating nature; they have all been purveyors of nature cures. Further, by virtue of subscribing to the principle that whenever recovery takes place, nature rather than the doctor is ultimately responsible, all would gladly accept as their credo "Nature cures!"

Historically, the ranks of nature cure have been thicker than is generally appreciated. In the 1850s a New York physician concluded his volume on *Quackery Unmasked* with an accounting of the "most prominent" unconventional practitioners that cited homeopaths, hydropaths, eclectics, botanics, chrono-thermalists, clairvoyants, natural bone-setters, mesmerists, galvanic doctors, astrologic doctors, magnetic doctors, uriscopic doctors, blowpipe doctors, the less than a decade old plague of "Female Physicians" (that is, women MDs), and "etc. etc. etc." The etceteras included Baunscheidtism, physiomedicalism, and yet other medical isms: and this was only the antebellum generation of natural healers. Following the Civil War, Christian Science, osteopathy, chiropractic, naturopathy, and new etceteras made their appearance. Still more approaches have become established in the United States during the twentieth century, particularly as Asian healing traditions have been brought into the country. By the end of the century, the census of alternative therapeutic and diagnostic methods had surpassed three hundred.[7]

The entries on the list enjoy varying degrees of recognition and acceptance from the orthodox profession. Some are thought of as silly, others regarded as at best alternatives one might try in place of conventional treatments for a particular condition. A few, however, are coming to be looked upon as complements to be used in conjunction with conventional care, and the term "complementary medicine" has gained much currency in recent years. More than a few readers might feel this book should therefore be subtitled *The History of Complementary Medicine*, or even *The History of CAM*, the widely used acronym for "complementary and alternative medicine." I nevertheless have elected to use "alternative," as it is still a more widely recognized term with the general public and a more suitable description of how unorthodox medicine has been perceived historically.

There are surely other readers who believe *The History of Quackery* would be the proper subtitle. The quackery label has in fact been consistently applied to unconventional medical systems from the outset. An English visitor to this country in the mid-1800s, astonished by the sheer number of unorthodox systems of cure, despaired that "daily some poor unfortunate falls a victim to these murderous quacks. Their deeds of darkness and iniquity fairly outherods [sic] Herod." In truth, many alternative methods of the last two centuries surely were inert or positively dangerous. Nevertheless, historically the word "quackery" has been used less to mean ineffective therapy and more to connote fraudulent intent on the part of the therapist. "Charlatanism," a respected orthodox practitioner of the mid-1800s remarked, "consists not so much in ignorance, as in dishonesty and deception." "The distinction between quacks and respectable practitioners," a British contemporary added, "is one, not so much of remedies used, as of skill and honesty in using them."[8] Practitioners of the systems of healing covered in this book have by and large been every bit as honest as orthodox physicians in their belief in their methods, and just as sincere in their desire to restore sick people to health.

In any event, my object is not to separate the quacks from the conscientious but rather to unearth the roots of a contemporary stage of medical evolution that has profound implications for the future of health care. Thus while I hope this book will be of interest to fellow historians, my greater concern is to provide a perspective on the past that will serve health professionals of all affiliations in their interactions today. I would wish as well that lay people interested in questions of health and healing find in this work some enlightenment on a subject as important for patients as for physicians.

In exploring the evolution of alternative medicine, I will not attempt to detail the development of every single unconventional system of therapy that has established a foothold at some point in America's past. Rather, I will select a few of the most significant programs of treatment to illustrate different modes of healing and to dramatize battles with mainstream medicine that had to be fought by all systems. Finally, as with my medical school course on alternative medicine, I intend the book to be neither a recommendation of individual programs of natural healing nor a condemnation of any. If I am taking a position, it is simply that of the first director of the Office of Alternative Medicine, speaking "not as an advocate of alternative medicine, but as an advocate for its fair evaluation." I would urge upon readers the same spirit of tolerance that was solicited by Walter Johnson, a nineteenth-century MD who converted to homeopathic practice. "If among those who cast a glance at these pages," he began his 1852 *Exposition and Defence* of homeopathy, "there be any who would fain subjugate reason to authority—who would impose upon the conscience of the many the dogmas of a few—who would empower halls and senates to fine and imprison, and to disqualify from public trusts all who dissent from their doctrines and repudiate their practice; if, among my readers, there be any who, in their hatred of medical heresy, scruple not to calumniate the moral character of the so-called heretics, and openly to term them pests of society—to all such I say, this work is not for you."[9]

Historians are heavily dependent upon the goodwill of librarians, and I feel blessed to have had three extraordinarily goodwilled custodians of books and documents to work with. First is Colleen Weum, acquisitions and collection management librarian for the University of Washington Health Sciences Library. I long ago lost count of the times Colleen has uncomplainingly set aside her own work to help me track down some book or periodical or to let me into the locked catacombs in which the library's older journals are stored. Without Colleen's help, I would no doubt be working on this book for some time to come, and I am deeply grateful for her assistance. Jan Todd, curator of the Todd-McClean Physical Culture Collection at the University of Texas, also made my task much easier during a week's research stay in Austin. Finally, Jane Saxton, director of the Bastyr University Library, was most generous with time and expertise on my research visits to her institution.

Other library staff have also gone extra lengths for me. I would particularly like to thank Kathleen Sisak, of the University of Washington; Susan Banks, of Bastyr University; Margaret Kaiser, of the National Library of Medicine; and Jane Brown, of the Medical University of South Carolina.

I have benefited as well, of course, from ideas and advice from fellow historians and from health professionals, both mainstream and alternative. I am indebted in various ways to Christina An, Bob Anderson, Pat Archer, the late John Bastyr, Kim Beckwith, Jack Berryman, Christian Bonah, Dan Cherkin, George Cody, Dean Crothers, Gary Elmer, Norman Gevitz, Greg Higby, Ron Hobbs, Rosalie Houston, Jennifer Jacobs, Mara Jeffress, David Kailin, Brenda Loew, James McCormick, Laurin McElheran, Ronald Numbers, Mary Jo Nye, Robert Nye, Melissa Oliver, John Parascandola, Joe Pizzorno, Lyndsey Rasmussen, Ron Schneeweis, Tom Shepherd, Lenore Small, Pam Snider, Mark Tonelli, Wendy Valentine, Lisa Vincler, and Susan Vlasuk.

I would also like to express appreciation to my editors at Oxford University Press: Jeffrey House, Edith Barry, Joellyn Ausanka, and especially copy editor India Cooper, whose painstaking reading of the manuscript eliminated more than a few errors and contributed a number of stylistic improvements.

Above all, I wish to thank my wife. Jackie has endured more than a year of books and papers piled and scattered about our shared office without protesting once (at least not within earshot). More, she has brought patience and understanding and love to our shared life. Without the fulfillment I find with her, writing this book would have been a far less satisfying endeavor.

PART I

The Nineteenth Century: Natural Healing

Physicians of the highest rank—To pay whose fees would need a bank—
Have pressed their science, art, and skill Into a dose of calomel.
Whate'er the patient may complain Of head, or heart, or nerve, or brain,
Of fever high, or parts that swell—The remedy is calomel.
When Mr. A. or B. is sick, "Go for the doctor; and be quick."
The Doctor comes with right good will, And ne'er forgets his calomel.
He turns unto the patient's wife, And asks for paper, spoon, and knife;
"I think your husband will do well To take a dose of calomel."
He then deals out the fatal grain, "This, ma'am, will surely ease the pain,
Once in three hours, at chime of bell, Give him a dose of calomel."
The man grows worse quite fast indeed, A council's called. They ride with speed.
They crowd around his bed, and tell The man to take more calomel.
The man in death begins to groan, The fatal job for him is done.
His falt'ring voice in death doth tell His friends to shun all calomel.
Now, when I must yield up my breath, Pray let me die a natural death,
And bid you all the long farewell Without the use of calomel.

"Calomel," a mid-nineteenth-century song

1

The Hippocratic Heresy: Alternative Medicine's Worldview

Walter Johnson, the homeopath quoted at the close of the preface, referred to his practice as a "medical heresy" and his colleagues as "so-called heretics." In fact, the members of all alternative schools of treatment have regarded themselves as heretics, as dissenters from the established gospel of medical theory and practice subjected to castigation and persecution for their heterodox beliefs. They thought of their heresy as "so-called," however, because all were confident that they possessed the one genuine gospel of health. Even so, each of the alternative systems has paid homage to the same source of inspiration revered by orthodox medicine, looking back to Hippocrates, the Greek physician of the fourth century B.C.E., as their doctrinal father. Indeed, so strong has this attachment been, one might think of alternative systems of medicine collectively as so many Hippocratic heresies.

For MDs, Hippocrates is the "father of medicine" primarily because of his introduction of a consistently naturalistic orientation to thinking about disease and cure, banishing gods and demons as agents of sickness and recovery. For alternative medicine's heretics, Hippocrates has been more important for his advocacy of certain other principles, principles that have persisted in alternative medical philosophy to the present. These principles are evident in particularly concise form in another alternative medicine cartoon, this one dating from the early 1800s. In 1834 *The Thomsonian Botanic Watchman*, a fledgling literary organ for a scheme of herbal healing known as Thomsonianism, spiced its inaugural issue with "An Illustration of the Difference Between the Regular and Thomsonian Systems of Practice." (Surviving copies of the cartoon, unfortunately, are too faded to reproduce clearly.) There a patient is shown mired in the Slough of Disease despite the ministrations of a "regular" doctor, as orthodox physicians styled themselves. The doctor is depicted standing upon the banks of the slough, with his left hand upon the patient's head, holding him in place, and his right raised and poised to descend with a club labeled "calomel." Clearly intent on bludgeoning the disease into submission with regular medicine's favorite drug, he assures the patient that "You must be reduced, Sir!" The MD's meaning is that calomel, the most commonly employed purgative in nineteenth-century practice, will reduce the disease by cleaning out the intestinal tract. The patient, contrarily, fears that he is the one being reduced, reduced all the way to the grave: "The Doctor knows best," he moans facetiously, "but send for the Parson." In the middle of the picture, an observer attempts to get the doctor's attention, to show him there is a better way: the way of the Thomsonian healer to the right, who rescues a second patient by pulling him up the Steps of Common Sense.[1]

Heroic Therapy Versus Reliance on Nature

This cartoon is a nutshell presentation not just of Thomsonians' views but of the core philosophy of all alternative systems of practice over the past two centuries. Specifically, it highlights three fundamental tenets of the Hippocratic heresy. First, by portraying the physician as one who treats the sick by beating them, the artist suggests that conventional medicine attacks disease so brashly as to indiscriminately overwhelm the patient too. Thomsonian remedies, on the other hand, are indicated to be gentle and, more than that, to be "natural," to support and enhance the body's own innate recuperative powers: "I will help you out," the Thomsonian doctor tells his patient, "with the blessing of God." He might just as well say "with the blessing of nature," since God and nature were implicitly one in nineteenth-century thought. Thomsonians did often state the matter explicitly, however: "The old school physician lifts his fatal club and strikes at random," one wrote a few years after the cartoon's publication, "the force of which oftener comes on the head of the only healing principle that exists in man, termed nature, than on his enemy, disease."[2]

Thomson's characterization of standard therapy as an assault on nature embodied a considerable amount of truth. Calomel, one of the most frequently prescribed drugs at that time, was a powerfully acting cathartic that physicians believed would flush morbid material from the body while also stimulating the liver to greater action. But as a mercury compound (mercurous chloride), calomel was toxic, and when given in repeated doses over a period of days or weeks it made the patient's mouth painfully swollen, causing cheeks and gums to bleed and ulcerate and teeth to become loose and fall out. In severe cases, the sufferer's jawbone could be destroyed. All too often, critics charged, "the mercurial treatment" left the sick "maimed and disfigured," subjects "of pity and horror . . . pitiable objects with distorted features." Such injuries were compounded by ptyalism, a profuse flow of viscous and foul-smelling saliva ("his tongue is protruded out of the mouth . . . and the saliva streaming out at the rate of from a pint to a quart in 24 hours"). But since salivation and its attendant oral damages were "the only index of the degree to which the mercurial impregnation of the blood is carried"—in effect constituted the proof that an adequate dose had been given—"this mark [salivation] is usually aimed at." Doctors then rationalized the side effects as necessary evils, much as oncologists today justify the damages done by cancer chemotherapy. "Salivation was a trifling evil," one argued, "compared with the benefit which was derived from it." Patients, understandably, dreaded a course of calomel treatment and "submitted to it," one doctor observed, "as an evil almost as formidable as the disease for which it was administered."[3]

Yet the great majority did submit, even as the size of calomel doses increased through the first half of the nineteenth century. This "Samson of the Materia Medica," as it was hailed, came in for particularly heavy use in the epidemics of Asiatic cholera that swept the country in the mid-1800s, by which time calomel prescribing had become virtually a reflex for physicians. The drug was often given, physician-litterateur Oliver Wendell Holmes joked, "on the same principle as that upon which a landlord occasionally prescribes bacon and eggs,—because he cannot think of anything else quite so handy." When doctors are "in doubt as to correct treatment," another skeptic suggested, they behave like card players—"*they play trumps.*"[4] Calomel was trumps.

Doctors nevertheless had lots of other cards in their therapeutic pack. Calomel was just one of a host of violent purgatives employed to scour the intestines, while the upper alimentary tract was cleaned just as thoroughly through the use of vomitive drugs. The most popular, tartar emetic, produced evacuations that one doctor described as "cyclonic" in action, while at the same time frequently resulting in antimony poisoning. The physical system in general, furthermore, was relieved of excess or unwholesome blood by venesection, or phlebotomy—Latin and Greek respectively for the cutting open of a vein. Incised veins were allowed to release a pint or more of blood at a time, and bleedings were repeated if improvement was not soon manifest.[5]

In most cases, improvement did occur. The great majority of patients recovered notwithstanding their treatment, and their survival only confirmed in physicians' minds that the therapies they administered, therapies that were suggested by medical theory, were actually being demonstrated to be effective by clinical experience. Even so, doctors often acknowledged the rigorousness of their treatments (which included more than a few other assaults, such as the application of blood-sucking leeches and the raising of blisters on the skin) by referring to them as "heroic therapy." Therapeutic heroism was the norm through the first half of the 1800s. "The practice of that time was heroic; it was murderous," an aging southern physician recalled of his novice days in the 1830s; "I knew nothing about medicine, but I had sense enough to see that doctors were killing their patients, . . . and that it would be better to trust to Nature than to the hazardous skills of the doctors."[6]

Trusting in nature was, in fact, a policy that a number of America's *orthodox* physicians adopted during the first half of the century. For reasons beyond present purposes, a minority of doctors, mostly younger members of the profession, came to doubt the efficacy of the traditional depletive therapies. "Boast as doctors will of *their* cures," a leader of the American profession wrote in the 1840s, the *"vis medicatrix naturae* is the chief doctor after all." *Vis medicatrix naturae*—the healing power of nature—was the Latin phrase that had been used for centuries to signify the agency first identified by Hippocrates, the inborn ability of the human body to respond to the insult of illness or injury and restore itself to health in most episodes of disease or trauma. Among the hallmarks of Hippocratic medicine, in fact, had been trust in the sick person's power to recover, without aggressive medication, and avoidance of treatments that might inhibit the *vis medicatrix*. The self-reparative powers of the body had ever since been held in high regard by physicians, though by 1800 that regard had become largely theoretical. Practitioners' true enthusiasm was for the heroic interventions that took the work of cure out of nature's hands and placed it in physicians'. Students of University of Pennsylvania medical professor Benjamin Rush, that most heroic of practitioners, recorded in their notebooks his advice to "always treat nature in a sick room as you would a noisy dog or cat drive her out at the door and lock it upon her."[7]

The early nineteenth-century revolt against the excesses of therapeutic heroism saw more than a few mainstream practitioners denouncing "the abominable atrocities of wholesale and indiscriminate drugging" and otherwise expressing their displeasure with the profession's neglect of the body's restorative power. Nature, in the eyes of these therapeutic reformers, was a "good, kind angel, hovering over the bed of sickness, without fee, and often without even any acknowledgment of her services," an angel who regularly saved "the life of many a poor patient, who is near being drugged to death by some ignorant quack, or some over-dosing doctor." In conjunction with such sentiments, there was developed the concept of "self-limited" diseases, conditions that would run their course for better or worse whether treated or not (much as the common cold will last a week if no medication is taken but be cured in seven days if drugs are used). In most cases, the advocates of nature maintained, the patient's best hope was in being given basic nursing care: nourishment, rest, and warmth—but little or no medicine.[8]

The resultant debate of "nature versus art" ("art" denoting the doctor's pharmaceutical armamentarium) was a hotly contested issue among America's regular physicians from the 1830s into the 1860s. But the fact that Oliver Wendell Holmes, the profession's most articulate spokesman for therapeutic humility, described "nature-trusting" as a "heresy" indicates that the majority of doctors denied nature's power to heal unassisted, and stayed on the side of active intervention. Some of the orthodox actually denied there was any such thing as the *vis medicatrix naturae*. ("Obscure and incomprehensible," one doctor called it; "only an inference—a theory," stated another.) Most acknowledged that when the body was attacked by disease it did make efforts to reverse the injury and reclaim health but believed that generally the aid of the physician was required nonetheless. To have concluded otherwise would have been a form of professional suicide, an admission that the doctor was redundant. Even Holmes and other nature-trusters hardly abandoned drugs altogether. They simply called for a more moderate and discriminating use of those that seemed to have some clinical evidence in their favor, rationalizing their use as agents that removed obstacles to nature's reparative activity. Judged that way, even calomel could be identified as a friend of nature; used judiciously, the purgative eliminated constipation, which might otherwise cause discomfort, weakness, and sleeplessness.[9]

Regular physicians of the first half of the nineteenth century maintained allegiance to their traditional drugs for other reasons as well. Doing something active in place of waiting for nature instilled confidence in patients that the doctor had power, and confidence stimulated recovery. Indeed, if the doctor did not take action, more often than not the patient or his family demanded it. "How often," one physician complained, was he "forced by patients and their friends to give medicine when it is not plainly indicated. . . . He must cure *quickly*, or *give place to a rival*." Finally, calomel, bleeding, and other heroic treatments were the very things that gave the profession its distinctiveness vis à vis unconventional healers. As these enemies became ever more strident in their attacks on traditional medicine, it was only natural for MDs to close ranks and cling more tightly to that tradition as a badge of professional identity, making depletive therapy the core of their self-image as medical orthodoxy. In brief, a fair amount of lip service was paid to nature by physicians of the mid-1800s, but when it came down to practice instead of philosophy, they sided with art.[10]

The Emergence of "Irregular Medicine"

Claiming to side with nature instead was the distinguishing therapeutic phi-losophy of those first alternative systems of practice that appeared in America in the early 1800s. *Systems* of practice is specified because while there had been a variety of methods available as alternatives to conventional medicine before the nineteenth century, the practitioners of folk medicine, the so-called root-and-herb doctors, the purveyors of Native American remedies, and other informally trained medicos had not been professionalized to any significant degree. They were often paid for their ministrations, to be sure, but they generally practiced alone, using what knowledge they had acquired in their individual ways. They did not band together with people of like mind to prescribe the same drugs and to swear allegiance to the same theory. They did not establish schools to train the next generation of practitioners, organize professional societies, or publish journals. The alternative healers who came onto the scene in the early nineteenth century did all those things, and that is what made their practices stand out as systems.

Siding with nature meant that the new systems of treatment that cropped up in the early 1800s were openly hostile to traditional depletive therapies and to the profession that employed them. The new breed of doctors boldly placed themselves outside the boundaries of conventional practice, defiantly proclaim-ing their independence from a pharmaceutical orientation they believed to be discredited by common sense and experience. From their vantage point, drugs were poisons, and one could never help the sick by poisoning them. "To walk through the streets of . . . any great town," a homeopath reflected, "and ob-serve the green and red lamps [of apothecary shops] with the idea that each is a perennial fountain of physic [drugs], whence the sick and suffering derive not solace and restoration, but aggravation of their misery," was an exercise to "make a humane man shudder, and read the sage another lesson upon the perversity of mankind!" Every drug shop, he remonstrated, and every drug therein "is an independent focus of disease which radiates through the entrails of humanity." A Thomsonian concurred, summarizing the history of orthodox medicine as "a series of blind experiments with the most deadly poisons," experiments whose only result was that "millions sleep beneath the clods of the valley."[11]

The point would be made again and again over ensuing decades; an osteopath of the early twentieth century, for example, shamed MDs for claim-ing descent from Hippocrates. "Hippocrates has a perfect right to deny the parentage imposed upon him by these children who so little resemble him," she objected; "modern medicine is more like a descendant of the Borgias than of Hippocrates." The first rule of the Greek healer, after all, had been to do the sick no harm, and alternative doctors have always touted the gentleness of their medicines as loudly as their efficacy. It is this emphasis that is captured by the common French term for alternative medicine: *médecine douce*, mild medicine. But alternative doctors so persistently disparaged conventional drugs not just because they regarded them as poisons but also because they believed that regular physicians most often used them simply to relieve symptoms without getting at the root cause of distress. According to the founder of naturopathy, Benedict Lust, regulars "have sought to cure disease by the magic of pills and potions and poisons that attacked the ailment with the idea of suppressing the symptoms instead of attacking the real cause of the ailment." (This position continues to be held by naturopaths and other alternative practitioners today, who joke among themselves that MDs behave as if a headache is nothing more than an aspirin deficiency.) On the other hand, non-pharmaceutical procedures, particularly surgery, have generally been accepted as effective (though overused) and ceded to the regular profession. Alternative doctors have sometimes laid claim to skill in setting fractures and healing wounds and burns, but for the most part they have willingly left more severe injuries to the care of surgeons.[12]

More than any other factor, it was the scornful repudiation of the drugs administered by traditional physicians that set homeopaths, Thomsonians, and like critics apart as alternative healers. Yet their practices were not called "alternative medicine," at least not in the nineteenth century ("alternative" would not become the standard label until the later 1900s). Rather, the common term employed throughout the 1800s was "irregular medicine." As one might guess, that designation was coined by mainstream practitioners, the members of the "regular" profession. For their part, the "irregulars" preferred another identity, putting themselves before the public as champions of "natural healing," healing that worked hand in hand with the *vis medicatrix naturae* to support and strengthen its activities rather than attacking and weakening nature with drug poisons. "Arrogant doctors are ready to take the place of nature at $2.00 to $5.00 per response," a naturopath of the early 1900s complained, "and you have to suffer the consequences, foot the bill and—fill the coffin." Whenever nature presumed to take the doctor's place, however, the regular physician was not amused. A homeopath of the later 1800s imagined a Doctor Dosem's reaction:

> 'Tis nature that does it—but what right has she
> To be round curing people without a degree?
> A man to be cured without sending for me!
> Without sending for any right licensed M.D.!!
> It's unscientific, irregular, mean—
> The shamefulest thing that ever was seen![13]

The different ways in which various irregulars justified their remedies and methods as "natural," and in the early twentieth century as "drugless," will be a major subtext of this book. Historically they have also—and this will be no surprise—insisted that natural methods be extended to childbirth, not only to disease.

Nature has been worshipped not just as the strongest therapy but also as the most effective prevention. Indeed, all alternative systems have sub-scribed to the philosophy that natural physiological integrity, maintained through proper diet, adequate rest, and other correct habits of life, is the *only* sure resistance to disease agents. That position was advanced with particular ardor in the late nineteenth century, in response to regulars' emphasis on microorganisms as the cause of most illness. In the terse summation of a physio-medical doctor, the "best antiseptic" was not the chemical drugs pre-scribed so exuberantly by MDs but "vital force."[14]

Identification of the body's resisting power as vital force points to another essential component of the Hippocratic heresy: vitalism, or the belief that the human body is activated and directed by a life force that is unique to living organisms and that transcends the laws of physics and chemistry used to account for the phenomena of the inorganic world. For some the vital force has been equated only with the *vis medicatrix*, and for others it has been understood to be the soul as well, but in either case it has been embraced as a repudiation of the trend within orthodox medicine to reduce the body to physical and chemical mechanisms. "The fundamental basis of the theory and practice of physio-medicalism," an early twentieth-century irregular stated, is "the doctrine of vitalism as opposed to the soulless idea of mechanico-biology."[15] As will be seen, alternative healing systems have carried the battle against the mechanistic, reductionistic orientation of mainstream medicine down to the present.

Empiricism in Irregular Medicine

Irregular practitioners have also divorced themselves from regular medicine in terms of epistemology, the method by which they discover their therapies. Returning to the Thomsonian cartoon of the 1830s for this second principle of alternative medical philosophy, the regular physician is shown with a di-ploma hanging from his coat pocket. Stamped "MD," it is emblematic of the abstruse theoretical training that he received in medical school and that dictates his practice. As the observer in the middle comments, the physician is "sci-entific with a vengeance," hell-bent on doing what theory tells him *ought* to work but unable to learn from experience and realize he is poisoning his patient. As one Thomsonian commented, physicians who learned medicine primarily from books came out of school "as ignorant of what is really useful in curing disease, as though they had been shut up in a cloister all the time." The founder of the system himself, Samuel Thomson, called for "the study of patients, not books—experience, not reading."[16]

That has in essence been the principle subscribed to by all the systems of alternative medicine from their nineteenth-century beginnings. One of the fundamental motivating forces for the first generation of irregular practitioners was the belief that orthodox medicine was overly rationalistic, placing too much confidence in theory and not trusting sufficiently in experience. The conventional orientation, it was maintained, was to hypothesize about the basic nature of disease and then deduce therapy from the resulting theory. Treatments were presumed to work because theory indicated they had to and because most patients did in fact recover. The truth, irregulars proposed, was that the patients who got better did so in spite of their treatment, not because of it; their survival demonstrated nothing more than the power of the placebo effect and the toughness of the *vis medicatrix*. The proper way to discover methods of healing was to evaluate clinical experience unbiased by theoretical preconceptions, knowing that nature would clearly reveal her therapeutic laws to those who listened humbly and with an open mind.

Listening to nature leaves room for intuitive discoveries of curative agencies, and irregular doctors have often claimed a special talent or knack for healing that comes from direct communion with nature and that could never be learned through science. That talent, they have maintained, is what makes one a true healer, instead of merely a technician, as most MDs are seen to be. Naturopathy's originator, Lust, asked, "Isn't that the way truth has always come into the world? *Doesn't it come, not through a cold process of reason, but by intuition or accident?*" To a considerable degree, alternative medicine has followed an alternative science, one requiring not sophisticated reasoning and abstruse theory, or expensive laboratories and extensive experimentation, but intuition, common sense, patience, and close observation. An important element of that alternative science, unorthodox healers believe, is the power to restore people spiritually as well as physically, through the ability to connect with an inner immaterial essence that is beyond the reach of cold laboratory science.[17]

While irregular healers listened to nature, MDs perverted it, it was asserted, by trying to force nature to submit to their theoretical musings. Facts obtained by observing patients had to come first. "Without facts," a Thomsonian pointed out, "it is as impossible to establish a correct theory as to commence building a chimney at the top." A major tenet of unconventional practitioners was their conviction that effective remedies were to be discovered only through adherence to strict empiricism, following the example of Hippocrates. Noble as that sounds, one is sorely taxed when reading accounts of the discovery of the different irregular methods to imagine how complex programs of treatment providing truly effective care could ever have developed from such crude clinical experimentation as marks the origin of many systems. The founders of osteopathy and chiropractic both, for example, as much as admitted they simply followed a hunch in performing their first spinal manipulations. Nevertheless, the skills of osteopaths and chiropractors in relieving musculoskeletal problems are now widely conceded, and similar observations can be made about the evolution of other unorthodox systems. (The terms "empiricism" and "empiric," incidentally, were used in contradictory ways in nineteenth-century medical discourse. Regulars and irregulars alike recognized the necessity of attentive clinical observation and believed they tempered their treatments according to experience. At the same time, mainstream practitioners decried reliance on observation alone, devoid of any scientific training to direct and interpret clinical experience, as "mere empiricism"; they scorned irregulars as "empirics," meaning they were so unsophisticated in their understanding of science as to be incapable of critical evaluation of experience. In short, "empirical" could be a compliment or a slur, depending on context.)[18]

There was a second facet of regulars' rationalist orientation that was equally upsetting to alternative doctors. It was not enough that conventional physicians made the sick even sicker with treatments that had not been validated by experience, it was objected, but they then compounded the error by absolutely refusing to consider the possibility that unorthodox remedies might be effective. Because of their blind devotion to scientific theory, regular practitioners simply dismissed irregulars' therapies out of hand because they could not be explained by the principles of orthodox science. "The magnetic phenomena rest on principles unknown," a nineteenth-century magnetic healer observed, "and therefore [they are] rejected as absurd; . . . they are so eccentric from every received idea, so extraordinary in their nature, that one passes for a fool, when he believes in them after having seen them, and for an impostor, when he succeeds in making others see them." More than a century later, virtually identical comments would be made, even by MDs, about Western physicians' reaction to acupuncture. The technique "is so foreign to everything he has been taught," an anesthesiologist stated, "that he has an almost Pavlovian reflex to refuse to believe it, if not to ridicule it." Even more recently, within the past decade, proponents of therapeutic touch have been instructed that they "must demonstrate some basis in reality for their theory. Then, and only then, can they move to the next step—proving its efficacy."[19]

In the mid-1990s I attended a lecture on the subject of "non-local manifestations of consciousness" in which there was discussed the accumulation of evidence in recent years that ill people who are prayed for have better rates of recovery than those who do not receive prayers. That evidence has met with a considerable amount of skepticism from medical scientists, of course, as the healing power of prayer is not a phenomenon readily explained by the laws of science. A common reaction, the lecturer related, has been the one voiced by a faculty member at a prestigious medical school: "That's the kind of crap I wouldn't believe even if it were true." Every alternative system of therapy has in fact been ridiculed by the medical establishment at first because it could not be rationalized by accepted theory ("such sublimated folly, such double distilled nonsense," an MD summed up "the humbugs of New York" in the 1830s).[20] From the alternative perspective, MDs have decided in advance that unconventional treatments are crap and they're not going to believe them even if they're true. Like the doctor in the cartoon, they are scientific with a vengeance.

In contrast, alternative practitioners have often contended that whether a therapeutic procedure can be explained is unimportant. If it works, they say, who cares why? Why not just accept it as a natural phenomenon that cannot be explained *yet?* The world accepted gravity, after all, long before Newton. An early nineteenth-century English acupuncturist epitomized the cavalier attitude of irregular doctors toward theory by happily accepting that the efficacy of his needles was due to "some of those mysterious operations of nature that will ever be beyond the reach of human ken." Physicians need to learn such humility, irregulars have argued, to come to see the light in the way an American doctor touring China did in 1972 after observing surgical procedures performed with acupuncture as the only anesthetic. "When you see these operations, you come out and you pinch yourself," he reported. "You wonder if you really saw what you saw. After you have seen it over and over, you have to give up what you thought in favor of what you saw." Alternative healers have always claimed to give priority to what they see over what they or others think. The moral of their story has been that of the man who in the mid-1800s had his ailing hip treated by a mind-curer and was enabled to walk comfortably for the first time in years. When a friend chided him that "people considered all these cures as humbugs," the man replied, "So did I . . . but here I am, and if humbug can work such wonders, glory be to humbug, say I."[21]

Another problem with how mainstream practitioners have thought about irregular therapies, it has been asserted, is that they have not recognized nature's simplicity and thus have rejected methods that have been seen to work not only because they could not be readily explained but further because they were so uncomplicated. "What!" a hydropath of the 1860s expostulated, "*water a remedy!* One of the most simple and common substances in nature, useful . . . for the purpose of diluting whisky and brandy . . . but, to make it a medicine to cure the sick is altogether too high a use for water. Something 'far fetched and dear bought' meets the ideas of people generally as a medicine; they are not willing to be cured by so simple an article. They had rather be sick and take a potion of delicious calomel . . . rather than to 'wash and be made whole.' " His point was echoed by a naturopath of the early 1900s, who submitted that "one of the reasons why Nature Cure is not more popular with the medical profession and the public is that it is *too simple*. The average mind is more impressed by the involved and mysterious than by the simple and common-sense." The Thomsonian doctor in the cartoon saves the patient by guiding him up the Steps of Common Sense, but as orthodox medicine has evolved over the last two hundred years, alternative practitioners believe, it has increasingly equated therapeutic potency with scientific complexity and technical sophistication, cutting itself off from common sense.[22]

Mainstream doctors' attitudes toward irregular therapies are dictated also, irregulars have frequently pointed out, by fear of being denounced and shamed by colleagues if they show any sympathy for unorthodox treatments. An early nineteenth-century French physician who was won over by magnetic healing spoke to the matter from firsthand experience: "He knows he must encounter the ridicule of many learned men for his profession of faith in this new power; his best friends . . . will express their regret that he has turned the energies of his mind to fantasies and to illusions; his enemies will be too happy to take his investigation as an engine by which they can depreciate him, and hold him up to public laughter and contempt as an idle dreamer, a wild visionary, and a dangerous physician." All those forces working together meant, as a late nineteenth-century spokesman for hydropathy stated, that the MD was always automatically opposed to healing discoveries made outside his profession, "fancying that abuse or sneers will suffice as an apology to his conscience for putting off the duty of learning or inquiry."[23]

Holism in Alternative Practice

A third principle shared by alternative medical systems throughout their history can also be found in the Thomsonian cartoon. The regular physician in the drawing appears to be restraining the poor man stuck in the swamp of disease; with his hand pressed against the patient's head, the doctor actually seems to be pushing him down to his death. The Thomsonian, on the other hand, is shown extending a compassionate helping hand to his patient, pulling him up to the safety of the shore. The Thomsonian doctor clearly cares for the man as a fellow human being and thinks of him as more than just another case of disease that needs to be conquered. From the very beginning, practitioners of alternative medicine have professed to deal with illness as a disorder affecting the patient as a whole and unique person. In the language of a later day, they have claimed to be holistic and have seen that commitment to holism as one of the chief virtues setting their method above the orthodox approach.

To MDs, all that self-congratulation for having a more profound understanding of illness and exercising a more humane handling of patients has come across as an irritating air of "holistic-er than thou" condescension. Irregulars' espousal of holism was particularly annoying to physicians of the early nineteenth century, because regular medicine had its own tradition of holistic practice running all the way back to the profession's origins in ancient Greece. For fully two millennia, it had been accepted that the understanding of any case of sickness required the healer to take into account the patient's inherited constitution, living environment and habits (diet, exercise, sleep, etc.), emotional state and stresses, and personality type and to incorporate the patient's subjective experience of illness into the analysis. In doing so, the doctor was paying his respects to Hippocrates, who had asserted that there are no diseases, only sick people.

During the second half of the eighteenth century, however, medical attention began to focus on the pathological changes that disease brought about in specific organs, and henceforward medicine would characterize each disease in terms of its localized organic pathology. The emphasis on illness as a condition unique to each individual steadily lost ground to the concept of a number of specific pathologies, each productive of a distinct disease that affected all its victims essentially the same way. Further, because the victims of any particular ailment were seen as suffering from the same organic lesions, physicians became more oriented toward the similarities between patients than the differences, making the client's subjective experience subordinate to the objective evidence of pathology discernible by the doctor. The search for the uniqueness of each patient was steadily displaced by the task of determining which disease pigeonhole to place her in. (Thus was born the old joke about the difference between illness and disease: illness is what a person has before she enters the doctor's office, disease is what she has when she comes out.)

Further, as diagnosis and treatment came increasingly to be predicated on the discovery of physical damage in individual organs and tissues, and eventually cells, medical practitioners necessarily concentrated more and more on the patient's parts, instead of his whole body and being, and on understanding and explaining his disease in the elevated terms of scientific pathology. Concern for what has been called modern medicine's "problem of the vanishing patient" was being voiced already by the mid-1800s. One sees it, for instance, in a novel by Oliver Wendell Holmes published in 1861. One of the main characters in *Elsie Venner: A Romance of Destiny* is a physician, "old

Doctor Kittredge," who voices his fear that science is beginning to replace sympathy in the physician's repertoire. Responding to a younger man's question about his proficiency in the latest medical science, the old doctor assures him that "I don't want to undervalue your science, Mr. Langdon. There are things I never learned, because they came in after my day, and I am glad to send my patients to those that do know them, when I am at fault." Nevertheless, he immediately adds, "I know these people about here, fathers and mothers, and children and grandchildren, so as all the science in the world can't know them, without it takes its time about it, and sees them grow up and grow old, and how the wear and tear of life comes to them. You can't tell a horse by driving him once, Mr. Langdon, nor a patient by talking half an hour with him."[24] Observe that Doctors Kittredge and Holmes were reproving scientific physicians for talking *only* half an hour with their patients.

Generosity with time and personal attention has been a strong suit of alternative medicine throughout its history and is often the reason patients select unconventional doctors still. Studies of the appeal of chiropractic at the present day, for example, have found that patients typically rate the care they receive from chiropractors higher than care from family physicians because they "perceived that their provider was concerned about them during and after the visit"; they observed that the chiropractor "does not seem hurried. . . . He uses language patients can understand. He gives them sympathy, and he is patient with them." After comedienne Gilda Radner was diagnosed with cancer in the 1980s, she saw a number of alternative practitioners as well as regular physicians for treatment and repeatedly expressed a preference for the former, not because she believed their therapies were more effective but because they were "taking me seriously" and were "paying attention to me."[25]

Conflict Between Mainstream and Alternative Medicine

Regular physicians' rejoinder throughout the past two centuries has been that while they may not talk with patients as long as irregulars do, at least they talk scientifically. The fundamental objection in the case against irregular practitioners has always been that there is no scientific merit to either their therapies or their theories. There is an unbroken two-century-long skein of amazement and exasperation among conventional physicians over the ability of alternative healers to attract patients with their unscientific ideas and methods. As an 1850 commentator on "the rascality of a mesmerist" put it, "that Hydropathy, Homoeopathy, and Mesmerism, those offsprings of deceit and humbug, should have found, not only believers, but enthusiastic supporters in the nineteenth century, will ever be a cause of wonder and regret to the sensible and unbiased portion of the community." How else to explain such things, others joined in, except as a demonstration of the unplumbable depths of human credulity? Irregulars promised a "perfect cure for all diseases," a physician wrote in the 1840s, giving them "a magnet of irresistible attraction. . . . So infatuated are men in contemplating a power which they fain would believe . . . to exist . . . that whoever raises such a standard is *sure* of having very many to flock around it." Often the point has been made more bluntly, as by a doctor of German extraction speaking against the licensing of osteopaths in New York State at the beginning of the twentieth century. "Vat ve vant," he explained, "is to veed them all oudt so they cannot humbug the public for ve know how easy it is to humbug the public." Those were the sentiments likewise of a 1920s Chicago physician who was convinced that "about ten per cent of the public insisted on being fooled. . . . Ten per cent of the American people and the people of the world will buy every gold brick that comes along."[26]

For irregulars, such rejections have only been further proof of the truth of their position. Time and again they have played what might be called the Galileo card, pointing out that Galileo's revolutionary insights were initially scorned by the authorities as gold bricks, and the scientist himself persecuted. Although Galileo has been far the most frequent example, Watt, Fulton, and many another great discoverer has been cited to demonstrate that every revealer of new truths is initially reviled. "Ye are the children of them which killed the prophets," a homeopath berated regulars in the 1840s. Conventional physicians in turn saw the Galileo argument as mere logical sleight-of-hand: scientific trailblazers have always been persecuted by entrenched authority; irregular doctors are now being persecuted by the established medical profession; therefore irregular doctors must be scientific trailblazers. "This subterfuge cannot avail," one of the regular profession's leaders objected in the 1830s. "Call himself by what name he will, a quack is still a quack—and even if the prince of darkness should assume the garb of heavenly innocence, the cloven hoof would still betray the real personage."[27]

Examples could be multiplied indefinitely, but it should be sufficiently clear already that our present-day spirit of cooperation between orthodox and unorthodox schools of healing is an extraordinary reversal of a mutual animosity that heretofore characterized relations between the two sides. What, a nineteenth-century physician asked rhetorically, should be the attitude of true medicine toward homeopathy? "It should be that of *abomination, loathing* and *hate*. It should be considered the unclean thing—foul to the touch, wicked and treacherous to the soul . . . as the death of every upright principle. . . . How can we endure their base betrayal and prostitution of our noble profession?" What, a nineteenth-century homeopath asked, should be his profession's orientation toward regulars? "Spurn them beneath your feet as foul and slimy reptiles," he answered. "Dogs may return to their vomit," a compatriot added, "and sows to their wallowing in the mire," but homeopathy must never return to orthodox methods, "the chaos from whence it came forth." Civilians caught in the crossfire between regular and irregular factions, not surprisingly, often wished a pox on both camps. Witness the French artist of the 1830s who presented a regular physician and a homeopath behaving as "rascals" (*polissons*), going for one another's gullet while the neglected patient expired.[28] Civility was alien to both sides' thinking until the last decade.

In short, there are two perspectives from which to recount the history of alternative medicine in America, if not two distinct stories to tell. The orthodox perspective is that alternative practitioners have subscribed to absurd theories and inane, sometimes dangerous, therapies and that, even when the remedies have been harmless, patients have often suffered and died because irregulars' ignorance of the science of diagnosis led them to treat serious conditions that could have been cured only by scientific medicine. The argument unquestionably contains a great measure of truth, particularly with regard to the early stages of development of alternative systems, when, all too often, crude therapies justified by simplistic and naive theories were employed by marginally educated practitioners and even outright quacks trading off a system's popular appeal. "Our profession has not unfailingly been a picture of beauty and innocence," a leader of chiropractic has admitted recently, and like confessions could be made by other alternative groups.[29] In the discussion of various systems in the chapters to follow, much attention will be given to the dubious elements of each, in part to demonstrate why the mainstream profession felt duty-bound to wage verbal and political war on irregulars.

One form of verbal warfare used in retaliation by irregulars was the word "allopathy." Coined two hundred years ago by Samuel Hahnemann, founder of homeopathy, it was taken from Greek roots meaning "other than the disease" and was intended, among other things, to indicate that regular doctors used methods that were unrelated to the disharmony produced by disease and thus were harmful to their patients. "Allopathy" and "allopathic" were liberally employed as pejoratives by all irregular physicians of the nineteenth century, and the terms were considered highly offensive by those at whom they were directed. The generally uncomplaining acceptance of "allopathic medicine" by today's MDs is an indication of both a lack of awareness of the term's historical use and the recent thawing of relations between irregulars and allopaths.

Throughout the book I will use "allopathic" to apply to the medicine practiced by MDs, along with designations such as regular medicine, orthodox medicine, conventional medicine, and mainstream medicine. Similarly, I will identify alternative medicine with both the negative and positive terms that have been used historically: irregular medicine, natural healing, medical cult-ism, drugless healing, fringe medicine, unconventional medicine, medical sec-tarianism, and holistic medicine. Employment of all those phrases will enhance the book's readability, I hope, by making it possible to avoid too frequent repetition of the same few terms. Use of both positive and negative adjectives will also serve to repeatedly remind that there are two sides to the story of alternative medical history.

From alternative practitioners' perspective, the story is that they have been well-intentioned healers fighting to rescue suffering humanity from the assaults of drugs and the knife, only to be rewarded with legal harassment from a hidebound profession fearful of their competition and determined to maintain its power and cultural authority. "Despite their vaunted concern for the public health and welfare," a twentieth-century chiropractor protested, "the medical sachems act toward chiropractic as any collection of businessmen being threatened by a rival concern which seems to have the kind of merchandise that customers prefer." Consequently, my coverage of each alternative sys-tem's development will give consideration to the allopathic profession's efforts to denigrate and eliminate the system, with the intent of conveying an appre-ciation for why present-day alternative practitioners feel they have been his-torically abused. Their resentment of allopathic medicine is backed by an enormous amount of historical momentum, a pressure that still sets off erup-tions such as the previously cited expostulation that allopathic doctors are not quite human beings. But it should also be kept in mind that until well into the twentieth century alternative practitioners were equally hopeful of elimi-nating the orthodox profession. "The day of powder and pill and knife is nearing its end," an osteopathic text predicted in 1903. "The world is becoming too intelligent to be drugged and hacked in a search for health when more agreeable methods can be obtained at the same price." (They hoped as well to eliminate one another. Until recently, at least, most alternative systems have seen themselves as the sole repository of medical truth and thus have been as critical of other irregulars as of allopaths. "They were very war-like," a prac-titioner of eclecticism observed of rival schools of practice in the nineteenth century, "pugnacious as snapping turtles." But, he allowed, "they had abun-dant cause for it; . . . every man's hand was against them, and they were inclined to turn their hands against other people.")[30]

The Question of Efficacy

Central to both stories is the issue of efficacy: do alternative medicines work? The question has begun to be energetically pursued over the last decade, but unequivocal findings are still limited, and in any event the question is not one to be answered by a historian. What history does reveal is an allopathic analysis of the clinical results of alternative treatments that has stayed consistent throughout the past two centuries. The patients of irregular doctors get better, first of all, because most sick people eventually overcome their ailments no matter what therapy they are given, or even if they are given nothing, thanks to the "tincture of time," the *vis medicatrix*. If one is given *something*, however, recovery is even more likely, because the efforts of nature will be enhanced by the placebo effect. It has long been appreciated that there is a symbolic significance to the mere act of clinical intervention in itself, whether with drugs, instruments, or words, that stimulates a healing response distinct from any specific pharmacological or physiological effects of the therapy. "The great stock-in-trade of the profession," famed clinician William Osler pronounced early in the twentieth century, is faith. "In one pan of the balance," he suggested, "put the pharmacopoeias of the world, all the editions from Dioscorides to the last issue of the United States Dispensatory; heap them on the scales . . . ; in the other put the simple faith with which from the days of the Pharaohs until now the children of men have swallowed the mixtures these works describe, and the bulky tomes will kick the beam." Osler was speaking of allopathic remedies, of course, but his insight applies equally to all alternative schemes of therapy.[31]

It has also long been apparent that the physician himself is the most powerful placebo of all, so long as his manner inspires trust in the patient. "An empiric oftentimes . . . doth more strange cures than a rational physician," Robert Burton wrote in his 1628 *The Anatomy of Melancholy*, "because the patient puts his confidence in him." (For that same reason, even "a silly chirurgeon [surgeon]" could accomplish cures.) Irregular practitioners thus have been branded confidence men of a special sort, peddlers of useless drugs who nevertheless get therapeutic results by pouring confidence and hope into their customers. Confidence unquestionably cures. A study published in the *British Medical Journal* in 1987 reported that patients affected by symptoms but showing no definite organic pathology recovered at a much higher rate (64 percent to 39 percent) when the physician provided a diagnosis and assured them they would be better in a few days than when the doctor professed not to know what they had or how long they would have it. In that way, allopaths have charged, alternative practitioners' lack of science is an advantage. Their medical ignorance, coupled with uncritical enthusiasm for their methods, allows them to promise wonders in cases where the conscientious MD can offer only limited hope. A commonly provided explanation of the popularity of chiropractic today is that patients "may be more satisfied with the confident and definite approach of chiropractors than with the less certain and more scientific approach of family physicians."[32]

The doctor's confidence is allied with another healing force, that of the power of suggestion and imagination. One of the classic demonstrations of the potency of suggestion is a device briefly famous as the Perkinean tractors. Elisha Perkins was a Connecticut physician of no particular unorthodox leanings until certain clinical experiences in the 1790s opened his eyes to the fact that all disease is due to "a surcharge of electric fluid in the parts affected." It followed that pain and illness could be relieved by discharging the electrical excess through metallic objects applied to the site of injury. Perkins verified this notion using items such as a penknife and an iron comb but was quick to realize that profits were not to be made promoting cures with materials already present in every household. Forthwith appeared his metallic tractors, three-inch-long rods shaped like carrots bisected lengthwise and available for only $25 the pair. Purchasers treated themselves or others by taking one tractor in each hand and making stroking movements over the affected part to draw the electrical surcharge out.[33]

The discovery of electrical traction was announced in 1795. Shortly after, early in 1796, the Connecticut state medical society expelled Perkins as a quack. At virtually the same time, however, the U.S. Patent Office recognized Perkins's invention with its first patent for a medical device, and sales took off. Several members of Congress purchased the new healing instruments, as did the Chief Justice of the Supreme Court and, it was rumored, President Washington himself. Testimonials to the tractors' power abounded, at least until Perkins died of yellow fever while selling his devices during the terrible New York epidemic of 1799. (Perkins now rests under Washington Square, which in his day was a potter's field.) The discoverer's demise seriously undermined confidence in the tractors, and they disappeared from the scene as suddenly as they had burst upon it; forty years later, when Oliver Wendell Holmes searched for a pair of tractors to illustrate a lecture on medical delusions, he found the instruments "now so utterly abandoned that I have only by good fortune fallen upon a single one of a pair."[34]

Holmes perhaps would have required less help from fortune had he searched in England, for even as the tractors' sun was setting in the New World, Elisha's son Benjamin had introduced the instruments to Great Britain and created an equal sensation there. Cures were reported by the thousands, of pets and livestock as well as people, and public contributions for the establishment of a Perkinean Institution to provide charity care exceeded the endowment of any London hospital of the time. Physicians were skeptical, to state it mildly, and soon were putting tractors to the test by treating patients with counterfeit devices made of wood, bone, and other non-conductors—and compiling just as remarkable a record of recoveries. Clearly "tractoration" did not involve the removal of pathological electrical fluid, and its effectiveness could indeed be explained by nothing other than the patient's imagination stimulated by the therapist's suggestion. As reports of success with sham tractors accumulated, Perkinism faded in England, too, but not before Perkins *fils* fattened his purse with the addition of ten thousand pounds.[35]

The tractors were nothing more than "galvanising trumpery," British physicians sputtered. Nevertheless, a few more astute observers pointed out that, call it what one might, the trumpery worked. As one writer reasoned,

> Why to be sure,
> If we by Fancy's aid can cure;
> Then why not use Imagination,
> A cheap and simple operation?

Why not? Because imagination is all in the mind, a nebulous and unpredictable entity instead of a physical agent explainable by the laws of chemistry and physics that govern other therapies. More than once, it will be seen, physicians have admitted that some unorthodox treatment apparently benefits patients but have immediately rejected it as useless because it operates only through imagination instead of by the chemical action or energy or other mechanism proposed by its advocates. Therapeutic facts have been shamed into disregard by their association with theoretic fallacies.[36]

The alternative practitioner's own imagination has often figured powerfully, too. The patient recovers after taking a treatment; therefore, it is supposed, he recovers because of the treatment. (Irregulars have not held a monopoly on such post hoc reasoning, of course; allopaths have been just as susceptible, as was demonstrated time and again with calomel.) In addition, heretic healers' enthusiasm for their particular system has often led them to proclaim therapeutic successes without sober evaluation of the data: "Some devotees of natural medicine," a naturopathic physician has recently observed, "are so enamored of the philosophy that the presence or absence of hard evidence seems to bore them." Alternative doctors readily admit that they rarely have the sort of hard evidence associated with the allopathic standard of proof, the controlled clinical trial. Yet they maintain there is equal certainty in their approach of "scientific empiricism." If a patient quickly improves under their care, after having suffered with the problem for a considerable time and received no benefit from orthodox therapy, then a genuine cure has occurred. The improvement is too rapid, they reason, and the history of illness too long, for the event to be explained by coincidence.[37]

This book's discussion of each alternative system will include reports of numerous cures by practitioners, some of which will border on the miraculous-sounding. They will be presented at face value, with the understanding that in many if not most instances the allopathic interpretation of what occurred was correct: most sick people get better with or without medical assistance, thanks to the *vis medicatrix;* all patients respond to some degree to the placebo effect and to suggestion; many patients have chronic conditions that have alternating periods of remission and relapse, and remission can coincide with treatment; many cases have been misdiagnosed by inadequately trained irregulars, resulting in spontaneous resolutions of minor complaints being passed off as miracle cures of cancer or other deadly ailments.

Yet unquestionably some reported cures were genuine. There is enough evidence from controlled clinical trials in recent years to support the claim that some alternative methods do indeed "work." These trials even include positive results for homeopathy, the system that historically has been regarded by regular physicians as the closest of all to the realm of absolute impossibility. It thus would be prudent to entertain the possibility that notwithstanding the placebo effect, the power of suggestion, and the healing power of nature, there may well be more things in heaven and earth than have hitherto been dreamt of in mainstream medical philosophy.

Philosophy and practice have not been the only points of conflict, for politics has been inextricably bound up with both sets of questions. Indeed, the history of alternative medicine is, almost by definition, the story of outsiders fighting the establishment, and, awkward though it sounds, there is considerable merit in another of the names that has been suggested for unconventional practice: "counterhegemonic medicine."[38] Irregulars' challenging of orthodox medical hegemony, and the political and legal battles that ensued, are elements of most of the chapters in this volume.

Some alternative doctors have found additional reason to protest allopaths' efforts to suppress them in the fact that their systems concentrate on treatments and problems that medical orthodoxy has not seriously bothered to deal with. MDs have in effect left certain ground untilled, much as tooth care was ceded to dentists, then objected when others moved in to cultivate the area. Medicine has been historically inattentive, for example, to psychological and emotional troubles. Many of the sick "have been driven into Christian Science," a Harvard medical professor pointed out in the early 1900s, by "the total neglect of rational psychotherapy on the part of many physicians." Consequently, "there can be no candid criticism of Christian Science methods that does not involve also an arraignment of existing medical methods." Musculoskeletal discomfort, especially back pain, has been another area disregarded by mainstream medicine. Yet over the centuries bonesetters, osteopaths, and chiropractors all developed methods to better address these problems. "The medical history of the future will have to record that our profession has greatly neglected this important subject," *The Lancet* editorialized in 1925; "the fact that must be faced [is] that the bonesetters had been curing multitudes of cases

by movement . . . and that by our faulty methods we are largely responsible
for their very existence." It is still the case that many chiropractic patients are
people who first consulted a regular physician for back, neck, or other musculoskeletal pain but were not helped.[39]

Both the prayer and positive thinking of Christian Scientists and the
manipulations of chiropractors and osteopaths had gained recognition by the
end of the twentieth century as useful approaches to dealing with illness and
pain. That development is emblematic of a broader process that perhaps will
soon bring an end to two centuries of struggle between medicine's ins and
outs. That will occur, however, only for those out-groups that can assemble
a persuasive scientific demonstration of the efficacy of their methods. Throughout the history of alternative medicine in America, orthodox physicians have
denounced the various systems as nothing more than therapeutic cults and
decried cultism as unscientific. "There are no sects in science," a physician
wrote in the *Journal of the American Medical Association* in 1913, "no schools
of truth." There could be temporary differences of opinion within science
"while facts of Nature are being studied out and until final certainty is attained
. . . but in ultimate truth there is an essential unity." Just as it was "unthink-
able" for there to be competing sects "of chemistry or astronomy . . . it is
equally incongruous in medicine."[40]

The following chapters will detail the history of alternative medicine in
America over the past two centuries with an eye toward clarifying how an
undoubted state of sectarianism that existed through the nineteenth century
and much of the twentieth has evolved into a situation at the present in which,
many believe, medical sectarianism is giving way to medical pluralism. In the
future, optimists hope, a range of approaches to healing will operate in conjunction with allopathic medicine on a basis of equality and mutual respect,
eradicating incongruity from medicine and achieving at last an "essential
unity" of medical truth. No turn of events could be more surprising to the
ghosts of those stalwarts who led the first generation of irregular practitioners
into battle in the early nineteenth century.

2

Every Man His Own Physician: Thomsonianism

The different systems of alternative medicine that appeared on the scene in the early nineteenth century took form in response to distinct trends in medical thought and practice, as well as in the broader culture. Eighteenth-century medicine had gone overboard in its reliance on highly speculative theoretical constructs as the basis for therapeutic decisions, suffering an imbalance that encouraged a search for more empirical approaches. The increasingly heroic therapeutic interventions that the theories encouraged likewise created a backlash, and the resultant desire to place more trust in the body's natural restorative powers was reinforced by the appeals of Romantic philosophers and poets to return to nature as the source of all truth and beauty. Further, the quickening pace of professionalization of American medicine that was evident by 1800 generated opposition. Eighteenth-century medical practice had been only loosely organized and regulated, an activity in which just about anyone was free to participate. But as medical schools were established during the second half of the century, and as medical societies were formed and medical journals launched, medical practice took on the lineaments of exclusivity, an endeavor restricted to those who had the right training and adhered to the right theories and practices. As medicine was transformed into a more tightly organized profession, it became a well-defined entity against which the medically disaffected could rally and mount alternative movements. They wasted little time, first into the field being the creator of Thomsonianism.

Origins of Thomsonian Medicine

Samuel Thomson (1769–1843, Fig. 2.1) allied himself with nature virtually from birth. He came into the world in the "almost a howling wilderness" of

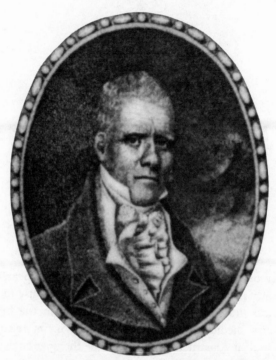

Figure 2-1. Samuel Thomson [Samuel Thomson,
New Guide to Health; or Botanic Family Physician
(Boston: Author, 1835), frontispiece]

backwoods New Hampshire. By the age of four, he claimed, he was doing
his part to help the family survive by watching over the cattle, a responsibility
that left him with lots of time on his hands in the fields and woods. An interest
in plants and their physical effects soon blossomed, and through random sampling of leaves, berries, and barks (as well as by accompanying a local herb
doctoress on her collecting excursions), the young Thomson became an herbal
pharmacy *Wunderkind*. Indeed, it was barely after his fourth birthday that he
discovered the drug that would serve as the foundation of a new system of
healing. Tasting the pods of a plant he had chanced upon while searching for
the cows, he found the "operation produced was so remarkable, that I never
forgot it."[1]

Nor would any of the thousands who would later take lobelia on Thomson's recommendation forget its operation either. His "Emetic Herb" (also
known as puke-weed, vomitwort, and gagroot) was described by an authoritative nineteenth-century pharmacology text as having a "pungent and acrid"
taste and causing, when swallowed, "a degree of nausea and depression which
amounts to anguish." Vomiting usually followed, "with great straining and

distress [and] an abundant outpouring of gastric mucus." As little as a teaspoon could be lethal (if the drug were not removed by vomiting): "The action of the heart is enfeebled. . . . Muscular weakness and trembling, shallow respiration. . . . and sometimes convulsions, have occurred. Death ensues from paralysis of the muscles of respiration—the action of the heart continuing after respiration has ceased." The young Thomson never knew what risks he ran. He in fact blithely made a practice of tricking other boys into eating it, "merely by way of sport, to see them vomit." For fully twenty years he used lobelia for practical jokes without suspecting anything of its medicinal virtue.[2]

In the meantime, Thomson was building an inventory of knowledge about other botanical remedies, along with a healthy skepticism about the therapeutic skills of regular doctors. At age nineteen, for example, he badly wounded his ankle with an ax, then worsened drastically after having the injury treated by a physician. His life now being "despaired of" unless he consented to amputation, he gave desperate directions for the preparation of a comfrey root plaster, had it applied to his ankle—and was soon on the way to recovery. That successful experiment with his amateur botanical knowledge was "a principal cause," Thomson wrote, of his taking up the practice of medicine.[3]

Another major source of motivation was the death of his mother in 1790. Mrs. Thomson developed a cough that spring that her physicians identified as "galloping consumption" and treated with mercury and opium: "They galloped her out of the world in about nine weeks." Thomson, meanwhile, was beginning to cough, too, but seeing how his mother was declining under orthodox care, he refused medication out of preference for "a natural death." When his mother finally passed away, he determined to "doctor myself" with botanical syrups—and galloped back to health. In less than two months he was robust enough to take a wife, and soon after to sire a child.[4]

The child's birth was occasion for Thomson to put still greater distance between himself and the doctors. His wife suffered a protracted labor, followed by convulsions, and the several physicians called to save her could agree on nothing except her likelihood of dying. Thomson finally dismissed them and summoned two nearby "root doctors," and under their ministrations the patient slowly improved. She never regained her health completely, however, and her recurring illnesses forced Thomson to give deeper consideration to trying his hand at medicine.[5]

One might continue at some length citing personal and family experiences that encouraged the farmer to become a healer, but they would only reiterate the already established theme: Samuel Thomson was an unlettered man whose common sense told him physicians were incompetent and who learned what he believed to be the effective way to cure through personal observations and practical trials. By the mid-1790s he had employed a regular doctor for the last time and was now himself being called by ailing neighbors who had heard of his soothing syrups and healing herbs. His list of botanicals had grown considerably, of course, through his years of self-experimentation, yet it was headed by one of the first discovered, the puking potion of his childhood days, lobelia. Thomson's medical epiphany, the realization that his favorite recreational drug was also a most potent therapeutic one, came in the early 1790s, while he was working in the fields. Still the joker, he induced a fellow field hand to taste some lobelia. The man broke out "in a most profuse perspiration, . . . trembled very much, . . . and laid down on the ground and vomited several times." He had to be carried into the house but partook of a hearty meal within two hours, then performed a good half-day's work that afternoon. When the man announced at the end of the day that he now felt the best he had in some time, Thomson's mind was made up: henceforth, the "Emetic Herb" would stand unchallenged as "Old Number One" in his system of practice.[6]

Thomsonian Theory

That system was rapidly expanded by testing of other botanicals, on himself and on ailing family members, until it came to embrace the administration of more than five dozen different plants. The virtues of the botanicals were discovered entirely by clinical "testing." (Like regular practitioners, Thomson was guilty of post hoc reasoning: patients got better after taking the plant; therefore the plant must have cured them.) But eventually he felt the need to make sense of his experiences by devising a theory of disease and drug action. He was particularly impressed by the fact that some of his most effective remedies had, like lobelia, an evacuative action on the body and that others had a spicy hotness to their taste. With a bit of analysis, it became clear to him that the human body is energized, infused with vitality and physiological function, by an elemental power of heat. For life to be sustained, an adequate supply of heat has to be generated by the burning of food fuel. The reason the stomach is a vital organ is because it is the body's fireplace, and like an ordinary fireplace it burns inefficiently if fed too much or improper fuel and becomes clogged with the ash and slag of inhibited digestion. Heat is then produced in too small quantity and not effectively distributed to the rest of the frame, resulting in the body being overcome by the power of cold. As cold gains control, this principle of inertness instigates "canker" and putrefaction throughout the body (the mechanism for this was left unexplained), culminating at last in death unless the routed forces of heat are renewed.[7]

That was why the "Emetic Herb" was a veritable panacea. Like a chimney sweep, it scraped the human fireplace clean and equipped it to burn undampened. That was why Thomson had found plants such as cayenne, black pepper, and ginger to be beneficial in all illnesses. Spicy botanicals were rich in heat, which they added directly to the body, sustaining motion and life until digestion returned to full power. Hot peppers promoted sweating as well, which served to dislodge and eliminate those impure products of canker and putrefaction. The same was accomplished by "injections" (in those pre-hypodermic days, "injection" always meant "enema"), which scoured the intestines, and by steam baths, which added heat to the body at the same time they flushed it clean with perspiration. All those disparate therapies found by trial and error were linked together by their opposition to cold and its morbific offspring and their support of nature's power of heat. Consequently, fever was regarded not as a pathological product of disease, as allopaths believed, but as the effort of the body—of nature—to sustain itself against the enfeebling effects of cold and so was to be encouraged. The great error of the regulars' practice of venesection, Thomson maintained, was that bleeding reduced fever; his rule, in effect, was that one should feed a fever and starve the cold. Feeding a fever with hot drugs, furthermore, was emblematic of all his therapies: all treated nature "as a friend; and not as an enemy, as is the practice of the physicians." His approach had "always been . . . to learn the course pointed out by nature," then to administer "those things best calculated to aid her in restoring health."[8]

The Thomsonian System of Treatment

Since his drugs assisted nature through a variety of ways, Thomson organized them into six distinct categories according to mode of action. The first, a division unto itself, was lobelia, needed to "cleanse the Stomach, overpower the cold, and promote a free perspiration." It was a remedy of "almost unlimited extent of friendly power," one "truly prepared to deal out death-blows to the hydra, disease."

> Th' Emetic number ONE's design'd
> A gen'ral med'cine for mankind,
> Of every country, clime, or place,
> Wide as the circle of our race.
> In every case, and state, and stage,
> Whatever malady may rage;
> For male or female, young or old,
> Nor can its value half be told.

Nor could the discomfort it caused be easily recited. Thomson reported one patient's description of its action, without disputing him, as twisting in his guts "like a screw auger."[9]

Being administered first, it was also the augur of worse things to come. Remedy group number two was designed "to retain the internal vital heat of the system and cause a free perspiration." It contained the hot drugs, among which the preferred was cayenne, employed as a powder, a snuff, a "Pepper-Sauce"—and in enemas (this despite Thomson's repeated castigations of orthodox physicians for applying blistering agents to patients' skin). Drugs in the third category were gentler but still were used "to scour the Stomach and Bowels, and remove the Canker." Marsh rosemary and witch hazel were representative specimens and were generally given as water decoctions, as teas or "coffees."[10]

These first three classifications fought against cold in part by evacuation, and even Thomson recognized they weakened the patient somewhat and had to be followed by restorative or tonic preparations. Number four, "Bitters, to correct the Bile, and restore Digestion," included poplar bark, goldenseal, and other botanicals and was followed by number five, a peach or cherry "Syrup for the Dysentery, to strengthen the Stomach and Bowels." Number six consisted of "Rheumatic Drops, to remove pain, prevent mortification, and promote a natural heat." Its recipe of brandy, myrrh, and cayenne indicates it would indeed promote a heat, natural or otherwise.[11]

Several additional remedies Thomson refrained from numbering completed the system: his "nerve powder" made from valerian; the "Composition," or vegetable powder of bayberry root, ginger, cloves, and cayenne; a skunk-cabbage-based "cough powder" a clover-derived "cancer plaster"; and other plasters, ointments, and salves. Listed individually, his botanical mainstays numbered sixty-five to seventy, depending on the list, and were administered almost as often anally as orally. Thomson put much stock in injections, especially for female complaints, and gave his warmest recommendation to an enema mixture of numbers one, two, three, six, and nerve powder. This injection, he suggested ominously, "must be repeated as occasion may require, till relief is obtained."[12]

Finally, there was steaming. The patient to be steamed would take a dose of number two, number three, or Composition, undress, and sit on a chair placed over a bucket of water. Stones taken glowing from the fire would then be placed in the water as needed, and the patient surrounded by a blanket to retain the steam. If the patient was too weak (from illness, lobelia, or previous steamings) to leave her bed, steam would be brought to her in the form of heated rocks or bricks wrapped in several thicknesses of wet cloth and placed in bed along her sides and at her feet. If that, and all the preceding, failed, the doctor tried again, and yet again. There is on record the case of a hardy Virginian who endured six months of treatment comprising "300 sweats" and sixty-six full courses of numbers one through six; he perhaps would have paused before endorsing Thomson's statement that his system was "about as perfect as it is possible to make it."[13]

Even a single course of Thomsonian therapy was a trial, if we can take the experience of a Philadelphian named Knappe as a guide. He was treated first by allopaths, who administered "an infinite number of remedies" yet "gave him up at last," leaving him to seek Thomsonian treatment as a final hope. (From the beginning, unconventional programs of therapy have grown in large measure by attracting the desperate cases that regular medicine has failed to help: a Virginia man in the 1830s explained that it was "the death of *seven* out of eleven in my family, under the treatment of Regular Physicians, [that] induced me to call a Thomsonian to attend the eighth.") In the hands of a Thomsonian agent, Mr. Knappe was subjected to at least eleven days of a regimen that involved a thirty-minute steam bath followed by some period of time in bed surrounded by hot bricks, then a dose of lobelia and other herbs in brandy, "after which warm water is drunk until there has ensued the most extraordinary vomiting." When the vomiting ended, he was given a second steaming and put to bed with bricks again for an hour. Two cayenne-and-lobelia enemas brought the day's treatment to a close.[14]

Knappe assured a worried friend that "this horse-cure" was not weakening him, even though on the previous day, his eleventh, the lobelia he was given both orally and anally "made me so sick that for three hours I gave no sign of life. . . . At the end of that time I vomited forth more than three gallons of bile, mingled with a sort of thick, heavy skin which would no end have astonished you." Still, there was a "last straw of that cure. Sick as I was, they made me take my steam bath!" A day later, "I am still spitting up matter and blood, but the pains are over and I feel a great deal improved." His doctor was certain he would recover, Knappe informed his friend: "Time shall tell us the rest."[15]

The Marketing of Thomsonian Medicine

Unfortunately, time tells us nothing more of the courageous Mr. Knappe; any records that might document his survival or destruction at the Thomsonian infirmary have long since been lost. His willingness to undergo the treatment, however, was certainly not due to its mildness. The allopath's leeches and calomel were only slightly more repulsive than lobelia and hot bricks. Thomson's success in attracting patients (an extraordinary degree of success, it will be seen) has to be accounted for by something other than the satisfactions of

cayenne enemas. He triumphed, in fact, more through marketing than medicine, through shrewd packaging and presentation that resonated with popular
prejudices against allopathic therapy and the allopathic profession.

The spearhead of Thomson's campaign was exploitation of public antip-
athy toward calomel. There was a highly vocal "anti-calomel part of the
community," a Massachusetts physician observed in the mid-1830s, that was
waging "a war for its [calomel's] utter and entire destruction and annihilation,
[a war] that rages in many parts of our country with as much venom, fury,
and heat, as ever did feudal war or party politics." Much of that fury and heat
was stirred up by Thomsonians, who portrayed calomel not as the "Samson
of the Materia Medica," as allopaths would have it, but as "the uncircumcised
Philistine of medical science," not a cure-all but a "kill-all," the "bane of life."
Thomsonian literature harangued the public to "resolve you will not be cal-
omelized any more" by "the Mineral Faculty" and attacked "the mercurial
craft" as "a monstrous bone rotting, tooth destroying, pain engendering, bile
vitiating, skin blistering, blood and life destroying system."[16]

Calomel was "the great bug-bear" in popular opinion, "the raw head
and bloody bones," an MD grumbled in 1838, not just because it inflicted such
damages upon patients but also because it was a mineral substance, representative of the complete spectrum of corrosive mineral compounds so dear to
allopathic practice. "With calomel," regular doctors complained, "all minerals
have been dragged in, and receive the same sentence of condemnation, for no
other reason but . . . for being found in bad company." Prejudice against minerals was fostered particularly by irregulars, who "have raised a hue and cry
against all minerals, and in the hope of throwing ridicule upon the profession
they term us 'Mineral Doctors.' They cry *mad dog*, and set upon the chase."[17]

In setting upon the chase, Thomsonians ignored the fact that some of
the most active drugs prescribed by orthodox practitioners were of vegetable
origin. They simply dictated that the world of medicine could be divided into
two realms, mineral practice and vegetable practice, and that the latter was as
safe and in keeping with nature's ways as the former was destructive and anti-
natural. The separating out of botanicals played effectively on popular enthusiasm for Romanticism, the philosophical and artistic movement that looked
to primitive society as the natural and purest state of human existence and
doted on the natural world as the source of beauty and spiritual inspiration.
Delicate, scented, colorful flowers and towering, leafy trees evoked the beauty
of nature in a way hard, sharp minerals never could, and plant products were
easily imagined to be wholly beneficent. One botanical healer spoke for all in
"ardently" longing to direct the sick "away from the rocky cliffs, the miney
depths, and the scorching sands of the mineralogical practice" and lead them
to the promised land of "fruitful fields, green pastures, and flowery banks of

sweetly-gliding streams and grassy fountain sides, to gather roots, and leaves, and blossoms, barks, and fruits, for the healing of the nations."[18]

Defenders of orthodox medicine reminded the forgetful laity time and again that nicotine, strychnine, and many other plant substances were deadlier than any minerals. Yet the vegetable creation was so infused with images of peaceful grandeur that toxicity was overshadowed by tranquility. "It is a very prevalent error," a regular doctor observed in the 1840s, that a remedy's being "composed entirely of vegetable substances, is a sure proof that it is innocuous, and that it can be used freely without any discrimination." "Let the pill be what it may," a colleague added, even "the most active, acrid, irritating poison, so it only be called 'vegetable,' no further questions are asked."[19] Substitute the word "natural" for "vegetable" in each physician's comments, and one will have warnings such as are issued all the time by medical scientists today.

Thomson repeatedly assured readers that his botanicals were fully safe because they were the progeny of fecund and beneficent nature. His son John took the argument still farther into mysticism, with the explanation that "the metals and minerals are in the earth, and being extracted from the depths of the earth, have a tendency to carry all down into the earth; or, in other words, the grave, who use them." Contrarily, "the tendency of all vegetables is to spring up from the earth. . . . Their tendency is to invigorate and fructify, and uphold mankind from the grave."[20] But neither Thomson, father or son, was the mush-minded Romantic such passages might suggest. On the contrary, they and their followers were the most unsentimental political realists, and it was through adroit exploitation of prevailing political values that Thomsonianism became so remarkably successful an alternative to regular medicine.

One of the most compelling elements of the cartoon discussed in the preceding chapter for the public of the 1830s was the Steps of Common Sense by which the Thomsonian doctor is pulling the patient out of the swamp of disease. Those steps appealed to the anti-intellectual sentiments that came to the fore in America with the election of Andrew Jackson to the presidency in 1828, sentiments that had a profound impact on attitudes toward medicine. Unlike the aristocratic sorts who had preceded him in that office (Washington, Adams, Jefferson, et al.), Old Hickory was a rough-hewn frontiersman, even a "barbarian," in the estimate of presidential rival John Quincy Adams. Not for him were the genteel breeding and fine education of East Coast elitists. What mattered were the qualities that were winning the West, the independence, egalitarianism, courage, industriousness, and perseverance against hardship and long odds that had opened up and secured the frontier. And to the extent that intelligence counted in that mix, it was the intelligence of common sense, the ability to solve practical problems, not the intelligence of abstract thought and high-falutin' language.[21]

Those were values shared by many Americans who had participated in, or at least applauded, the expansion of the frontier. And as restrictions on voting were relaxed over the first quarter of the nineteenth century, more and more men of common standing were enfranchised and made able to express their values in the polling booth. Ultimately, in 1828, they succeeded in electing one of their own, bringing on a Jacksonian age that elevated the common man to cultural preeminence. For the next two decades particularly, American society indulged in a self-conscious celebration of mediocrity, extolling hard work over genius, folksiness over refinement, and humble origins over high position.

Jacksonian attitudes affected the entrenched profession and promoted popular support for irregular medicine in two ways primarily. First, Jacksonianism was synonymous with anti-intellectualism, with suspicion of book-larnin' as a useless affectation and hatred of any person or group that requested special recognition or favor on the basis of educational attainment. The 1830s were rocked by a wave of ridicule and criticism of professionals—lawyers, bankers, even clergymen. Of course doctors, with their college degrees, fancy language, and etherial theories, received their share and more.

But it was not just their learning that brought condemnation down upon physicians. A second major tenet of Jacksonian philosophy was economic freedom. In a democratic society, it was accepted, all citizens (white Protestant males, at any rate) should have equal opportunity to make their way in the world, to rise as far as their unstinting labor and common sense would carry them. The corollary was that no one should be granted a competitive advantage by government or other agency; special privilege belonged in the benighted monarchies of the Old World. In this area, the medical profession was in violation on all counts because of its advocacy of legislation to require all practitioners of medicine to be licensed.

For most of America's colonial period, a license had not been needed to practice the healing art. Health problems were so rampant and formally trained practitioners so thin on the ground that people had to accept medical care wherever they could find it. The identification of a select few as legitimate doctors was a luxury society could not afford. By the later 1700s, however, a number of American physicians had been educated at European universities, more had been trained at the first American medical schools, and there was at last a sizeable corps of men possessing credentials that were distinctly superior to the attainments of the lower rank of would-be healers. Pleading protection of the public from incompetents, accomplished doctors called for legislation prohibiting the unschooled from practicing: "A just discrimination should be made," the physicians of Massachusetts argued in 1781, "between such as are duly educated and properly qualified for the duties of their profession, and those who may ignorantly and wickedly administer medicine whereby the health and lives of many valuable individuals may be endangered." The provincial legislature of New Jersey became the first to establish licensing restrictions for medical practitioners, in 1772, and several other states followed that lead by 1800.[22]

The professionalization of medicine continued apace through the first third of the nineteenth century, with the opening of many more medical schools, the founding of more professional societies and journals—and the enactment of more state licensing laws. By 1830 an aspiring doctor in virtually any state in the country had to qualify to practice by graduating from a medical school or by passing an examination administered by the state medical society; either way, it was orthodox medicine that had to be mastered. Yet while these laws do not seem to have been rigorously enforced, and in many instances imposed no more severe penalty than denial of the right to sue for uncollected fees, irregular practitioners found them intolerable. To begin, licensing legislation gave the stamp of government approval to a single form of medicine, while inhibiting the freedom of those with different beliefs to pursue the calling of their choice. Similarly, it interfered with the rights of patients to select the type of medicine they preferred. From the Jacksonian perspective, licensing requirements looked more like persecution of the people than protection of them. Further, the laws conferred an economic advantage on a professional group—in effect, a medical monopoly—on the basis of education, the book-larnin' so despised by Jacksonian democrats. In short, the presentation of Thomsonianism as common sense (as in the cartoon described in the previous chapter) delivered a powerful political message; irregular schemes of practice generally, in fact, originated in significant part as reactions to the professionalization of regular medicine and its spreading political hegemony. At the same time, the growth of alternative systems was assured by the Jacksonian public's distaste for learned professions and its respect for those who fought for the rights and freedoms of the common man.

The Battle for Medical Freedom

"Fought" is hardly too strong a term. The political context of the cartoon was the campaign mounted by Thomsonians to repeal the licensing laws that gave regular doctors their anti-democratic monopoly. They, among all the groups of irregular practitioners, were the leaders in a battle carried on in state capitals throughout the country, a heated struggle turgid with Jacksonian rhetoric tarring allopathic doctors as parasites and exploiters of the masses and calling for the abolition of anachronistic legislation granting unearned privileges to an educated and arrogant elite. "Mankind should be left to judge for themselves who treats them best," state legislators were reminded, "and not have absurdities forced upon them, merely because they are dictated by men who have got Diplomas . . . earned principally by fees, and some years attendance on absurd and insipid lectures at Medical Rooms." Even so, the struggle was not easy. In New York, Thomson's son John fought against the licensing law for more than a decade. When at last he prevailed, in 1844, it was only after collecting thousands of signatures on a scroll nearly a hundred feet long, then wheeling the petition in a barrow, engulfed in fanfare, down Albany's State Street to the capitol. A state legislator took over at that point, declaiming that "the people of this state have been bled long enough in their bodies and pockets" and telling them "it [is] time they should do as the men of the Revolution did: resolve to set down and enjoy the freedom for which they bled." New York's licensing law was "swept with indignation" from the statute book. By 1850 all but two states' licensing statutes had been swept from the books, so that, as one defender of orthodoxy despaired, "any one, male or female, learned or ignorant, an honest man or a knave, can assume the name of a physician, and 'practice' upon any one, to cure or to kill, as either may happen, without accountability. 'It's a free country!' " (American physicians have always felt that alternative medicine flourishes here more luxuriantly than in other nations because of our attachment to political freedom: as the author of *Medical Heresies* complained in the 1880s, "in this country, where the utmost freedom abounds, there is no law to prevent a man from being a fool himself, or patronizing one in any business in which he may choose to engage.") It was primarily thanks to Samuel Thomson, his disciples rejoiced, that "the Apocalyptic Beast [of] the Medical Inquisition" had been slain and "a dark chapter in American history . . . brought to an end."[23]

Thomson's image as champion of the common man was polished in other ways. First, he was the archetypal common man himself, veritably the Old Hickory of medicine. Born into poverty (beans and potatoes were all the family could afford to eat), subjected to early hardship by a stern father ("a man of violent and quick temper"), Thomson had perforce attended the "University of Hard Knocks" that common folk suppose to provide the only genuine and worthwhile education. ("God, in his wisdom," one Thomsonian proclaimed, "has adapted important truths to the capacity of feeble intellects.") What was needed to be a healer was not intellect but common sense and intuition. "I am convinced myself that I possess a gift in healing the sick," Thomson modestly allowed, "a natural gift" that no amount of schooling could provide.[24]

Thomson's demeanor reflected his lack of formal education. An early portrait (see fig. 2.1) depicts a man of blunt and sober countenance with a sizeable wart on the side of his nose—and that seems to have been just who he was, an unretouched, unceremonious sort who presented himself warts and all, take him or leave him. His autobiography (widely circulated as the preface to his guide to botanical medicines) was as unpretentious as it was long-winded, devoid of the incomprehensible jargon that doctors used to dumb-found patients. He called diseases by colloquial names folks could understand: canker, scalt head, salt rheum, itch, rattles, spotted fever, numbpalsy, the relax, and mercury sore. Educated readers might be put off by his insufferable martyr complex, but men of coarser fiber saw in his autobiographical record of insults endured and setbacks overcome a life saga that inspired empathy and respect. Forever being slighted, deceived, cheated, left unpaid, and otherwise mis-treated, Thomson was just the sort of hard-luck maverick who would one day become the hero of country music ballads. Nor were his working-class cre-dentials damaged by the fact that his persecutors were mostly men of higher station, his social betters—physicians.

The Popularity of Thomsonian Medicine

Thomson's appeal to the masses came partly from his demonstration that any commoner could practice medicine. It was due more, though, to his making it possible for every commoner to practice medicine. "Every man his own physician" was the democratic goal of Thomsonianism, a goal toward which the first step was taken in 1813. Weary of being harassed by envious regulars (who were now campaigning for stricter licensing legislation to suppress the botanical heresy) and fearful of having his discoveries stolen by inept imitators, Thomson decided to protect himself by obtaining a patent on his system of practice. Patent rights to medical innovations were rather freely granted at the time; Thomson's was the twenty-sixth since the Patent Office had opened in 1790. The patent gave him the exclusive right to practice—or to sell to others the right to practice—his special course of therapy. That second provision was the critical one for the future of Thomsonianism. Its discoverer had re-sorted to patent protection, he avowed with typically plaintive self-congratulation, "in order that I might reap some benefit from my discovery, to support me in my old age, having by a long series of attendance on the sick . . . become almost worn out." Why wear himself out further, particularly since his medicines were as simple to use as they were effective? Why not offer individuals the knowledge and the legal right to cure themselves safely and inexpensively in exchange for a reasonable sum to recompense Thomson for his years of experimentation, service, and adversity? The details of the scheme were to take still more years and adversity (and a second, stricter patent, obtained in 1823 and renewed in 1836) to work out, but by the mid-1820s the essential features were in place.[25]

The Thomsonian health care delivery system was a pyramidal structure with Thomson at the apex (with headquarters in Boston) and the American public—the common folk among them, at least—providing the base. In between were liaisons, Thomsonian "agents" who purchased from the founder the right to sell to individual families the right to dose themselves with numbers one through six. These agents, who eventually numbered close to two hundred, held botanic franchises, so to speak, which carried the privilege of vending botanical medicines and literature. Agents quickly took it to mean they were allowed to administer the medicines as well, to operate infirmaries where they might treat people reluctant to treat themselves. It was at such a place that Mr. Knappe had taken his cure—or met his end. The inmates of these Thomsonian institutions, regular doctors scoffed, were subjected to "the violence of the external and internal treatment to which this sect of quacks resort . . . until they either run away before they have become its victims, or are quietly buried from the infirmaries."[26]

The agent's primary function, however, was to take medicine to the people and teach them—nay, exhort them—to be their own doctors. A Vermont agent, to illustrate, opened his textbook with an address "To the farmer, the mechnic [sic], and the non-professional reader in general." The book, he explained, "is designed for you. It has been taught, and believed that common people—nature's real nobility—have not a proper right to study medicine. That is utterly false. Would you be slaves? No! Arouse, then, to your sense of reason and humanity, and take charge of your own bodies. Your abilities are equal, yea, better, for the task, than the faculty. . . . Yourselves do know that rejecting the physician has sometimes saved life and limb. We know it has hundreds. Be your own physicians! No one can supply your place. It will not only save your LIVES but your MONEY." At the same time, becoming one's own physician contributed money to Thomsonian agents, for the agent was above all a peddler of "Family Right Certificates," licenses for individual families to use cayenne and Composition in the privacy and convenience of their own homes. Each certificate cost twenty dollars; the agent kept ten dollars from the sale, and Thomson got the rest. The "puke doctor," as regulars called him, had indeed found a way to support himself in his old age.[27]

Everybody won at this game, in fact, for the owner of a Family Right Certificate was entitled to treat himself and all members of his household with the Thomsonian course of steam and botanicals. Each Family Right holder also became automatically a member of his local Friendly Botanic Society, in which he could exchange therapeutic experiences and advice with certificated neighbors. He was entitled as well to obtain his lobelia and other drugs from licensed Thomsonian pharmacies, where he could be confident there were stored no toxic mineral drugs to contaminate the precious herbs. Finally, so that certificate buyers could use their pure cayenne wisely, for only two dollars more Thomson supplied each with a manual outlining the proper use of his drugs. (People had long relied on such handbooks of "domestic medicine," though these had as a rule been authored by regular physicians; even so, Thomson's guide fit into a tradition with which the public was familiar and comfortable.) Through the Family Right Certificate, America's humbler citizens were empowered to realize the dream set out for them by the sometime poet Thomson:

> We wish every family apart
> To understand the healing art,
> Without so many forms and rules
> Coined and practiced by the schools.[28]

Twenty dollars was no trivial expenditure for a working man of the 1820s or 1830s, even if the lobelia system was (as a Virginia agent gushed) "next to the Christian religion the greatest boon that has ever been granted by indulgent Heaven to the sons and daughters of affliction." Yet in 1839 Thomson calculated that he had sold "upwards of one hundred thousand family rights" and that about three million Americans had adopted his system. (Apparently more than a few people were taking lobelia without paying for the right.) The national population in that year was just approaching seventeen million, so if Thomson's figures were correct, nearly 20 percent of the country had given up calomel for botanicals. There is every reason to suspect Thomson of inflating his figures—when did any advertiser do otherwise? Yet independent estimates also indicate high levels of popular support. In 1835, for example, the governor of Mississippi announced that half the citizens of his state were Thomsonian. About the same time, the regular physicians of Ohio (the third most populous state in the country) red-facedly admitted that probably one-third of the public there preferred Thomsonian remedies. (According to a Thomsonian speaking in the early 1840s, at least one-third of the entire country had "converted to common sense," even though not that many years before Thomsonian self-doctors had been "nearly as scarce as white crows.") The lobelia-and-steam regimen was evidently more popular in the South and Midwest than in the Northeast. (Ohio supported forty-one Thomsonian agents in 1833, Tennessee twenty-nine, and Alabama twenty-one, while New York had only eight, Massachusetts five, and Pennsylvania three.)[29] Nevertheless, if fully a third of Ohio went botanical, the overall national average might well have approached Thomson's guess. Even half that figure, 9 or 10 percent, would have been a showing that would gladden any of today's alternative medical groups.

The exact number of converts can never be known, but the political-cultural profile of Thomsonians is sharp and clear. Thomsonian medicine was blue-collar medicine. It was a continuation, on a higher plane, of the domestic medicine, or folk practice and self-care, historically used by people for whom professional medicine was inaccessible or too expensive or mistrusted. Its simple theory seemed reasonable to the farmer and mechanic; its straightforward therapy clearly accomplished what theory said it should. A man could feel his innards being scrubbed by lobelia and could hardly doubt after a cayenne enema that heat had been added to his body.

Thomsonian medicine was democratic medicine par excellence, medicine tailored to fit the desires and biases of the newly enfranchised masses. It drew those masses with a marketing blitz that, though not actually disingenuous, was very carefully orchestrated to exploit Jacksonian sentiment to the utmost. The whole wide expanse of Thomsonian publications—Thomson's own books, those of his agents and apostles, and periodicals such as *The Thomsonian Recorder, The Botanic Watchman, The Lobelia Advocate,* and *The Boston Thomsonian Manual and Lady's Companion*—fairly dripped with folksy egalitarianism. As if Thomson had not made enough of his log cabin upbringing in his autobiography, his supporters vied to see who could make the greatest bumpkin out of him. That "illiterate farmer," that "mere plough-boy [who] spent his life among the clods of the valley, and [was] himself but little superior to the dust he walked on," that "rude and uncultivated" backwoodsman nevertheless had "discovered *facts* which are destined to overturn the *visionary theories* of his predecessors."[30]

The anti-intellectualism appealed to by such characterizations could be milked as well by attacks on allopaths' use of unintelligible language, much as today's critics of the medical profession strive to "demystify" medicine for the laity. Thomson's opening remarks in his *New Guide to Health* were snide comments about doctors who kept "the knowledge and use of medicine . . . concealed in a dead language," and he never let pass an opportunity to accuse physicians of enslaving patients in the bonds of bewildering terminology: "They have learned just enough to know how to deceive the people, and keep them in ignorance, by covering their doings under an unknown language to their patients. There can be no good reason given why all the technical terms in medical works are kept in a dead language, except it be to deceive and keep the world ignorant of their doings, that they may the better impose upon the credulity of the people."[31]

A second component of present-day natural health philosophy presaged by Thomson is the principle of demedicalization of pregnancy and labor. The natural way to give birth is to do it at home rather than in the hospital, with the assistance of a lay midwife rather than the supervision of an obstetrician eager to impose pharmacological and surgical interventions. Thomson happened to mature during precisely the period when midwifery, the method of centuries, was beginning to be displaced by obstetrics, at least in the cities. The distinctive feature of early obstetrical care, what made it appealing to those who could afford it, was that it was administered by a trained physician who was presumed to be more knowledgeable than any midwife about the mechanics of birth and was skilled in the use of manual and instrumental techniques for repositioning and extracting refractory fetuses. Thomson regarded such procedures as unnatural and consequently dangerous. His own wife had experienced extended torture during her first labor (attended by physicians), and his sister-in-law's first confinement had ended in tragedy. In that instance, family members had gone against Thomson's wishes and called in a doctor, who, after seven hours of fruitless attempts to deliver the child, summoned a second physician. This latter at once got out his forceps and applied "the instruments of death" with force "enough to have drawn an hundred weight!" The infant was soon withdrawn—but with its head crushed, "murdered." The mother's condition was nearly as low, and Thomson was no longer able to stand silently by. "Had it been at my own house," he swore, "I think I should . . . have pitched the monster out at the window." Instead, he dismissed the doctors, placed the woman under botanical care, and brought her back to health. Two years later, she gave birth to a vigorous child.[32]

His sister-in-law had been only one victim among thousands, and a lucky one at that. In the good old days of midwifery, of natural childbirth, "there was scarce an instance known," Thomson fatuously imagined, "of a woman dying in child-bed" or losing her child; "but at the present time these things are so common that it is hardly talked about." Why was that? Because midwives "used no art, but afforded such assistance as nature required." Forceps "forced nature." Artificial expansion of the birth canal made the fetus stop its "natural progression" and draw back, requiring it then to be snatched forth by instruments "as the dog catches its game." The physician, Thomson could not refrain from pointing out, was the dog.[33]

The old method of relying on nature could nevertheless be improved by botanical assistance, lobelia being as good for babies as for adults, by Thomson's reckoning. His recommendations for "Treatment in the hour of Travail" included a tea of hot water, sugar, Composition, nerve powder, cayenne, and a "large tea-spoonful of brown emetic." With that kind of aid, "your children will be born naturally, as fruit falls from the tree, when ripe, of itself." They would also be born inexpensively. Another thing Thomson deplored about obstetrics was its escalating costs. Midwives still charged a dollar, but physicians had increased their fees from an original three dollars in the late 1700s to anywhere from twelve to twenty dollars. "If they go on in this ratio," Thomson forecast, "it will soon take all the people can earn, to pay for their children."[34]

With a Family Right and its perpetual protection costing no more than one obstetrician-delivered baby, the lobelia system was a medical idea whose time had come. In the heady days of the 1830s, as Family Rights sold as quickly as they could be printed, Thomsonian practitioners rejoiced at their prospects. "The world is wakening round you," they taunted regular physicians.

> Botanic Doctors (sounding the majesty of truth)
> Gain ground: the mercurial craft declines!
> Thick darkness flies before Thomsonian light,
> Bursting in glory on a long benighted world![35]

Allopathic Opposition to Thomsonianism

In truth, what would soon burst was the Thomsonian bubble, for by 1850 the epidemic of medical democracy was rapidly abating. Regular doctors liked to think that the demise of Thomsonianism was their doing. They had, after all, tried mightily for decades to suppress what they saw as a life-endangering heresy. Thomsonians saw those efforts in a different light, objecting that allopaths had "persecuted and pursued" their leader "with all the malice of demons," that they had "hunted [him] down like a wild beast," and not because he was a public danger, but "because of his extraordinary success in curing disease, which has tended to enlighten the people, and do away their blind confidence in the infallibility of doctors."[36]

By Thomson's own telling, the persecution began early, as soon as he left his permitted sphere of treating his own family and a few neighbors. The herb doctor's successes could not be kept secret, and as word steadily spread beyond his hometown, appeals for help came back from surrounding hamlets. As his influence rippled outward, Thomson found enough doctoring business to be able to abandon the farming he had hated since childhood. From 1805 onward he was usually to be found on the road to Portsmouth or Hillsborough or Woodstock, carrying the miracle of lobelia and steam to all who needed it. Their number seems to have been legion. The recurrent theme of this segment of his autobiography is a drama in which Thomson arrives in a town to find a horde of gravely ill people whose various ailments have been worsened by calomel. The local regulars have given them all up as incurable, so they have nothing to lose by accepting Thomson's offer of rescue. He then proceeds to save nearly one and all, the rare failures being laid to the patient being too far gone already, whether from disease or allopathic abuse. In Beverly in 1808, for example, he attended "many desperate cases; in all of which I effected a cure, except one, who was dying before I was called on."[37]

No wonder regular doctors were so spiteful and malicious. When *they* lost patients it was *their* fault, and their occasional recoveries were, so Thomson said, due to nature's outlasting their worthless medicines. No wonder they called Thomson "steam doctor" and "puke doctor" and "old wizzard" and attempted to frame him for murder. When in 1809 one of Thomson's patients died (after ignoring the instructions he had been given for recuperation after lobelia), a Dr. French succeeded in getting the herb doctor indicted and thrown into jail. There Thomson languished for a month, his food nothing but stale bread and coffee, his bed a pile of straw overrun with lice ("enough of them to shingle a meeting-house"), and his cellmate a convicted child molester. But when his case finally came to trial (after forty days of imprisonment, he emphasized, the same period that another maltreated dispenser of salvation had spent in a wilderness), he was promptly acquitted, the jury needing only five minutes of deliberation before deciding he was the victim of an allopathic plot. Further vindication came when one of Dr. French's accomplices in carrying out the plot, a Mr. Pecker, "had a stroke of the palsy, and has remained ever since, one half of his body and limbs useless." Thomson immediately filed a slander suit against French, and though in this instance he lost, and even had to pay court costs, there was still a measure of satisfaction to be had in the fact that his nemesis was shortly after arrested for graverobbing. "Most of those that have been instrumental in trying to destroy me and my practice," Thomson rejoiced, "have had some judgment befall them as a reward for their unjust persecutions and malicious conduct towards me."[38]

Regular doctors continued to risk judgments befalling them, keeping up a steady stream of ridicule to discredit Thomsonianism with the public. Not only was it "the most stupendous system of quackery and the most insulting offering ever tendered to the understanding of a free and enlightened people," it was blatant hypocrisy to boot, congratulating itself for overthrowing the orthodox medical monopoly while succeeding through use of the most monopolistic device of all, a federal patent. The Thomsonian agent, MDs scoffed, was an "ignoramus" whose total medical education consisted of reading "a small duodecimo volume containing the whole of medical science—the plan of steaming." If this simple-minded system were true, "what a perfect relief it brings to all the uncertainty of medicine! Away then with all care-worn experience, and all study! Keep up a constant fire of lobelia, red pepper, and steam, and you will certainly kill the disease at last—at least if you do not kill the patient." The agent was laughed at as a "knight of red pepper," "a veritable Don Quixote" setting off to rescue the world with his "homicidal quackery," his "incendiary treatment" that "exterminat[ed] patients and the disease at a single blow." It was thus with an easy conscience that a Mississippi regular took satisfaction in the hangings of "two celebrated steam doctors" in his neighborhood when they were found to have been members of a group plotting a slave uprising. The Thomsonians' botanicals, he joked to his wife, "were found to avail nothing against hemp."[39]

As proof of incendiary treatment, regulars presented cases such as the unfortunate Mr. Sherburn, a Vermont gentleman who underwent one too many courses of steam therapy. According to the 1841 report of the county attorney, the patient's remains were nearly unidentifiable, his head "swelled to double size—black, tongue out, eyes stand out of sockets, blood running from the nose, blistered in various places . . . thighs blistered, one leg seemed par-boiled, no feature of the face or body that would be recognized. . . . Inside of stomach appears to be ironed over as with a hot iron as likewise is the lower parts of the intestines, probably scorched with hot drops of Cagerin [sic] pepper." The mistreated man's Thomsonian therapist, meanwhile, had "left town hastily."[40]

Not all botanical doctors managed to leave hastily enough. In 1837, to cite one example, a Thomsonian named Frost (strange name for a heat-promoting doctor) was arrested for the death of one Tiberius French (fitting name for a lobelia victim, given Thomson's persecution at the hands of Dr. French a quarter century before). The indictment of Frost accused him of "feloniously and willfully" assaulting the "body and bowels" of French with a cayenne-and-lobelia enema and just as feloniously injuring "the breast, stom-ach, belly, and back, head, legs and arms" of the victim with "a certain noxious and injurious hot vapor called steam," with the result that the patient "then and there died." The jury returned a verdict of "guilty of manslaughter," but even when they won, regular doctors lost. Frost was found guilty only in "the fourth degree," mercy was recommended, and the convicted man was allowed to go free. And in the middle of the trial, when a defense witness acclaimed the vegetable kingdom for containing "all the necessary remedial agents" and wished "mankind would get their eyes open to the difference between the vegetable and mineral practice," he was answered with "great applause." The decision in favor of the regulars was evidently a grudging one. But the fact that Dr. Frost and other agents were arrested at all was, for Thomsonians, an "everlasting scandal," a demonstration that allopaths could not win patients through "skill and wisdom," only through "fines, prisons, dungeons, chains and death."[41]

*Fragmentation of the Thomsonian System: Physio-Medicalism
and Eclectic Medicine*

As it turned out, Samuel Thomson's own death struck a more crippling blow
at the botanical system than anything MDs did. Thomsonianism had only
grown from strength to strength until 1843, when the founder suffered a
sudden attack of "the relax" brought on by a fit of "worriment" over the loss
of a sizeable sum of money. For nearly two weeks he took lobelia and enemas,
swallowed canker tea and nerve powder, had steaming stones placed about his
feet and back and brandy-soaked flannel applied to his body. But nature's fire
was low and flickering, and he finally "dropped away like going to sleep. He
died [in Boston] highly respected and lamented."[42]
    Various fault lines had already appeared within Thomsonianism. There
had been a good bit of internecine squabbling, for instance, over the operation
of infirmaries by agents, a practice that smacked of the allopathic model of
taking care out of the hands of the people. Even more controversial were
proposals by some agents to establish schools to train the next generation of
infirmary directors. What was that, disciples of Thomson wanted to know,
but the imposition of book-larnin' and intellectual elitism on a practice derived
from common sense and intended for the comprehension of the common man?
There were disagreements over just which botanicals should be used as well,
and all the issues were exacerbated by the dictatorial and difficult personality
of Thomson himself. There was a consensus that the founder was "illiterate,
coarse in his manners, and extremely selfish," even "an old avaricious churl."
Once the leader's controlling hand fell from the helm, the botanical system
fragmented into any number of small groups seeking identity in esoteric names
that utilized nearly every possible combination of "Botanic," "Reformed,"
"Improved," "Independent," and similar revised Thomsonian terminology.
More intent on discrediting one another than overcoming regular medicine,
most had disappeared by the time of the Civil War. "As certain sagacious
quadrupeds are said to quit a sinking ship," an MD commented, "so Thomsonian doctors one after another abandoned their craft."[43]
    Thomsonians actually began to abandon ship as early as 1832, when an
Ohio agent named Horton Howard published a treatise that purported to be
an *Improved System of Botanic Medicine.* Howard promptly organized his own
group of "improved botanics" and set about promoting a system that added
another forty-two botanicals to Thomson's list of herbs and rested "upon a
new combination of principles . . . in harmony with the . . . operations of Nature." Typically, Thomson responded with threats of legal action, but when
Howard died in a cholera outbreak the next year, the improved botanic movement quickly passed away as well (Howard's death was no doubt seen by

Thomson as another of those judgments visited upon his enemies; during his career as an agent, Howard had sold eighty thousand dollars' worth of Family Rights and refused to give Thomson even a penny of his half share). A more enduring offshoot appeared in 1838. In that year, Alva Curtis, another Ohio Thomsonian (by way of New York and Virginia) and editor of *The Thomsonian Recorder*, withdrew from the U.S. Thomsonian Convention, the system's national professional society, and launched an organization he called the Independent Thomsonian Botanic Society. The schism came about over the issue of education, Curtis and his followers believing that the science of botanical healing was too complex for just anyone to learn on his own. In open defiance of Thomson's goal of medical democracy, Independent Thomsonians called for the establishment of formal medical training for botanical doctors. One "must deplore the presumption of ignorant men," an editor harangued readers, "who imagine that by purchasing a Thomsonian book, and reading over a mass of heterogeneous nonsense, the sum total of Botanic medical practice is obtained." For these reformers, original Thomsonianism was nonsense both in the disorganized way its teachings had been presented by the founder and in the childish faith it placed in the intellectual abilities of the common man: "The miraculous power of transforming farmers and mechanics into doctors in a moment, is doubted in the present day." Curtis even went so far as to argue that educated botanical doctors should be licensed the same as regulars.[44]

A year later, in 1839, Curtis opened the first chartered school for his independent group, the Literary and Botanico-Medical Institute of Ohio, in Columbus (He had been running an unchartered school in that city for three years by then.) In 1841 the institute was moved to Cincinnati, where it underwent a series of name changes until finally achieving permanency in 1850 as the Physio-Medical College. The name was the outcome of much debate among practitioners over the best way to capsulize their healing orientation. "Physio-medicalism" ("which signifies . . . curing according to nature," Curtis explained) expressed the group's commitment to using nature's plants to assist the life force: their object was to "remove every obstruction to the full, free and universal action of the vital principle," much the same as Thomson's had been. The botanical products they used were much the same as Thomson's, too (lobelia, cayenne, and steam baths remained favorites), though there were a number of additions, and they were used skillfully enough that the physio-medicals were able to survive in practice, and indeed to grow, through the rest of the century. There would be another dozen physio-medical colleges established, eight prior to the Civil War and the last as late as 1902. Curtis's college lasted until 1880, and the final school closed its doors in 1911, no longer able to finance the expanded training required by the scientific revolution that occurred in medicine in the late nineteenth century. It has been estimated that there were never more than 2,500 physio-medicals at any one time in America.[45]

Far more numerous were the members of another botanical healing group, one that originated independently of Thomsonianism. Eclecticism was exactly what its name implied, a system that borrowed freely from all schools of practice, taking anything that experience showed to be effective and safe. Thomsonian remedies were quite popular among eclectics, but so were items taken from Native American and other botanical traditions, as well as non-mineral drugs from the allopathic armamentarium. Guided by the rule of *vires vitales sustinete*, or "sustain the [patient's] vital forces," eclectics abjured all strong depletive treatments, which meant lobelia as well as calomel and bleeding.[46]

Eclecticism had its origins in the work of Wooster Beach, an 1825 graduate of a regular medical school who soon grew suspicious of the safety of orthodox remedies. As early as 1827 he opened a school in New York City to educate students in the full range of gentle botanical medicines, and as public dissatisfaction with medical orthodoxy grew over the next two decades, eclecticism became one of the more widely patronized systems. Its botanic materia medica was steadily enlarged and refined, its educational system expanded to more than twenty institutions, and more than sixty journals were founded. Part of eclecticism's appeal was its unusually pragmatic approach. Alone among irregular systems, it made no attempt to rationalize the operation of its medicines with a theoretical superstructure. "Use anything that works" was its only principle, a rule that allowed practitioners considerable leeway to do as they pleased and regular doctors wide scope for derision. "The Eclectics keep themselves alive by swallowing everything which happens to turn up," *The Medical and Surgical Reporter* commented, "until they have become like Macbeth's cauldron." In the eclectics' "extraordinary conglomeration" of therapies were to be found "all the 'ics,' 'lics,' 'isms,' 'cisms,' 'ists,' and 'pathies' " of all the other alternative systems.[47]

Because of their insistence on freedom from the dictates of authority, eclectics often identified themselves as the American school of medicine. In medicine as in society, of course, American freedom meant room for disagreement, and the history of eclecticism was in fact a turbulent one. But however pointed internal dissension became (one skirmish, a faculty dispute over control of a school in Cincinnati, was settled with a cannon), eclectic medicine remained one of the more popular alternatives to allopathy until the early twentieth century. Then, like physio-medicalism, it faded from the scene, its last school, Cincinnati's Eclectic Medical Institute, closing in 1939.[48]

Thomsonianism, incidentally, found its way in the 1830s to England, where its message of medical freedom and equality briefly gained some footing among the working and farming classes, despite the surnames of its leaders, John Skelton and Isaiah Coffin. But while the system was short-lived abroad, it has survived to the present in Thomson's native country. As recently as 1978 the chapter on herbs in a popular *Holistic Health Handbook* praised lobelia as "the best muscle-relaxant herb there is" and suggested combining it with cayenne ("the most powerful natural stimulant") to accelerate the circulation (improve body heat distribution?). The author's recipe for "Composition Powder" ("to be used hourly during the acute stage of disease") differed from Thomson's only in the proportion of ingredients and by the addition of white pine to the original mix of bayberry, ginger, cloves, and cayenne. Finally, the first name on the list of Caucasian contributors to the botanic tradition was that of the "old wizard" himself.[49]

3

Dilutions of Grandeur: Homeopathy

S illy as they considered Thomson's steaming-and-puking regimen to be, nineteenth-century physicians thought of another irregular system as still more unlikely. Indeed, homeopathy's practices were so remarkably at odds with all accepted notions of how nature worked, of how nature conceivably *could* work, that they were only to be regarded as utterly impossible. It was "a stupendous monument of human folly"; it represented "the crowning exploit of pseudo-scientific audacity"; it constituted a fabric of "astounding absurdities" and "nonsensical trash." "This horrid disgrace of the human mind" was such "a confused mass of rubbish" as to make sense only to "simpletons" possessed of "imbecile credulity." All in all, "the fact that men of sense and character should become its dupes, is one of the most striking exhibitions of intellectual stupidity and moral obliquity which the history of fanaticism itself can furnish."[1] Homeopathy was also the most popular of all alternative systems of practice from the 1850s to the beginning of the twentieth century.

Origins of Homeopathy

The system's founder, the German Samuel Hahnemann (1755–1843; Fig. 3-1), got his start as a regular MD, obtaining the degree at Erlangen in 1779. Afterward, he practiced in a succession of small towns in Germany but steadily lost confidence in the efficacy of the treatments he had been taught to provide. "I sank into a state of sorrowful indignation," he related, after coming to realize "the weakness and errors of my teachers and books." Medicine, he decided, was "founded upon *perhapses* and blind chance," its professed remedies nothing but "*Pferdecuren* [horse cures]." Thinking of himself as "a mur-

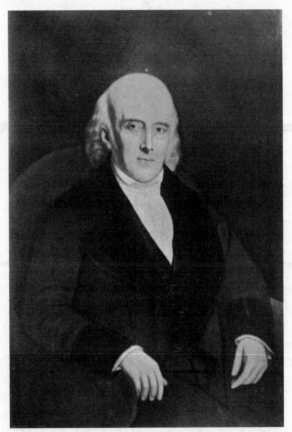

Figure 3-1. Samuel Hahnemann [Thomas Bradford, *The Life and Letters of Dr. Samuel Hahnemann* (Philadelphia: Boericke and Tafel, 1895), frontispiece]

derer" was "so fearful and distressing" that he soon abandoned medical practice and "occupied myself solely with chemistry and literary labours."[2]

Among his literary labors was the translation of foreign medical works into German, and it was through that activity that Hahnemann arrived at his interpretation of nature's way of healing. During his first year of work as a translator, in 1790, he encountered a passage in a text authored by a celebrated Scottish physician that addressed the action of the drug cinchona. The dried bark of a South American tree of the madder family, cinchona contains quinine and had been used in Europe since the mid-1600s to treat malaria and other fevers. As one of the handful of drugs with unquestioned therapeutic value, cinchona was a substance of more than ordinary interest to doctors, and Hahnemann must have been disposed to take special care in translating a foreign expert's pronouncements on the drug. One of Professor Cullen's opinions struck him as questionable: the proposal that cinchona countered fever by means of a tonic effect on the digestive system clashed with Hahnemann's own experience using the drug, which had left him nauseous. So he put the matter to the test by taking a standard dose of cinchona for several days and observing its effect on his stomach. He soon realized he was onto something much more significant than a translator's footnote correcting the statement of a renowned authority, for as the twice-daily four-drachm experimental dose took effect, "my feet, finger tips, etc. at first became cold; I became languid and drowsy; then my heart began to palpitate; my pulse became hard and quick; and intolerable anxiety and trembling [followed] then pulsation in the head, redness of the cheeks, thirst." What had happened, he realized, was that "all the symptoms usually associated with intermittent fever appeared in succession."[3]

Intermittent fever was the eighteenth century's synonym for malaria, the disease that cinchona cured. The very drug that relieved a certain disease in a sick person, therefore, had produced the disease, or at least a close facsimile of it, in a healthy person. Rephrased, a drug that in a healthy person generated certain symptoms relieved the same symptoms in a sick person. "By the observation of nature and my own experience," Hahnemann had discovered the principle of *similia similibus curantur*, that likes cure likes. (In Hahnemann's original formulation, the principle was expressed as *similia similibus curentur*, let likes be cured by likes, but the *curantur* formulation eventually became standard.) To be sure, Hahnemann at first believed only that the similar disease produced by the cinchona "*probably*" cured intermittent fever; but before long, "after mature experience, I add, not only *probably*, but *quite certainly*."[4]

An approach to healing based on this "law of similars," Hahnemann decided, should be called "homeopathy" from the Greek roots *homoios* (like) and *pathos* (suffering). Yet whether spelled "homeopathy" or "homoeopathy" (a version popular in the nineteenth century and still encountered occasionally), the notion that like cures like was not an entirely new concept. As a hunch about nature's way of healing, it is as old as the human race and has been applied in every form from the ancient Roman's faith in the power of raw dog's liver to ward off rabies to the seventeenth-century Englishman's use of pomegranate seeds to relieve toothache to the eighteenth-century American's trust in yellow mustard seed as a preventive of yellow fever. For that matter, the still popular recommendation of "the hair of the dog that bit you" as the surest hangover remedy might be thought of as homeopathy.

Hahnemann's homeopathy, however, was different from these various folk practices by virtue of arriving at similarities between drug and disease not on the superficial basis of common origin (the dog, for example) or physical appearance (toothlike shape, yellow color) but as a result of experimental determinations of likeness. Experiment had uncovered the first example of a drug producing symptoms similar to those it would cure (cinchona), and if the law of similars was to be generalized so that the full range of human afflictions could be treated naturally, many more drugs would have to be tested to learn what symptoms they produced. Hahnemann soon began such tests on fellow villagers, then advanced to administering drugs to people suffering with symptoms that tests had shown the drug to produce and, he believed, curing them. Within a few years he had developed his homeopathic method to the point that he felt confident announcing it to the world (in a 1796 article) as a new system of healing derived from a law "dictated to me by nature herself," the law that "when homoeopathically selected" a drug "will imperceptibly create in the patient an artificial condition, bearing a very close resemblance to that of the natural disease, and will speedily and permanently cure the sufferer of his original complaints."[5]

Conventional medicine followed a different rule, Hahnemann pointed out, seeking to overcome disease through "the use of such medicines as are capable of producing in the healthy body a *different* . . . affection from that exhibited by the disease to be cured." Was there ever, he asked, "a more ridiculous pretension? a more recherché piece of stupidity?" than this presumption that disease had to be neutralized with something different or opposite to it, rather than duplicated? Well versed in classical languages, Hahnemann coined a label for the conventional approach: "allopathy," from Greek roots for "unlike" and "suffering." Allopathy had acquired its misguided faith in opposites rather than similars by trusting in theory over experience. It had fed on "the sweet baby-food of hypotheses and pleasant figments" and been "stunted in [its] growth by the eternal swaddling clothes of authorities that discountenance all investigations." Allopathic epistemology was "useless trash," and allopaths themselves bound in "the trammels of ignorant credulity." Worst of all, the therapeutic premise of "other than the disease" worked against the healing efforts of nature. Hahnemannian practitioners "abjure Allopathia for this," a mid-nineteenth-century American homeopath stated; "she ignores nature and her powers [and] in her practice violates her." The title of this doctor's book said it all: *Homoeopathia and Nature and Allopathia and Art*.[6] By the mid-1800s all irregular practitioners, not just homeopaths, would be using the epithet "allopathy" with exactly that same understanding.

Homeopathic Provings

Homeopathic practice, based on the administration of remedies that produced effects similar to those of the disease, required that potential drug materials be tested on people to determine just what effects they produced and thus what symptoms they would cure. These experiments to discover symptoms were called "provings" in English, from the German *Prüfung*, for a trial or test. Hahnemann personally conducted provings on a total of ninety-nine drugs over the course of his lifetime. Other homeopaths carried out provings as well, bringing the sum of remedies studied to more than seven hundred by the end of the nineteenth century.[7] Materials to be tested as drugs were selected from all three kingdoms of nature. There were minerals such as natrum muriaticum (table salt; homeopathic remedies were given Latin names), arsenicum, and cinnabaris. Animal products included lachesis (snake venom) and pediculis capitis (head lice). But the largest category consisted of botanicals: veratrum album, datura stramonium, nux vomica, rhus toxicodendron, pulsatilla, and many more.

Hahnemann took considerable pains to ensure that the findings in his trials were valid. First, he employed only healthy volunteers in the provings. Unhealthy ones would be experiencing symptoms of illness that might get confused with any symptoms produced by the drug; the law of similars, furthermore, specified that drugs relieved the same symptoms in the sick as they produced in the *healthy*. "Our trials have been made on persons enjoying perfect health," Hahnemann declared, "and living in contentment and comparative ease."[8]

Once healthy volunteers were recruited, they were instructed to take regular doses of the item being tested and to keep detailed records of all unusual sensations they experienced while doing so. "Provers" were ordered to practice moderation in diet ("as free as possible from spices") and drink ("not of a stimulating kind"), to avoid excessive physical or mental exertion, and to deny themselves "the excitement of sensual excesses." If any event causing unusual merriment, anxiety, or other emotional perturbation occurred during the trial, no symptoms were to be recorded afterward, "in order to prevent spurious symptoms being noted as genuine." Genuine symptoms had to be evaluated in depth by "the experimenter assum[ing] various postures, in order to observe if the sensation is increased, lessened, or made to vanish by motion of the affected part; by walking in the room, or in the open air; by standing, sitting, or lying; or whether it returns when he assumes the original position." Provers were expected to determine whether any symptom was affected "by eating, drinking, talking, coughing, sneezing, or some other bodily function." The time of day or night at which each symptom tended to occur was, Hahnemann instructed, to be given "particular notice."[9]

Drugs had to be proved by people of all ages and "by males as well as by females, in order to discover what effect is produced with regard to the sex." Finally, provers "should possess the requisite degree of intelligence, to enable them to define, and to describe their sensations in distinct expressions." Only after taking the drug for an extended period, several weeks at least, and reaching a point where no new symptoms were being experienced could provers report back to Hahnemann with their records. He then "examined every prover carefully about every particular symptom, continually calling attention to the necessary accuracy in expressing the kind of feeling, the point or locality, the observation, and the mentioning of everything that influenced their feelings, the time of day, etc. When handing their papers to him, they had to affirm that it was the truth and nothing but the truth."[10]

With all those precautions in place, Hahnemann was certain that his experimental results were accurate indications of the effects produced by each tested drug and of the symptoms they would cure. Orthodox physicians thought otherwise. Indeed, the provings were one of the chief elements of homeopathy they had in mind when they sneered at the system as a "monument of human folly." To regular doctors, the provings appeared to be unscientific and naive, because, as we would say today, they included no control subjects. The reactions of provers testing a drug were not compared to the sensations experienced by a similar group of people not taking the drug; the several provers of each drug, furthermore, did not all experience the same symptoms themselves. How could Hahnemann be sure that the symptoms reported to him had been produced by the drug rather than being some of the random occurrences of day-to-day living? Many of the reactions he ascribed to drug action, after all, were things that everyone experienced on a regular basis, whether taking any "drug" or not: pimples, hiccups, sneezing, and snoring, for example, were repeatedly credited to drug action. (A much later commentary, a cartoon from the 1990s, shows Snow White making the acquaintance of the dwarves. "Sneezy, Dopey, Sleepy, Grumpy?" she says. "I take it no one here's ever heard of homeopathy?") Hahnemann brushed aside such objections with the assurance that "the drug being taken in pretty large quantity, no disturbance can take place in the organism which is not the effect of the drug." To him, provings were the only way to "a true Materia Medica," one that "should exclude every supposition, every mere assertion and fiction; its entire contents should be the pure language of nature, uttered in response to careful and faithful inquiry."[11]

So confident was Hahnemann that he was listening to the pure language of nature, he chose the title *Materia Medica Pura* for the volumes in which he recorded his own provings. There, and in similar works produced by converts who oversaw additional provings, were listed all the effects found to occur in healthy volunteers when they took one or another drug. For each remedy, symptoms were organized with regard to body area affected, progressing from the head down to the feet. Mental and emotional reactions were included as well, giving the homeopathic practitioner a highly detailed and specific guide to matching up drugs with patients' symptom complexes.

To regulars, these "true materia medicas" were collections of absurdities. How, they wondered, could anyone maintain a straight face when confronted by lists of symptoms that ran anywhere from ten to fifty pages for each drug and that included such effects as "yawning and stretching," "easily falls asleep when reading," "weakness of memory," "excessive liability to become pregnant," "rage, at the time the menses made their appearance," "voluptuous itching" of the penis "when walking in the open air," and "excessive trembling of the whole body, when dallying with females," not to mention heartburn, flatulence, bad breath, and vomiting during pregnancy? What was one to make of the several drugs that produced both constipation and diarrhea or, as with opium, that caused "excessive erection" and "impotence" alike and that led to "diminution of the sexual desire" while also inducing "excitation of the sexual instinct" and "nightly amorous visions"?[12]

There was much attention given in the homeopathic materia medica to both erections and nightly visions. Long before the clinical testing of Viagra, one fortunate prover found that arnica montana produced "violent sexual desire, and continued erections (in a weak old man)." Dreams, which occurred with virtually every drug proved, were often "amorous" (sometimes ending with "an emission"), or else they were frightening: there were "anxious dreams about murderers and robbers," for instance, and "frightful dreams about falling from a height," "dreams that a horse is biting him in the upper arm," "dreams about curious cats assailing him," dreams "that the world is perishing by fire." There were even dreams "that all his teeth are falling out." Sometimes the frightful dreams came true. One woman was made "weary of life and inclines to drown herself," while a man "throws himself from a height. Jumps into the water."[13]

Regular doctors were particularly amused by the extraordinary detail with which symptoms were characterized. "Painful piercing pushes in the right side of the penis" were periodically produced by one drug; others caused such difficulties as "copious flow of urine, accompanied by distortion of the eyes, and spasmodic contraction of the feet," "catarrhal affections during a cold, dry, northwest wind," and "pressure and tearing in the tips of the fourth and fifth finger [sic] of the right hand." Headaches were particularly common in provers, and for some reason they were described in the most minute detail of all. Aconite alone could produce a remarkable gamut that ran from "sense of fulness and heaviness in the forehead, as if a weight were pressing out there, and as if the contents of the head would issue from the forehead," through "headache, as if the eyes must fall out," "headache, as if the brain were pressing out," "headache, as if parts of the brain were raised up," "headache in the forehead when walking," "burning headache, as if the brain were moved about by burning water," "lacerating pain in the left temple, with roaring tingling in the ears," and "headache, throbbing on the left side of the forehead, with paroxysmal hard shocks on the right," all the way to "headache, as if the skull were externally laced by a band and drawn tightly together," and several others. Similarly detailed attention was given to emotional symptoms. Just a few of the effects ascribed to nux vomica, for example, were "she is anxious, solicitous, and inconsolable, weeps, complains, reproaches, moans, her cheeks being very red and hot, without thirst."[14]

Those minute details that regulars found so nonsensical were for Hahnemann the distinguishing virtue of the homeopathic approach. Allopathic characterizations of disease were much too general, he believed, completely lacking in the nuances of illness that made each sick person's case unique. The conventional orientation was to presume the existence of a finite number of disease states, each defined by certain broadly identified symptoms such as fever, weakness, abdominal pain, skin rash, etc. All cases of any particular disease were regarded as more or less the same and were to be treated with the same drugs: "Almost every disease pretended to be described," Hahnemann scoffed, "is as like another as the spots on a die." His interpretation of the enormous range of drug symptoms discovered in provings was that sickness could express itself in any number of ways. There are "innumerable varieties" of suffering, he wrote; the "psychico-corporeal microcosm" was subject "to an infinity of modifications and shades of difference!" Diseases were therefore "as diverse as the clouds in the sky." To define a case of sickness in such broad terms as fever and fatigue was akin to describing a person's face by saying he has two eyes, a nose, and a mouth. "The key to the individuality of each patient is not found in the symptoms he has in common with others," as allopaths presumed, "but in those which distinguish him from others. It is not the possession of a nose which renders a person distinctive, but the particular shape of this organ."[15]

If for Thomson every man was to be his own doctor, for Hahnemann every man was his own disease. And whereas the allopath would ask the patient, "Where does it hurt?" the homeopath knew that it hurt just about everywhere, including the psyche and the soul. He knew further that it hurt differently in every area, that there was a "complexity of the pains composed of various kinds of sensations, their degrees and shades," and that exactly how it hurt everywhere had to be determined precisely before treatment could be prescribed. Then, however, the patient could expect a remedy specific to her case, tailor-made by nature to address every symptom down to its finest subtlety, instead of the "thoughtless routine," the assembly-line, everyone-the-same treatments administered by orthodox MDs.[16] The latter reflexly bled and purged whether the patient had chapping of the upper lip or the lower one and whether painful pushes were in the right side of the penis or the left.

The proof of the provings, the demonstration that all those little details truly had meaning, was in the superior recovery rates of homeopathic patients. Hahnemann was certain from his own clinical experience that homeopathic treatments cured, and that could be true only if the provings were legitimate. The similar drugs worked, however, only if they were prepared in a very particular way. This method of preparation was an unexpected finding to which Hahnemann was led by a purely empirical approach; it was also the second aspect of homeopathy that struck regular physicians as absurd, seeming even more implausible than the data obtained from provings.

Preparation of Homeopathic Remedies

At the time Hahnemann announced his discovery of homeopathy to the public in 1796, he was treating patients with ordinary-sized doses of drugs, of the order of several grains. With experience, however, he realized that when remedies were administered according to the principle of similars, ordinary doses magnified the sick person's symptoms, sometimes to a life-threatening degree. Consequently, he began to prescribe smaller doses and found with these that he could get curative effects without aggravation of symptoms; indeed, the less he gave, Hahnemann learned, the better the result. By 1800 he was recommending doses of a millionth of a grain, and soon he would push the level much lower.[17]

One millionth of a grain of anything is too small to be seen or handled, so how was Hahnemann administering his drugs? He did it through a method of dilution of drug material that made it possible to easily supply even infinitesimal quantities—and infinitesimals were in fact what he came to believe in. There were several variations of the dilution procedure, but the basic method was to mix 1 grain of drug with 99 grains of lactose (milk sugar), a substance Hahnemann believed to be inert with respect to producing homeopathic symptoms and therefore an ideal diluent. The two compounds would be finely ground by mortar and pestle and intimately mixed to give a medicine to the first dilution. Then 1 grain of that mixture (containing 1/100 grain of the drug) was mixed and ground with a second 99 grains of lactose to reach the stage of the second dilution. A grain of that mixture (now harboring a mere 1/10,000 grain of the drug) would be blended with another 99 grains of milk sugar, and the process repeated another twenty-seven times, to give a medicine of the thirtieth dilution. At that point a grain of the diluted mixture would theoretically contain $1/10^{60}$ grain of the active drug. In reality, as could be calculated by the second half of the 1800s, a random grain was extremely unlikely to contain even a single molecule of the drug. The second major variation on the theme of dilution was to mix a drop of a saturated alcoholic solution of the drug with 99 drops of alcohol and briskly shake it ten times per dilution. This method too was carried to the thirtieth dilution.[18]

Actually, the thirtieth was a norm that Hahnemann proposed but that many homeopaths exceeded. Some went into the hundreds, a few into the thousands, and one as high as sixteen thousand. Hahnemann experimented with somewhat high dilutions at first, treating an elderly woman with epilepsy, for example, with a ninetieth dilution: "Within an hour afterwards she had an epileptic fit, and since then she has remained quite free of them." But again, experience demonstrated the thirtieth dilution to be quite adequate, and Hahnemann came to insist on that as a standard of practice: "I do not approve of your potentizing medicines higher" than the thirtieth, he reprimanded one follower; "there must be some end to the thing. It cannot go on to infinity."[19]

Homeopathic Theory

Effectiveness from even a thirtieth dilution, Hahnemann recognized, was an "extraordinary discovery," a "hitherto unknown and undreamt of" phenomenon, a truly "astonishing" one. But if such a result was "incomprehensible to the man of figures," the theory-enslaved allopath, its reality was not to be doubted, because it had been demonstrated by clinical experience.[20] What Hahnemann had discovered through his therapeutic trials was not only that drugs act according to the law of similars but also that they act through some medium other than their matter. How else could the effects of a thirtieth-dilution preparation be interpreted? There was no drug matter present to act, so some non-material agent must be at work, some "spirit," in short.

The conclusion that drugs must exert their healing effects at the spiritual level made profound sense to Hahnemann. In his understanding of the human body, he was a confirmed vitalist. He believed that the body was endowed with life and that its physiological functioning was governed by a non-material vital force or vital spirit, a "dynamis," that operated beyond the realm of chemistry and physics: "During the healthy condition of man this spirit-like force (autocracy), animating the material body (organism), rules supreme as *dynamis*. By it all parts are maintained wonderfully in harmonious vital process, both in feelings and functions, in order that our intelligent mind may be free to make the living, healthy, bodily medium subservient to the higher purpose of our being." The vital force was responsible for maintaining health, and disease was nothing more than a disturbance and weakening of the vital force by agents such as "excesses in sensual enjoyment, or deprivation of the same; violent physical impressions; exposure to cold; overheating; excessive muscular exertion; physical or mental excitement, etc." Further, since this source of vitality was not a material entity, it could not be acted upon by material agents but only by "the dynamic [spiritual] influence upon it of a morbific agent inimical to life."[21]

It followed that a vital force disordered by disease could likewise not "be reached nor affected except by a spirit-like (dynamic) process," so if drugs restored the force to normality, they did so only by operating "dynamically," through spiritual activity. When looked at that way, the necessity of the process of drug dilution became perfectly clear. The procedures of grinding and shaking stripped away the particles of matter that bound and inhibited the drug's dynamic, or spiritual, potency. When drugs were properly diluted, there occurred a "disembodiment and spiritualization of their medicinal powers," a "development and liberation of the dynamic powers of the medicinal substance so treated" that was so "great and hitherto unknown and undreamt of . . . as to excite astonishment." (Grinding and shaking worked to release a drug's dynamic power, Hahnemann suggested in another instance, in the same way that two pieces of metal rubbed together release the immaterial entity of heat stored inside their atoms.) It was an error, Hahnemann argued, to think of matter as "something inanimate," for "astonishingly great powers can be developed from its inmost depths by trituration."[22]

To this point, Hahnemann had advanced purely by the empirical means of provings and clinical treatments. He had arrived, however, at conclusions that excited "astonishment" and so felt compelled to explain how such extraordinary things could be. "In the process of a homoeopathic cure," he conjectured, the prescribed drug "implanted upon the vital power" an "artificial morbid affection" that not only duplicated all the symptoms of the natural ailment but was also "somewhat stronger" than the disease. Being stronger, it displaced the natural disease from the body according to "that homoeopathic law of nature" which held that "in the living organism *a weaker dynamic affection is permanently extinguished by a stronger one if the latter . . . is very similar in its manifestation to the former.*" Substituting a stronger disease for a weaker one might seem to be throwing the vital force from the frying pan into the fire, but in fact the force was *"now only excited to stronger effort by the drug-affection,"* and since that affection was "very transient . . . on account of the extreme minuteness of the dose," it "vanishes easily and quickly" when confronted by the "increased energy" of the vital force it has stimulated. "For the purpose of *complete* recovery," in short, "the vital force needs to make but a slight additional exertion to overcome the effects of the medicine, after the extinction of the disease for which it was given."[23] This was, of course, a process of natural healing, of stimulating the body's own recuperative power to achieve the return to health.

Hahnemann clearly appreciated that his theory was highly speculative, but he was not particularly troubled by the fact. "I . . . place but a slight value upon an attempt at explanation," he shrugged, because all that mattered was that homeopathy worked. It had "been verified to the world by every pure experiment and genuine experience," so "a scientific explanation of its mode of action is of little importance." He considered the theory he had offered merely "the most probable one"; theoretical certainty was not a concern.[24]

Nevertheless, Hahnemann's modest attempt at explaining the action of his drugs is reflective of a pattern common to virtually all alternative systems of medicine historically. All evolved from empirical beginnings, but at some point after experience revealed a particular method to be nature's rule, there arose an impulse to make sense of the discovery, and theoretical rationalizations were soon forthcoming. (With Thomson, for instance, the discovery that hot drugs and emetics were curative spawned the concept that disease is due to a loss of heat from the body.) Alternative practitioners, in other words, generally reversed the process they attributed to allopathic medicine. Instead of formulating a theory, then deducing therapy from it—the alleged allopathic way—they discovered a therapy, then deduced a theory. Invariably, the theoretical principle that followed was that the therapy in question worked by eliminating some obstacle to the free functioning of the body's innate healing power.

The principles of homeopathy were presented most thoroughly and systematically in Hahnemann's classic text *Organon der Rationellen Heilkunde*, first published in 1810 and soon rendered into English as the *Organon of Homeopathic Medicine*. The year following the *Organon*'s appearance, Hahnemann moved to the medical center of Leipzig to offer lectures on the new style of healing; "a raging hurricane," as students described him, he "poured forth a flood of abuse against the older medicine." The old medicine poured abuse back, of course, and though Hahnemann endured regulars' attacks for a full decade, even his patience had limits. In 1821 he withdrew from the fray and retired to the quiet village of Köthen. Now in his mid-sixties, Hahnemann intended to live out his years as a semi-reclusive sage, treating a few patients, admitting some disciples to sit at his feet for a while, keeping up a voluminous correspondence with younger homeopaths, yet standing apart from the nasty strife between medical orthodoxy and his heresy. When his wife of nearly fifty years passed away in 1830, Hahnemann's schedule of withdrawal was quickened—only to be shattered five years later when a thirty-five-year-old French woman attracted to Köthen by the revolutionary philosophy swept the eighty-year-old Hahnemann off his feet and carried him back to Paris as her groom. Eight years of high living, including the publicizing of homeopathic doctrine among the French aristocracy, left Hahnemann world famous and worn out. When he passed away in 1843, his system of medicine had achieved a solid foothold throughout Europe—and was well along on establishing one in the United States.[25]

Introduction of Homeopathy to America

Homeopathy was first brought to America in 1825, by Hans Gram, a Bostonian who studied medicine in Denmark, was won over by the system of similars, and returned to teach it to several apprentices in New York. Within a few years, however, the Philadelphia area emerged as the first true center of homeopathy in this country, thanks to the efforts of several German homeopath-immigrants. Far the most influential of these was Constantine Hering (1800–1880; Fig. 3-2), a German medical student who converted to homeopathy in the early 1820s, then joined a botanical expedition to South America to carry out provings on a host of plants and animals. The strength of his commitment to the new medicine is evidenced by his introduction into practice of lachesis, the homeopathic preparation of venom from the New World's largest poisonous snake, the bushmaster (of the genus *Lachesis*). Hering heard stories about this dreaded serpent in July of 1828 while encamped with his wife on the upper Amazon. Reasoning that venom lethal in ordinary doses must be beneficial in infinitesimal ones, he paid locals to capture a bushmaster, from which he then—having with "grip of steel" seized behind its "reared head and flaming eye, forked tongue and naked fang"—collected its "deadly saliva." Diluting the saliva with lactose, he conducted a proving on himself, with Frau Hering recording his reactions of fever, delirium, and "the frantic struggle for breath." Lachesis was strong medicine. The list of symptoms it induced would eventually stretch beyond nearly all other homeopathic remedies. Yet even with its myriad indications, the ten drops of venom collected by Hering served to meet the world's needs for forty years. Incidentally, Hering was buried fifty-two years to the day after he had survived the trial with the viper, having succumbed to a heart attack several days earlier. By then, he had distinguished himself in homeopaths' eyes as "the Hercules, who cleansed the fouler than Augean Stables of Medical Science, and encountered and slew the Nemean Lion of Medical Orthodoxy." (It might be noted that Hering carried out other risky provings, testing the newly discovered explosive nitroglycerine in the late 1840s and determining that among its many symptoms were "contraction" and "oppression" of the chest; some three decades later, nitroglycerin would be adopted by allopathic practitioners for treatment of angina pectoris, the oppressive chest pains associated with heart disease.)[26]

Hering brought lachesis (as well as the bushmaster, preserved in alcohol) to Philadelphia in January 1833. There he found a handful of homeopaths

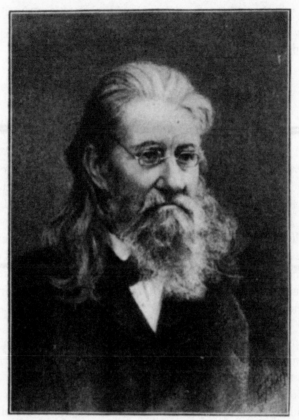

Figure 3-2. Constantine Hering [William King, editor, *History of Homeopathy and Its Institutions in America*, 4 volumes (New York: Lewis, 1905), volume 2, frontispiece]

already in practice in the German immigrant community and quickly organized them into the Hahnemannian Society, the first homeopathic medical organization in the country. He next engaged them in establishing a school, the North American Academy of the Homeopathic Healing Art, in Allentown, Pennsylvania. This Allentown Academy, as it came to be known, opened its doors in 1835 on Hahnemann's eightieth birthday and was the first homeopathic medical school in the world. Yet even though Hering was president and chief instructor, the school was not to last long, financial difficulties leading to its closure in 1842. It nevertheless blazed a trail of sorts, what graduates it had being of the evangelistic variety who felt chosen to carry the gospel abroad. When the Allentown Academy opened, homeopathy existed in only two states. By the time it folded, there were new-style practitioners in sixteen states, and Allentown graduates were largely responsible for all fourteen of the additions.[27]

Hering's was also the guiding hand behind the establishment of the system's second school, the Homeopathic Medical College of Pennsylvania, which opened in Philadelphia in 1848. Nearly twenty years later he resigned from that faculty and organized a rival institution, Hahnemann Medical College, the best and most long-lived of homeopathic schools. (It survived as a homeopathic institution into the 1950s, then became a wholly allopathic one.) By the end of the nineteenth century, more than twenty homeopathic medical schools were in operation.[28]

In the meantime, the Allentown faculty had undertaken a translation of the *Organon* into English. It appeared, with a preface by Hering, in 1836, making the new system much more accessible at a time of growing uncertainty within allopathic medicine. The 1832 invasion of Asiatic cholera, the first appearance of that dreadful infection ever in the western hemisphere, had made regular physicians particularly mindful of their therapeutic impotence. There were still sporadic occurrences of the disease at the time the English *Organon* appeared, and more than one MD turned to infinitesimals, and stayed with them, after futile efforts to cure cholera with bleeding and purging. (Since cholera kills by dehydration, evacuative therapy abetted it even more decidedly than it did other ailments.) Such defections would be much more numerous when epidemic cholera returned in 1849, and there occurred "a widespread desertion from orthodox ranks." In the South, yellow fever was also frequently the cause of a change from standard to homeopathic practice; the early expansion of homeopathy was in large measure due to such conversions of frustrated regulars. Still other physicians of the mid-1800s, it might be noted, switched allegiance to hydropathy (a system of water-cure to be discussed in the next chapter) and other alternative systems. The perfidy of these turncoats only further inflamed the mainstream profession in its hatred of irregular practice: "We desire not to see a poorer piece of humanity," one steadfast MD protested, "of prostituted manhood, than is seen in the conversion of a regular, well-educated physician, to the ranks of any of these popular theories of medicine." For their part, homeopaths often "regretted that so many Allopathic physicians are dabbling with Homoeopathic remedies, and pretending that they can practice Homoeopathy," seeing them as too often guilty of "serious mischief" and "bungling misapplication."[29]

The ranks of homeopathy expanded steadily. By 1860 the number of homeopaths in America had surpassed the two thousand mark, constituting something more than 5 percent of the number of regular practitioners. (Indeed, public demand for treatment with similars had grown "so great, that the country is becoming flooded with Homoeopathic quackery.") Hering, meanwhile, was staying busy editing a journal (albeit a German-language one), publishing books such as his 1837 *Wirkungen des Schlangengiftes* (*Effects of Snake Poisons*), and helping found a national professional association, the American Institute of Homeopathy, in 1844. (The American Medical Association would not be organized until three years later.) The first president of the American Institute of Homeopathy was, of course, Constantine Hering.[30]

Popularity of Homeopathy

The appeal of homeopathy derived not just from its apparently greater success against cholera. Homeopaths advertised better cure rates for all diseases (at the minimum, they did less to inhibit recovery than did allopaths, with their bleeding and calomel), and one could get cured more cheaply. Even with the labor involved in preparing remedies to the thirtieth dilution, homeopathic medicines cost less than allopathic ones. They also had a far more pleasing taste and produced no evacuations or other disagreeable reactions, making them especially adaptable to younger patients. Allopathic therapy, daunting enough to adults, was repulsive and terrifying to children. Hahnemann's infinitesimal globules, on the other hand, were sugar pills, virtual candy. "We no longer need to promise pieces of money or cookies," Hering chuckled, "to get the child to drink the nasty dose." He then related the story of an elderly Philadelphia woman who, "when her grandson jumped up around the [homeopathic] doctor and wanted to have all the medicines, said, 'Now I believe a new age is coming and wonders and miracles happen, *children ask for medicine.*' "[31]

She wasn't the only parent who found it easier to entice the kids into a candy store than force them into a torture chamber. And since women bore the brunt of responsibility for taking children to the doctor, a disproportionate number of women discovered homeopathy and became sugar pill patients themselves. The American Institute of Homeopathy estimated in 1869 that two-thirds of all adult homeopathic patients were female, and just a few years later discussion at the national convention of the American Medical Association brought forth the discomfiting admission that a number of allopathic doctors had wives who patronized homeopaths. (It was also true that a much higher percentage of homeopathic practitioners were women than was the case with regular medicine.)[32]

The style of homeopathy was as attractive as its substance. In truth, this may have been the system's chief attraction, for the selection of the proper drug for each patient required a type of clinical interaction that a century later would come to be celebrated as "holistic." The Hahnemannian interpretaton of illness, after all, stressed that all a patient's symptoms had to be taken into account ("the totality of the symptoms must be regarded by the physician as the principal and only condition to be recognized and removed by his art") and that mental and emotional disturbances had to be accorded as much importance as physical ones ("the state of the mind is *always* modified in so-called physical diseases; and hence the state of the mind . . . is to be noted, in order to secure a reliable record . . . of all diseases presenting themselves for treatment"). For Hahnemann, every case of illness was an expression of malfunctioning of the patient as a whole ("all parts of the organism are so intimately connected as to form an indivisible whole in feelings and functions"), and each took form as a condition unique to that individual whose particular vital force had been disordered (there were "millions of morbid cases that occur perhaps but once in the world"). The homeopathic clinical examination thus involved an attentive and lengthy listening to the patient's complaints in which the practitioner recorded every single symptom as something to be taken seriously, then inquired more deeply about the intimate details of each item on the list.[33]

That patients appreciated such careful individual attention is evidenced by scenes in a popular novel of the 1850s, *Delia's Doctors*. Having received no benefit at all from her family's allopathic practitioner, the mysteriously ailing Delia calls in Dr. Liston, the new homeopath in town. Her family is at first skeptical that any good can be accomplished by "diminuative doses" seemingly intended "for an infant Lilliputian"; her father suspects that "homeopathy must be a hoax," and her mother that "Dr. Liston is an idiot." But once the new doctor takes his patient in tow, attitudes change. "Dr. Liston . . . commenced a more formidable list of interrogatories than had ever before been propounded to the young lady. Producing pencil and notebook, he carefully recorded all her answers" to questions about her constitution, diet, reactions to food, other living habits, and so on. "At least, one hundred questions" were asked, and all the family agreed that "the homeopathist was evidently a close observer." He was a wise one as well, as was demonstrated when Delia's mother asked what her daughter's disease was. "Absence of sound health," Liston replied, voicing the homeopathic principle that while every disease is unique to the sufferer and cannot be pigeonholed by allopathic labels, all cases are fundamentally the same in the sense that they represent a dysfunction of the vital force.[34]

Giving the patient so much time and attention was not a mark of conventional medical practice, homeopaths maintained. Allopaths were "routine practitioners," Hahnemann charged, who placed quantity above quality; they were "celebrities who knock up two pairs of horses daily in swift-rolling gilded chariots in order to pay visits a couple of minutes' duration to sixty, eighty, or more patients." Further, those hasty visits resulted in essentially the same prescriptions for all, a "barbarous olla-podrida full of disgusting smells and tastes." Homeopathic patients received but a single drug, the one substance in all creation whose effects closely duplicated the complete constellation of the sufferer's symptoms.[35]

Homeopaths also attracted patrons by taking a leaf from Thomson's book and giving the public the power to treat themselves. To be sure, they did not promote self-care as an ideology and demand, as Thomson had, that patients assume full responsibility for their recovery. They were motivated rather by practical considerations, seeing self-treatment as only an occasional recourse to be taken if the complaint was mild or no homeopathic physician was available. Hering led the way in the development of self-care options with *The Homeopathist or Domestic Physician* (volume 1, 1835; volume 2, 1838), a work that listed the most common symptoms of the most generally useful drugs and that was sold in conjunction with a "domestic kit" of vials of forty homeopathic remedies. For five dollars (or only four for those who purchased the German version) a person could have available a detailed guide to the identification of the best drug for virtually any common illness, and the drugs too. The remedies, incidentally, were not identified by name—no need to confuse customers with mysterious Latin terms. They were labeled instead with numbers, so all the sufferer had to do was record his symptoms, find a corresponding symptom complex in Hering's catalogue, then take the numbered preparation recommended. (As in professional texts, however, symptom complexes were defined in hairsplitting detail, so that the search for a match must have occupied the better part of some illnesses. Number four, for example, was specific for headaches characterized by "pressing pain above the nose, mitigated by bending forward; pressing from within outwardly, shooting, throbbing; tearing in the forehead, as if a nail were driven through the head, piercing boring deep into the brain, with nausea, darkness before the eyes, aversion to light, pale countenance, much colorless urine; . . . the patient being very much affrighted, inconstant, or taciturn and dejected.")[36]

Hering's *Domestic Physician* was the first homeopathic materia medica of any sort published in the United States. It passed through fourteen American editions and thirteen German ones and was translated into French, Danish, Swedish, Hungarian, and Russian. Other domestic guides and kits followed, some outselling the original. Frederick Humphreys marketed two sizes of kits, selling twelve million of the smaller one by the 1890s. A rival version sought to reduce remedy selection to a science by listing each of the 2,467 most common symptoms on a separate slip of paper. Beneath each symptom there followed 127 drugs capable of treating it, with each remedy assigned an efficacy score from one to four. The patient had only to collect the slips for all his symptoms, determine the cumulative score for all listed remedies, and take the medication with the highest total.[37]

Such full provisions for self-treatment notwithstanding, domestic kits were intended not to liberate people from physicians but to lure the public into practitioners' offices. From the allopathic viewpoint, the kits were the homeopaths' Trojan horse, a harmless-appearing little box that gave the new medicine entry to thousands of households and started the slow ferment of conversion. "Multitudes" were converted, "especially the *female* multitudes, who practice in their families with their little boxes filled with little phials of little globules, with a little pamphlet of directions." The domestic kit, one allopath scoffed, "gives the ignorant, who have such an inveterate itch for dabbling in physic, a book and a doll's medicine chest, and lets them play doctors and doctresses without fear of having to call in the coroner."[38]

Homeopathy's appeal did not stem entirely from practical considerations, however. The system had as well a sophisticated theory that intrigued the intellectually aware. By the 1840s many well-read Americans were troubled by the direction science seemed to be taking. Ever since Newton had laid down his laws of motion in the late seventeenth century, the universe had been transformed steadily into a mindless, material machine. In the early 1800s the French physicist Laplace had boasted that given the precise position and momentum of every atom in the universe, a "Divine Calculator" could mathematically determine the entire past and future of creation. Reduction of the universe to a billiard table, even an almost infinitely complex one, was disturbing for its removal of God and free will and chance from existence and for the threat that even human life might be analyzed entirely by the equations of physics and chemistry. Much as bioenergeticists of the late twentieth century have reacted against the physical reductionism of modern medicine, many late eighteenth-century scientists, particularly in Germany, demanded that renewed attention be given to the non-material and non-quantifiable components of nature and that vitality be recognized as a mystery that transcends the physical sciences. Hahnemann's concentration on the body's vital force and the drug's dynamic power were reflections of the revived study of non-material agents in nature. Interest in the immaterial spilled over into several popular enthusiasms. The 1840s in America witnessed spurts of educated infatuation with animal electricity and animal magnetism, with Swedenborgianism and its mystical theories of soul as universal driving force, with communication with the spirits of the departed. Homeopathy, with its effusions over human vital force and the spiritual essences of drugs, was made to order for fashion-conscious intellectuals enthralled with the integration of spirit and matter.[39]

There were other factors that won homeopathy a more sympathetic ear from the upper classes than from the less educated. Most of its early practitioners were cultured immigrants from that most philosophical of nations. Their medicines were all identified by impressive Latin names, and their dedication to eliciting each delicate shading of a patient's physical and emotional experiences of discomfort no doubt was more fascinating to literati than to no-nonsense, let's-get-on-with-it commonfolk. The same went for therapy. Thomsonianism's vomiting and rectal blistering were fine for rough-and-ready frontiersmen, but for the refined and genteel they were just a bit undignified. Thus if Thomsonianism was the "radicalism of the barnyard," as it had been called, homeopathy was "the quackery of the drawing-room" or, as another allopath jested, "the Aristocracy of Quackery": "As a psychological experiment on the weakness of cultivated minds, it is the best trick of the century."[40]

The Consultation Clause

Partly because their patients were better off financially, partly because they enjoyed a more favorable ratio of practitioners to patients, homeopaths on average commanded a higher income than regular practitioners: "While the Thompsonian [sic] is satisfied with a small compensation for his liberal dosing, the infinitesimal doses of the Homoeopathist are generally paid for with fees very Allopathic, sometimes fairly 'heroic.' " Those fees, furthermore, came from patients who otherwise would have reimbursed conventional practitioners. Competition between the two groups of doctors, an Ohio regular noted in 1851, "has been brought to a very [high] pitch," so that "even the longest established and most estimable physicians have yielded large and lucrative portions of their practice to homoeopathy." That was reason enough to attack Hahnemann's followers, perhaps, but the bulk of allopathic opposition was based on homeopaths' principles and practice. Indeed, operating from the position that homeopathic theory and therapy were patently unscientific, the orthodox profession attempted to suppress the upstart system through enforcement of a provision in the American Medical Association's code of ethics. One of the first acts of the AMA on its founding in 1847 was to adopt a set of rules to govern physicians' relations with patients and colleagues. One element of this ethical code was a clause encouraging physicians to consult with other qualified practitioners in difficult cases. The "consultation clause," as it became known, nevertheless made a point of denying the privilege of consultation to doctors lacking the proper credentials. In truth, professional cooperation with irregulars had already been condemned any number of times, both as an injustice to patients, who deserved only qualified attendants, and as an insult to the profession, whose public image would be tarnished by association with medical impostors. Just a few years earlier, for example, a critic of mesmerism (Chapter 5) had declared that "any practitioner who sends a patient with any disease to consult a mesmeric quack, ought to be without patients for the rest of his days." The American Medical Association's code of ethics, however, now made it official, stipulating that "no one can be considered as a regular practitioner, or a fit associate in consultation, whose practice is based upon an exclusive dogma, to the rejection of the accumulated experience of the profession." In brief, irregulars generally and homeopaths most particularly could not be thought of as fit associates, and any professional cooperation with them constituted a breach of professional ethics. A regular physician might ethically consult "with foreign physicians, doctresses [women physicians]," even "colored physicians . . . provided they are regular practitioners." But if the would-be consultant was a dogmatist, even a native-born white male one, "justly exclude him as unsuitable for fellowship with those who profess to love all truth."[41]

From the 1850s onward, the consultation clause was used effectively by state and local medical societies to squash homeopaths' efforts to win practice privileges in publicly funded medical institutions. Homeopathy's supporters contended that as a therapeutic system patronized by a significant percentage of the tax-paying population, it should be represented in public institutions. Yet whether the issue was the appointment of homeopaths to municipal hospitals, to the faculties of state medical schools, or to military medical departments during the Civil War, the homeopathic argument was nearly always denied in favor of the majority profession's position that conscientious physicians could not ethically participate in such arrangements: the suggestion that homeopathic practitioners be granted positions in the Union Medical Corps was regarded by one allopathic commentator as "perhaps the most frivolous [notion] which has ever enlisted the thoughts of a rational creature." (A few homeopaths, as well as eclectic doctors, did win appointment to the Union's medical staff, incidentally, but only because they could present diplomas from orthodox schools and did not divulge their true affiliation to examiners; their practice was restricted to the drugs approved and supplied by allopathic supervisors, of course.) In addition, regular practitioners who were caught cooperating in any way with irregulars were punished with expulsion from their professional organizations. In one case, a Connecticut doctor was dismissed from his county medical society for collaborating with a homeopath who happened also to be his wife: "Had he consulted with another man's wife upon topics not purely medical," a bemused observer commented, "his error might have been overlooked" by his ethics-conscious colleagues.[42]

Allopathic Ridicule of Homeopathy

Allopaths also attempted to destroy the Hahnemannian heresy with ridicule, to the extent that the anti-homeopathic diatribe constituted a major class of medical literature from the late 1840s into the last years of the century. It was, moreover, a body of literature that was as paradoxical as it was voluminous. Its repeatedly expressed premise was that this "Humbug, of the Genus Germanicus, Species Homoeopathia," was much too silly a concoction for anyone to take seriously. Hahnemann himself was "little less than a lunatic": "We challenge all mankind to name another instance . . . where a man has asserted similar nonsense, and has not been considered fully entitled to a place in the lunatic asylum!" Likewise, his system was "one of the wildest vagaries that ever disturbed the mind of man," a set of ideas "so attenuated as to produce no sensible effects . . . except upon feeble intellects."[43] Then, as soon as Hahnemannism had been tossed aside as not worth a second thought, critics refilled their pens and plunged into lengthy dissertations aimed at rewinning the masses who had taken homeopathy seriously nevertheless.

Rarely has vilification been so merry. After all, wrote the 1851 winner of the Rhode Island Medical Society's fifty-dollar prize for best refutation of homeopathy, "when things are exceedingly laughable, it is a little unreasonable to demand of us an imperturbable gravity. When Homoeopathy conjures up its ridiculous fantasies to play before us like so many harlequins, it is hard to be denied the privilege of laughing at them. . . . If a little pleasantry suffice to demolish an error, it surely is an unnecessary waste of power to attack it with strong and sober argument. It were folly to deal sturdy blows at bubbles which can be dissolved by the slightest touch." It was in that spirit, therefore, that regulars evaluated the fundamental rule of homeopathy, the law of similars. "The patient has swelling about the throat that renders breathing very difficult," one hypothesized; "he gasps for breath, his lips are blue. Just tighten his collar, or tie a cord around his neck, and you will cure him if homeopathy be true." The patient with inflamed eyes should have cayenne pepper rubbed into them (by a Thomsonian perhaps?), and quick recovery would follow "if homeopathy be not a humbug." And as for the patient whose skull had been fractured by a stone: "Hit him again with a brickbat. Similia similibus!"[44]

Similia similibus necessitated provings, those "experiments" in which "the common accidents of sensation, the little bodily inconveniences to which all of us are subject, are seriously and systematically ascribed to whatever medicine may have been exhibited." Thus, another physician joked, if the prover's "face is flushed, the medicine has produced it—if he is inclined to sleep, the medicine has produced it—if he dreams, it is the medicine—if he is cold, it is the medicine—if he is warm, it is the medicine—if he is timid, it is the medicine—if he is courageous, it is the medicine—if his head, or eyes, or ears, or teeth, or limbs ache, or if he laughs, or cries, or whatever else takes place in his person or feelings, it has been produced by the medicine."[45]

As a result, every homeopathic medicine had a number and variety of symptoms attributed to it that struck regular doctors as ludicrous. Chamomile, for example, an herb long used as a folk remedy for digestive upset, had been found by Hahnemann to generate hundreds of effects, including toothache whose pains were on "one side, with violent, nightly exacerbation, creeping, darting, tearing, pricking, digging up, corroding, grumbling, drawing." To MD Worthington Hooker, it seemed that "if one who knew nothing about chamomile should read over the three pages of the effects attributed to it, he would be justified in supposing it to be a fit agent for inquisitorial torture, instead of being the innocent thing which all nurses and old women think it to be."[46]

Homeopathic medicines could be seen as agents of torture in other ways. If, for example, remedies increased in potency as they were shaken, country practitioners who hauled their medications about in saddlebags "will have to calculate what the effect of a hard day's ride over a rough road, on a trotting horse, may have on their physic." Surely all that shaking would so potentize a preparation that it would immediately "destroy any patient to whom it might be administered." A regular who had retired from practice told a story of being present when a homeopath gave a patient twenty pills to be taken one each day. "That must be very powerful medicine," the allopath observed, "if so small a quantity can effect any change." "It is very powerful indeed, sir," the homoeopath replied. What, the former physician asked, would be the consequences if the patient took two pills at once? "It would endanger his life, sir," said the homoeopath, "and if he should take three at a time it would most certainly kill him." The regular doctor "then grasped the whole lot in his hand, put them in his mouth and swallowed them, . . . remarking, 'now Dr. according to your story I am a dead man.' But not so," he laughed when recounting the event many years later.[47]

Another topic for mirth was the elderly Hahnemann's belief that drugs could work by "olfaction." A drug's "dynamic property," he had asserted, "is so pervading, that it is quite immaterial what sensitive part of the body is touched by the medicine." Hence one could get as full an effect by smelling as by swallowing the remedy. "A single olfaction" of a thirtieth dilution, he reported, "will restore a morbidly desponding individual, with a constant inclination to commit suicide, in less than an hour to a peaceful state of mind, to love of life, to happiness, and horror of his contemplated act." To allopaths, it mattered not that most homeopaths had quickly disavowed the concept of olfaction. "It is not unreasonable to suppose," they chortled, "that the air which we breathe every day, brings on the wings of the wind, from the noxious plants of India, and the venomous serpents of Peru, poisons, which after their thousand attenuations and succussions, would be sufficient to destroy all mankind, if there was any truth in Hahnemann's doctrines."[48]

If there was any truth to the idea that dilution continually augmented a substance's powers, then, one regular doctor suggested, farmers should stop using oxen to plow their fields and yoke up insects instead. One might, another envisioned, use homeopathy to eliminate starvation, for "is there not [in homeopathic practice] as great an exception to all the hitherto received laws of nature as in the miracle of the loaves and fishes?" Hahnemann could claim that his miraculous-seeming rules were all derived from carefully evaluated experience, but to allopaths it was all "unadulterated and arrogant dogmatism. . . . In the entire history of medical doctrines, there is not one in regard to which the proof of their soundness derived from experience is so entirely defective and unsatisfactory, as it is here." (Several physicians reported experimental trials that attempted to reproduce the findings of homeopathic provings or the claims of cure but failed completely.)[49]

Examples of contemptuous jests could be multiplied to homeopathic levels of repetition. It will suffice, however, to mention only a final category of ridicule, what might be called the calculus of homeopathy. This was the application of mathematics to Hahnemann's grand dilutions. Regulars delighted, even competed, it seems, in doing calculations, the more ingenious and outrageous the better, of such things as the length of time required to dilute all of a single drop of drug tincture to the thirtieth potency. At one shake a second, a person working ten hours a day, seven days a week, would be occupied for "661 quadrillions, 822 trillions, 919 billions, 336 millions and 1050 decillions of years. . . . Just think of it! If Adam had begun this agitation the day God made him, . . . he would still be shaking away below the tenth dilution." And just think of how many pills all that shaking would result in, another allopath proposed. "It would supply every inhabitant of the earth with a septillion of doses," and even if everyone took three globules a day, it still "would require very nearly a sextillion of years to use up the whole grain."[50]

Another computation might demonstrate the volume of alcohol needed for the same complete dilution of a grain. Oliver Wendell Holmes, whose 1842 address "Homeopathy and Its Kindred Delusions" was the most thorough demolition job of all the attacks on homeopathy, observed that by the seventeenth dilution the homeopath would have added alcohol equivalent to ten thousand Adriatic Seas: "Trifling errors must be expected, but they are as likely to be on one side as the other, and any little matter like Lake Superior or the Caspian would be but a drop in the bucket." If carried all the way to the thirtieth, another calculation determined, the alcohol "required to attenuate a single drop . . . would be more than sufficient to fill the orbit of Saturn, to blot out the sun and quench the stars." Even the minuscule amount of sulfur "existing in one humming bird's egg," a third estimated, "is more than enough to impregnate millions of hogsheads of the 40th dilution, and not only sufficient to supply all the Homoeopathists in this world, but in all the worlds if they were filled with Homoeopathists."[51]

These calculations of impossibility were mathematically correct but also totally beside the point. Homeopaths never attempted to carry the entire original drop or grain of drug through thirty dilutions; for the first twenty-seven or twenty-eight stages it was enough to dilute just a single grain of the hundred-grain drug-lactose mixture. Reserving full dilution of all one hundred grains of drug-lactose for just steps twenty-nine and thirty would still yield ten thousand pills, and use not much more than a pound of lactose. Just as irrelevant were the recipes for homeopathic soup (made from the shadow of a starved pigeon's wing, Abraham Lincoln joked), the reminders that a pinch of drug dropped into the Great Lakes would yield a more concentrated preparation than homeopaths administered, and all the other computations of the virtually nonexistent quantity of drug matter present in a thirtieth-potency preparation. Homeopaths claimed their drugs worked not through matter but through dynamic forces that, Hahnemann had written, were "incomprehensible to the man of figures."[52]

Yet the men of figures' humor masked no inconsiderable amount of hatred of homeopathy, "that common sewer of the Profession." Regulars' loathing of the infinitesimal system stemmed from disdain for its principles and practices, from anger at its success at winning patients and fees and converts from orthodox medicine, and not least from the arrogance perceived in the epithet "allopathy," a "title . . . impudently bestowed upon us." Orthodox medicine's view of homeopathy and other alternative schools of practice was that all were narrow systems in which every case was treated with the same remedies (be it lobelia and steam or infinitesimals or some other "false hobby") and in which all the phenomena of disease and cure had to be explained by a single simple theory; all appeared to be merely different expressions of fanatic medical sectarianism. This was much the same view that irregulars had of mainstream medicine, of course, but regular doctors insisted they were not bound to a single theory and therapy for everything and thus deeply resented their practice being called allopathy, as if it were any old "pathy," just one more close-minded system. "Homeopathists and other empirical sects are wont to talk loudly about ALLOPATHY," a New York physician complained, but "the legitimate profession repudiates the term," indeed "scorns" it, as an attempt to "enroll [regular medicine] in the regiment of *pathies* and *isms*." He had no objection at all "if empirics of all kinds, names and grades, should see fit to form one regiment, and tune their bass drums, tin kettles, French horns, and Yankee pumpkin vines, to one syren chorus." But he and his colleagues would have "no alliance with that marauding army" and were determined that "the standard of legitimate medicine will never be unfurled in that troop." His sentiments were repeated to an echo. As late as the beginning of the twentieth century a popular guide for the young doctor entering the profession warned him to "remember that the term 'Allopath' is a false nickname not chosen by regular physicians at all, but cunningly coined, and put in wicked use against us, in his venomous crusade against Regular Medicine by its enemy, Hahnemann. . . . 'Allopathy' applied to regular medicine is both untrue and offensive and is no more accepted by us than the term 'Heretics' is accepted by Protestants, . . . or 'Niggers' by the Blacks."[53]

Influence of Homeopathy

"Who can blame a man," Oliver Wendell Holmes asked, "for being satisfied with the argument, 'I was ill, and am well,—great is Hahnemann!'? Only this argument serves all imposters and impositions. It is not of much value, but it is irresistible, and therefore quackery is immortal." Yet if homeopathy was despised as quackery, and Hahnemann and his minions as detestable, it still had to be admitted that the system of similars had taught legitimate medicine a valuable lesson. The point of Holmes's remark was that most sick people recover no matter what medication they take, due to the restorative efforts of nature. The effects of homeopathic infinitesimals in particular, allopaths believed, could be explained in no other way. "In reality," a Boston physician explained, homeopathy "waits on the natural course of events . . . producing in the living body no other effects than those which charlatanry has in all ages produced in the minds and bodies of imaginative patients." Homeopathy's "cures" were all due to nature and the placebo effect; indeed, infinitesimals were "placeboism etherealized," and homeopathic practitioners would be just as successful "were the similars left out and atoms of taffy or sawdust . . . substituted, to give their patients room to exercise their faith, and nature time and opportunity to do the work." No doubt the poet was right in proposing that "If it be good in all complaints to take a dose so small,/ It surely must be better still, to take no dose at all."[54]

But giving nature time and opportunity was precisely what many allopathic physicians needed to do. Even though Hahnemann's "whole scheme . . . is frail as a spider's web, and must fall to atoms and be blown away by the wind," a New York practitioner observed, "yet, after all, perhaps Hahnemann did not live wholly in vain. . . . Through the use of his empty and inert means, we have been enabled to see what the innate powers of the animal organization can accomplish without medical interference. We have been taught to rely more upon these, and less upon art, and have seen the wonderful influence which the mind has over the bodily functions." Consequently, he predicted, physicians in the future "will look more carefully to the recuperative energies of nature, and from the darkness and confusion which Hahnemann spread around, a clearer light may shine upon the path of medical practice."[55]

In fact, heroic therapy's worst outrages against nature did come to be abandoned during the second half of the nineteenth century. To be sure, the melioration of allopathic drugging resulted from several developments, not least the discovery of new drugs to replace the old. But doctors of the time believed that one important factor in the decline of therapeutic heroism was the example of homeopathy. As early as 1857 Oliver Wendell Holmes gave homeopathy the credit for the fact that "the list of specifics has been reduced to a very brief catalogue, and the delusion which had exaggerated the power of drugging for so many generations has been tempered down." Thus, he added on another occasion, "the dealers in this preposterous system of pseudo-therapeutics have cooperated with the wiser class of practitioners in breaking up the system of over-dosing and over-drugging which has been one of the standing reproaches of medical practice. While keeping up the miserable delusion that diseases were all to be 'cured' by drugging, Homeopathy has been unintentionally showing that they would very generally get well without any drugging at all."[56]

Regulars saw a sweet irony in all this, that "unwittingly and unwillingly" Hahnemann had labored "through a long life in aid of that very system that he wished to overthrow and demolish." The new moderation in orthodox medicine, they believed, was drawing patients back from homeopathy and other alternative systems and ensuring a future in which the sick would avail themselves only of scientific therapies. They rejoiced that "when every vestige of Hahnemannism shall have passed away 'as the baseless fabric of a vision,' . . . even then, mankind may be indirectly benefited by this ineffable delusion."[57] As will be seen in a later chapter, however, the demise of Hahnemannism was not nearly as imminent as anticipated.

4

Physical Puritanism: Hygeiotherapy

I n the early 1850s Catharine Beecher, the sister of Harriet Beecher Stowe and a well-known promoter of exercise for women, was initiated into hydropathy, or the water-cure, a system of therapy recently arrived from Europe. "At four in the morning," she recorded, she was "packed in a wet sheet" and "kept in it from two to three hours." She was next taken "in a reeking perspiration" to be "immersed in the coldest plunge-bath. Then a walk as far as strength would allow, and drink five or six tumblers of the coldest water. At eleven A.M. stand under a douche of the coldest water falling *eighteen feet*, for *ten minutes*. Then walk, and drink three or four tumblers of water. At three P.M. sit half an hour in a *sitz*-bath of the coldest water. Then walk and drink again. At nine P.M. sit half an hour with the feet in the coldest water, then rub them till warm. Then cover the weak limb and a third of the body in wet bandages and *retire to rest*. This same wet bandage to be worn all day, and kept constantly wet."[1]

That was the condition of everyone who underwent the water-cure: constantly wet, inside and out, and for extended periods of time. (Beecher repeated the experience every day for three months.) Before examining the details of its multiple forms of wetness, however, it is necessary to distinguish hydropathy from the older tradition of "taking the waters" that had long been an accompaniment to mainstream European medicine. Spa therapy, which involved patients soaking in warm springs and swallowing the water of mineral springs, had never constituted more than a limited portion of regular practice, even in its heyday in the seventeenth and eighteenth centuries. Further, while taking the waters was presumed to be of some value for just about any ailment, it was strongly recommended for only a small number of conditions (rheumatism, gout, and bladder stones, for example). The water was administered in only two forms: patients drank it or dipped in it, and that which they dipped in was warm rather than "the coldest." Nor were the waters regarded as sufficient in themselves, the taking of them generally being supplemented with other therapies such as bleeding and purging. Finally, many of the "patients" at spas such as Bath and Spa were not so much driven there by the pains of any illness as drawn by the pleasures of dancing, drinking, gaming, and seducing that abounded at watering places.[2] Hydropathy, on the other hand, was all business. Its patients were deadly earnest about recovering their health and allowed no frivolity or self-indulgence to distract them from the goal. Hydropaths forswore any substance other than water, they applied that water in a great variety of ways, and they believed themselves capable of curing any disease or debility whatever with applications of nature's universal fluid.

Origins of Hydropathy

That water could be made a panacea was the discovery of Vincent Priessnitz (1799–1851; Fig. 4-1), an Austrian farmboy who learned of the curative powers of cold water through childhood self-treatments, then by experimentation on farm animals and family members. By 1829 the adult Priessnitz had perfected a scheme of water therapy that he called "hydropathy," which was then introduced to the world through the hydropathic institution he opened in his hometown of Graefenberg. Within ten years the hitherto sleepy village would be renowned throughout the western hemisphere as the home of the cold water-cure, with hundreds annually making the trek to the hydropathic fount of healing.[3]

The therapies administered at Graefenberg, and subsequently at hundreds of hydropathic institutions throughout Europe and America, were essentially the ones described by Beecher. The patient's day began at four each morning, when he was wrapped in the *Lein-tuch*, or wet-sheet. Made to lie upon a water-drenched sheet stretched over a stack of four blankets, he was rolled up tight in the sheet, with each of the blankets then wrapped around in turn, and left to soak and perspire for thirty to sixty minutes. ("It is no unfrequent occurrence," a British commentator noted, "for the liquid perspiration to be streaming on the floor"; Mark Twain joked that when he was given a wet-sheet treatment, "I perspired so much that mother put a life preserver to bed with me.") Simple though it sounds, hydropaths believed the *Lein-tuch* had "far outstrip[ped] all other therapeutical improvements ever made in the healing art" and was effective in just about any situation—"in acute diseases and in chronic ailments—in fevers and inflammations—in shivered nerves and palsied bowels— . . . in infancy and in age—in the weak and in the strong—

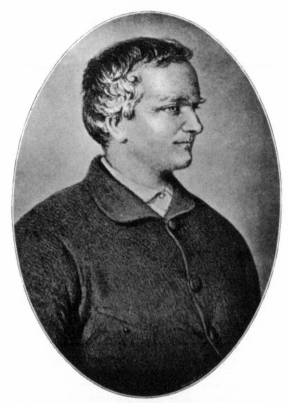

Figure 4-1. Vincent Priessnitz [Richard Metcalfe, *Life of Vincent Priessnitz* (Richmond Hill, England: Metcalfe's London Hydro, 1898), frontispiece]

in cottages and in palaces—in courts and in camps— . . . in all climates and seasons—shivering at the poles or scorching in the tropics," and so on, no matter the complaint or conditions. "Reader," one patient asked,

> did you ever Take a wet-sheet pack,
> Rolled up like a mummy, Lying on its back;
> Wet cloth on your forehead, Bottle at your feet [a hot water bottle],
> You would truly find it A hydropathic treat.

The wet-sheet likely was less of a treat in winter months. A Bostonian reported one evening seeing a sheet "spread out on the snow before my window, frozen stiff as ice" only three minutes before he was wrapped in it. The whole process was "so fearful that I almost catch my breath and shiver all over to think of it," he admitted, yet he still believed it "has done me great good."[4]

When a sufficient quantity of perspiration had streamed forth from the wet-sheet, the patient was unwrapped and treated to a cold full-body plunge bath, then sent outdoors to walk as many miles and drink as many tumblers of water "as strength would allow." One outdoor experience was particularly demanding, that of the douche bath, the shower of the coldest water that Beecher stood under for ten solid minutes. It was the douche above all that caused "many, on hearing the subject of the Water-Cure [to] shudder with horror, and think it another name for certain danger or sudden death." Scattered about Graefenberg's forested grounds were five open-topped enclosures (three for men, two for women) divided into two compartments. Ambulatory patients were expected to visit a douche hut twice a day, there to disrobe in the first room, then to stand for ten minutes or more beneath the shower in the second. The douche might as accurately be described as a cataract, for it was a stream of mountain water conveyed through pipes several inches in diameter that released the water anywhere from ten to twenty feet above the patient's head. In the days before people were accustomed to even ordinary showers, the douche must have been a formidable initiation: "It is indeed no child's play, to have such a torrent of liquid ice pouring down, in a stream of arctic temperature, . . . upon your tender epidermis." Having spent some time myself under *warm* douches in Baden-Baden, I can easily believe the reports of patients that "it is no rare thing to see a subject who at this first shower betrays actual terror, shouts, struggles, runs away, experiences frightening suffocation and palpitation." Beginners could be flattened by the force of the stream: "The water came roaring through the pipe like a lion upon its prey," an English patient recalled, "and struck me on the shoulders with a merciless bang, spinning me about like a teetotum. . . . It knocked me clean over like a ninepin." In another instance, an Englishwoman who hoped to soften the blow by standing on a chair and decreasing the height of the water's fall was dumped to the ground anyway when the chair itself was bowled over.[5]

The douche held additional terrors during the winter season, for not only was the water even more frigid, but icicles could form on the shower spout and eventually break loose and fall: blood was drawn from an English bather, in fact, when a wayward icicle stabbed him in the back. Much worse might have happened. A Bostonian who took the Graefenberg cure during the winter wrote his family that the weather had lately been so cold "that ice has formed around my bath, into which I plunge twice a day; and ice, at this moment, hangs around the *Douches*, in masses from ten to fifteen feet in length, and larger than a man's body"; one can only hope that those icy masses were frozen too solid to fall. In short, one understands why a Royal Navy admiral, "who blew Turks about like sparrows" when on the high seas, "struck his colour before the first discharge of the Douche." Hydropaths were undoubtedly right when they insisted that "if morbid matter can be broken, scattered, dissipated, and altogether put to flight, by the agency of water, . . . you are sure to be divorced by the douche from all your diseases."[6]

Though notably less intimidating, sitz and foot baths were also required therapy for all. Was pathology more concentrated in those nether regions? Were the morbid humors there more difficult to put to flight? The rationalization is less than clear, but the practice was for every patient to soak his or her feet and rump for fifteen minutes twice a day. Specific painful or infirm areas of the body were also given cold water treatment. Patients with arthritis bathed their joints, those with indigestion their stomachs; those with migraine took head baths, and exhausted roués got additional sitz baths. There were also cold water enemas and sundry wet bandages and packs such as Neptune's girdle, a special wet binding for the abdomen. All treatments considered, the author of "Confessions of a Water Patient" must have been all too typical: "I emerged at last from these operations . . . blanched and emaciated—washed out like a thrifty housewife's gown."[7]

Finally, almost as much water was poured into patients as over them; Priessnitz ordered the consumption of a minimum of ten to twelve tumblers a day. (Englishman James Wilson claimed to have taken thirty glasses before breakfast each day of his Graefenberg sojourn.) Priessnitz's attempts at explaining the efficacy of all these procedures included a pass or two at sophistication—vague propositions about cold water's relief of inflammation, its stimulation and toning of body systems, or its reestablishment of suppressed secretions. In the end, though, he fell back on the most intuitive and rudimentary theory, the supposition that disease resulted from contamination of the body by peccant matter. Water was presumed to dissolve these malefic particles and carry them to the skin, where they could be sweated and washed away through pores opened by the stimulus of cold baths: water, Priessnitz is reputed to have said, "brings 'bad stuff' out of the system."[8]

Introduction of Hydropathy to America

Hydropathy quickly spread from its Austrian source through the rest of Europe, becoming established in England in 1842, when James Wilson opened Graefenberg House in Malvern (and issued "Graefenberg flasks" to patients so they could imbibe thirty times before breakfast, too). "Hydros," as the British called their hydropathic institutions, were soon attracting not only thousands of ordinary people but the most intellectually eminent in society. Carlisle, Dickens, and Darwin all underwent the water treatment for a spell, and Tennyson swore that thanks to the Priessnitz regimen, "much poison has come out of me, which no physic [drugs] ever would have brought to light." America's first hydropathic institution opened its doors in 1843, and a second appeared in spring of the following year. Both were in New York City and were operated by disillusioned erstwhile allopaths. "Water-cures," the term preferred in America, soon numbered in the dozens; more than two hundred would be opened over the next half century, though many lasted only a few years. Hydropathic newsletters and journals sprang up: *American Water-Cure Advocate, Illustrated Hydropathic Quarterly Review, New York Water-Cure Reporter, Green Mountain Spring*, and more than a dozen others. The leading publication, *The Water-Cure Journal*, achieved a circulation of more than fifty thousand by the early 1850s, that number eventually rising to nearly a hundred thousand (including, it was claimed, more than a thousand subscribers from regular medicine's ranks). Hydropathic medical schools were opened, and in the United States a national professional association was established in 1850, only three years after the founding of the American Medical Association.[9]

The majority of water-cures were situated in rural areas, alongside lakes or rivers, both to ensure an ample supply of water and to immerse clients in restful and inspirational surroundings. Their advertisements promised "scenery on every hand of the most romantic and beautiful kind," "charming views," and "most varied and beautiful scenery." The Glen Haven, New York, cure, "on the rocky side of a green-clad hill," was "a cool retreat, as wild and sweet, as ever was trod by fairy feet." Water-cures, which also attempted to buoy patients' spirits with entertainments such as musical evenings and sleigh rides, were often large establishments, a Massachusetts one, for instance, having more than one hundred rooms. (Most were patient rooms, but there were also rooms reserved for treatment and for social purposes.) Rates typically ranged from five to fifteen dollars a week, depending on the type of room and the treatment required. This meant that only the middle and upper classes could comfortably afford to attend a water-cure for any length of time. (In the 1850s, the average farm laborer made less than fifteen dollars per month, and city laborers only about twenty dollars.) A certain number of charity cases were accepted, however, and most institutions offered a "clergyman's price" of $2.50 per week.[10]

One got more for one's money at American water-cures, as this country's hydropaths were ingenious innovators who greatly extended the range of water applications. An American introduced the wave bath, for example, a treatment taken in a pond in which waves were created by the turning of a millwheel; wave bathers were advised to anchor themselves in the current with a rope connected to shore. Best of all, America's water-curers were willing to allow warm, or at least tepid, water baths, utilizing all degrees of temperature from the forties up to the seventies depending on the patient's age and condition and the effect desired.[11]

American hydropaths were innovators in theory as well. Many were recruits from allopathic ranks, and because of the formal training in science they had received, their understanding of the source of illness was considerably more sophisticated than the "bad stuff" imagined by peasant Priessnitz. They identified any number of impurities that could invade the body from without, while also emphasizing that much poison originated within, since the vital activity of every organ generated waste. (Even mental activity was presumed to release products of decay; were dirty thoughts more contaminating than ordinary ones?) Only when the body became unable to purge itself at the same rate it was fouling itself, however, did hydropathic treatments have to be instituted. And then the bad stuff came out. When water-cure therapy was begun, the doctor handling a case of "Michigan fever" reported, "the foul matters of disease, laid up for years, exuded sensibly from every pore of his body. It filled the room, stained and saturated the clothing, and colored the water in which he was bathed. There could be no mistake about it, and no one who was not crazed with a hypothesis [read allopath] could deny it."[12]

American hydropaths devised their own complicated hypotheses to explain how water could cure everything (even, one proponent implausibly asserted, hydrophobia). "Cold water taken internally," it was proposed, "operates first to dissolve and thin the morbid accumulations in all parts of the system, and thus prepare them for ejection through the skin, lungs, kidneys, and bowels." Further, "cold water is a *tonic* . . . It operates to give stronger action to the minute capillaries, and this, like the exercise of the muscles, gives increase of vigor." There were still other effects of internal administration, while "cold water applied *externally*, in baths," likewise "operates in several ways." Cold baths stimulated the nerves; applied to specific areas of the body, they would "draw the blood from one portion of the body where there is an excess, to another part where there is a deficiency and consequent debility"; by removing heat from the body and thus quickening "the action of the capillaries," cold water "hastens the process of *change* which is going on all over the system in sending off old, decayed matter, and replacing it with new material furnished by the lungs and stomach."[13]

Even osmosis (a process clarified by chemists in the 1830s) was called upon to account for water's therapeutic action. How could the wet-sheet work its prodigies of healing if not because the blood of the sick person, thick with impurities, coursed through the capillaries of the skin, there moving across a very thin membrane separating its own contaminated fluid from the pure water of the sheet? By the action of osmosis, impurities dissolved in the blood would pass through the membrane into the water pressed against the skin until they reached the same concentration on both sides. If the wet-sheet was then replaced by a fresh one, and the process repeated, blood impurities would soon be eliminated. (Such were some people's impurities, though, the wet-sheets were sometimes "varnished" with a "thick coating of slimy matter," a "quantity of foul matter [that] is beyond belief.")[14]

Ridding the body of foulness and rejuvenating it with pure blood was, of course, nothing more than natural healing. The skilled hydropath, it was maintained, "has so educated his faculties that he is able to recognize promptly the indications of nature [and] is always ready to assist her, by the active interference of his favorite art." Water-cure, practitioners claimed, "recognizes the recuperative or healing power of . . . the 'vis medicatrix naturae,' [and] makes its medical prescriptions in harmony with that power." Indeed, water alone was capable of "awakening all the vital powers to their greatest restorative capabilities" and "unchaining all the powers of the constitution, giving nature a genial impetus, and leaving uncurbed her desire and efforts to heal." Water was thus "a conqueror without bloodshed . . . a divine and universal remedy." A representative practitioner, Philadelphia's Charles Schieferdecker, claimed that he had "*not lost one* patient out of the hundreds of desperate cases I have treated" and foresaw that hydropathy "will give men the age of 150 to 200 years, and that marasmus senilis [old age] alone, or accident, ought to end the life of a human being, but not disease." Hydropathy could even cure inadvertently, as was attested by the preacher who was suddenly and permanently relieved of his long-standing rheumatism after performing a series of baptisms in an icy river.[15]

Water lent itself to recognition as nature's mode of healing in an even more fundamental way. It was a very special substance, after all, the chief component of the human body and of human blood, an indispensable nutrient. It nourished the earth as well, its rains and rivers constituting the life's blood of all creation. Water possessed a powerful Romantic attraction, an intrinsic association with life and nature that hydropaths tapped again and again. "What is there in nature so beautiful as water," one mused. "In the form of genial spring showers, that fertilize and render fructiferous the earth—in the opening flowerbuds—in glistening dew-drops—in sparkling fountains—in rivulets—in spring streams—in cascades—and in the delicate teardrop that moistens the cheek of woman, how beautiful is this agent, everywhere so abundant—pure, simple water!" In short,

> Go wash in pure water, 'twill gladden thy soul,
> And make the diseased clayey tenement whole;
> 'Twill nerve thee for life's deepest trials, and bring
> A zest with each joy that around thee may spring.
> Wash often—wash daily—'twill save thee from ills,
> That long dreary catalogue dire disease fills;
> 'Twill quicken thine energies, strengthen thy frame,

> Yea, yield thee rich blessings too many to name. . . .
> Go wash in pure water—'tis plenteous and free,
> All o'er the wide earth flows this blessing for thee;
> Then use it most freely—for thus wilt thou prove
> Thy maker designed it in wisdom and love.[16]

Another basic tenet of American hydropathy was that the maker had employed wisdom and love in designing the human body, too. That principle of belief exerted a powerful transformative influence on water-cure in the United States, redirecting it toward what one practitioner described as "Physical Puritanism," the worship of the "PURE BODY—a body free from all foreign and unassimilable substances—a body washed and cleansed from all corruption and putrefaction." Hydropathy as Physical Puritanism was not just intent on washing all inner filth away but equally determined to deny new filth entrance into the body.[17]

The Grahamite Health Reform Movement

In adopting that latter ideal, hydropaths were inspired by the precepts of a slightly earlier alternative health movement, the health reform campaign known as Grahamism. A Presbyterian preacher who enlisted in the anti-alcohol crusade of the early 1830s, Sylvester Graham (1794–1851; Fig. 4-2) soon came to recognize that alcohol can be as bad for the body as for the soul and, broadening his perspective, to see that there were many other habits of life as physically self-destructive as drinking. He was hardly alone in this realization. Any number of his contemporaries despaired of Americans' seeming determination to dig their own graves with self-indulgent behavior: "In the pursuit of pleasure," a Vermont health advocate marveled, "the people have been endeavoring to see how far they can venture down the whirlpool of disease without being irretrievably caught by its eddying force, drawn down into the vortex and dashed at last upon the rocks of death." Where Graham stood apart, however, was in translating health rhetoric into a program of action, what he dubbed the "Science of Human Life." Through books, magazine articles, and popular lectures, Graham worked to persuade people to turn their backs on the temptations of pleasure's whirlpool, to teach them the laws of health, and to convince them that all illness could be prevented by proper hygiene. (Graham addressed "hygiene" through the nineteenth-century definition of the term. "Hygiene" derives from the Greek word for health, and historically, up until the last hundred years or so, it has been used to designate all the habits of life—food, exercise, sleep, dress, etc.—that provide the basis for personal health. Not until the end of the 1800s, as the germ

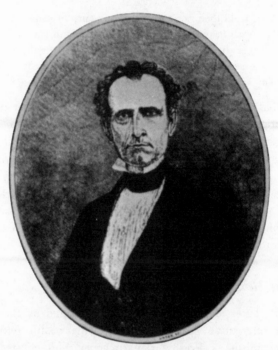

Figure 4-2. Sylvester Graham [Sylvester Graham, *Lectures on the Science of Human Life* (New York: Fowlers and Wells, 1858), frontispiece]

theory stimulated such anxiety about dirt, did "hygiene" acquire the very specific meaning of attention to bodily cleanliness that everyone accepts as its definition today.)[18]

By Graham's analysis, medicine was not needed (was, in fact, injurious), because right living prevented illness from ever occurring. His "science" consisted of rules governing diet, physical activity, clothing, sexuality, and various other activities, including bathing for cleanliness. Those hygienic regulations were drawn, however, not from scientific observation but from the former minister's pious logic based on two unquestioned premises: there was first the Puritanical conviction that all pleasurable sensation was Satanic temptation in disguise, and second the certainty that any behavior that was immoral had to be unphysiological, unhealthful, as well. An efficient God would not have designed things any other way. In practical translation, this meant that any activity appearing to be stimulating, to emotions as well as physical organs, was potentially pathological.

But it was not enough that the laws of physiology had to be congruent with the commandments of scripture. The Grahamite gospel extended farther, to the belief that those laws were "indeed nothing less than the application of Christianity to the physical condition and wants of man . . . the means which God has ordained for the redemption of the body."[19] In that light, every human being had a moral duty to her or his creator to understand the structure and function of the body, God's gift, and to adopt the diet, activities, dress, and other habits that keep the body working at its maximum disease-thwarting, God-glorifying efficiency.

Graham's line of reasoning constituted a radical departure from the traditional medical interpretation of hygiene. Since the days of Hippocrates, the golden rule of health had been moderation in all things. Virtually any activity was acceptable so long as it was not carried to a level of excess. (Excess included too little as well as too much.) Thus alcohol, for example, was regarded as actually beneficial to health when enjoyed in moderation; it was only drunkeness, and to a lesser extent teetotalism, that injured. But by Graham's reckoning, many activities were dangerous in any amount, because they were immoral: there could be no compromise with evil. What set his campaign apart as alternative medicine, as hygienic extremism, was these qualitative distinctions, as opposed to the traditional quantitative orientation of physicians. For Grahamites, even moderation had to be practiced in moderation, for abstinence was usually the rule. Theirs was a Victorian physiology that was the antithesis of the twentieth century's "Playboy philosophy": if it feels good, Graham might have said, don't do it! Those who did do it, who drank whiskey, for example, or smoked tobacco, were condemned to suffer a stimulation-induced inflammation in the immediately affected organ that could pass through the nervous system to all other parts of the body and show up as disease anywhere.

It was not only alcohol and tobacco that were condemned as dangerous in even the smallest quantity. The list also included all drugs and medicaments, coffee, tea, and, in fact, all beverages except water. Spices, the stimulants of appetite, were rejected. Even warnings about impure air were colored by the fear of stimulation: the crowded surroundings stagnant with carbon dioxide that people were told to avoid were ballrooms, theaters, and gaming halls, never churches. Since sex felt best of all, it particularly was not to be done, at least not outside wedlock or without a partner. The "social vice" (pre- and extra-marital sex) was presumed to be as damaging to the body as to the soul, and the "solitary vice" (masturbation) to be particularly deadly. Even within the Christian confines of marriage, where procreation was a moral injunction, sexual exertion had to be limited: a once-monthly indulgence was permitted for young and robust couples, but not even that for the older or weaker. Above all, though, Grahamism meant vegetarianism, the diet indicated by Genesis 1:29 as the original, God-appointed diet of humankind. Graham and comrades were responsible for introducing into the vegetarian movement the argument that meatless diet was superior for *physiological* reasons, not just for the *moral* advantages that had hitherto provided its chief justification.[20]

Grahamite vegetarianism was selective, however. It did not countenance such vegetable products as coffee and spices, as we have seen, and it most particularly did not condone consumption of the white bread that was just then coming into fashion. Through an argument too convoluted to pursue here, Graham rejected white flour as stimulating. He also regarded it as unnatural. During the human race's early centuries, he explained, food was received "from the bosom of nature, with very little or no artificial preparation. Flouring mills and bolting-cloths . . . were then wholly unknown." But eventually those engines of refinement made their appearance, and "mankind . . . began to put asunder what God has joined together," until now, Graham moaned, "human ingenuity" truly "tortures the flour of wheat." (Fortunately, this first prominent champion of natural foods was not long-lived enough to see the oxymoronic travesty of a modern American cereal company marketing "artificial Graham flavor" as one of its selection of instant oatmeals.) Untortured wheat, whole wheat flour, was the only acceptable substrate for nourishing bread, and it was from this natural wheat that the health crusader perfected the recipes for Graham bread and Graham crackers that have kept his name alive to the present. Whole wheat was the item most clearly associated with Graham by his contemporaries, too; his followers were laughed at as "the bran bread and sawdust pathological society."[21]

Graham hoped to be remembered for much more, as indeed nothing less than the savior of American society. His expectation was that as everyone adopted the principles of his science of human life, disease would be eliminated, and as improved health was passed on to offspring, human life expectancy would, over the course of generations, return to its original standard, the eight hundred and more years of Methusaleh and other biblical patriarchs. Further, because of the divinely wrought sympathy between body and soul, physical purity would necessarily promote moral purity and eliminate all inhumanity and mistreatment of others. Correct hygiene was the prescription for the millennium, a new Christian world in which all would live for centuries in sinless vigor. Physiology, in short, was the ultimate morality. Even as the storm clouds of approaching civil war darkened the skies of the 1850s, hydropath and Graham sympathizer Russell Trall would proclaim that the issue of North versus South was inconsequential next to "hog v. hominy" and "chicken v. whortleberries." It would not be the election of Lincoln or Douglas but the selection of corn and fruit over ham and drumsticks, vegetarianism over flesh eating, that would hammer "spears of blood and carnage into prunning [sic] hooks for the new Garden of Eden."[22]

Grahamism never converted more than a few thousand adherents, even during its peak period in the 1840s. But to be fair, it did include much good common sense. Its index of prohibitions included not only white bread but gluttony, slothfulness, neglect of bathing, and women's wearing of tight-laced corsets. And although it originally denied the need for any kind of therapy, regular or irregular, it was a natural ally for the curative program of hydropathy. Graham trusted in the body's power to restore itself when put on the right regimen, worshipped water as the only non-stimulating beverage, and advised daily cold water baths. Except for details of content and emphasis, that was Priessnitzian philosophy. Drug-hating Grahamites could accept hydropathy because water was not a medicine; it was a natural substance, a physiological essential. Hydropaths attuned to therapy could still appreciate Grahamism's preventive orientation: it employed the same bathing and exercise for *sustaining* body purity that they used to *achieve* body purity. The two sides quickly and happily merged once hydropathy arrived in the United States in the 1840s. After Graham's death in 1851 (and the conversion of his house into a tavern), the best presentations of health reform teachings were to be found in hydropathic journals and at the water-cures themselves. At length, water-cure came to place as much faith in diet and exercise—in Grahamite hygiene—as in water (sometimes more), until in the end American hydropathy became "hygeiotherapy."

The Formulation of Hygeiotherapy

The metamorphosis of hydropathy into hygeiotherapy is easily followed through the pages of the profession's chief periodical, *The Water-Cure Journal.* The journal began publication in 1845, and before that first year was out editor Joel Shew, who had opened the country's first water-cure (1843), felt readers were ready to hear *"that the best part of hydropathy—incomparably the best, is the preventive part."* Only when people had been persuaded to exercise, eat wholesome food, and breathe pure air—in addition to bathing daily—"do we accomplish what hydropathy is destined to bring about." This view of water-cure's destiny took such hold of practitioners' thinking that when they formed a national organization in 1850 they named it the American Hygienic and Hydropathic association. "Hygienic" preceded "Hydropathic" in the Association's name in "formal recognition of the principle, that the highest duty of a physician is the preservation of health—the prevention, rather than the cure of disease." Soon, the very name of the Priessnitzian system of cure was being subjected to reconsideration. Various names in which *hygeio-* was substituted for *hydro-* were debated in the 1850s. The simplest change, "hygeiopathy," had considerable backing, as did "hygeio-medicine." But in the end "hy-

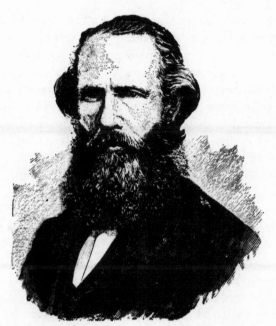

Figure 4-3. Russell Trall [*Food, Home and Garden*, May–June 1891, 21]

geiotherapy," with its direct statement that hygiene could treat and cure, as well as maintain, won out.[23]

The chief proponent of that last name was Russell Trall (1812–1877; Fig. 4-3), who better than any other water-curist exemplifies the way hydropathy was restructured to make water just one among several equals. Although he was trained in allopathic medicine, earning the MD in the 1830s, Trall showed little patience with conventional methods. The ink on his diploma was barely dry, it seems, before he began experimenting with botanic and homeopathic remedies. When hydropathy, the latest alternative system, came to his attention in the early 1840s, he gave that a try and finally settled down. From then until the very week of his death, in 1877, he was one of the busiest and most successful practitioners of hydropathy—rather, hygeiotherapy. The water-cure he founded in New York City in 1844 was the second in the country, and when he transferred operations to then-rural New Jersey in 1867, his Hygeian Home became instantly one of the country's most desirable havens for health seekers. He assisted Shew in editing *The Water-Cure Journal* for several years, until assuming full responsibility in 1849. (In 1862 he changed the publication's name to *The Hygienic Teacher and Water-Cure Journal*, and the following year to *The Herald of Health;* both names are indicative of his orientation toward hygiene.) Trall was the dean of his profession: crusading editor, prolific article writer, touring lecturer, head of hydropathy's leading educational institution (the Hygeio-Therapeutic College), and author of numerous popular books, both texts on water-cure (*The Hydropathic Encyclopedia, Water-Cure for the Million*) and guides to hygiene (*The Scientific Basis of Vegetarianism, The Complete Gymnasium, Home-Treatment for Sexual Abuse*).[24]

Hygeiotherapy was in essence holistic medicine at a time when the word "holistic" had not been thought of yet. The hygeiotherapeutic interpretation of illness required practitioners to elicit much detail from patients about their living habits and also their mental and emotional condition. (One of the key components of hygiene historically was a category denominated "passions of the mind," meaning psychological stresses that might affect health.) As with homeopathy, the patients of hydropaths received much time and personal attention from their physicians, and their emotional complaints were taken as seriously as their physical ones. Time and personal attention carried over from examination into treatment, for wrapping patients and supervising their baths were extended procedures that involved physical touch and intimacy.[25]

When the word "holistic" was introduced into medicine in the 1970s, it at first denoted only the specific meaning of treatment of the whole person. "Holistic" was immediately embraced by practitioners of alternative therapies as an ideal that distinguished them from conventional medicine, and in short order the word's meaning expanded to incorporate other distinctive emphases of alternative systems: the use of "natural" therapies, reliance on preventive measures, and determination to educate patients about health and encourage them to assume a significant degree of responsibility for their own recovery. Hydropathy expressed all those connotations of holism in the mid-1800s. Its self-perception as natural healing has been discussed above. Water-cure was equally dedicated, it has been noted, to preventing the return of disease through strengthening of the *vis medicatrix* with proper hygiene, beginning with daily exercise. Thus at Trall's Hygeian Home, walking about the spacious grounds above the Delaware River, all that would have been expected of patients by Priessnitz, was not enough. Invalids had to rejoice in their returning strength by riding horses, sailing and rowing boats, sawing and splitting logs, and/or digging in the garden. (The last was recommended for the ladies, who generally were treated more delicately. Shew's advice on preventing consumpton, or pulmonary tuberculosis, was that men should hike, ride, and swing dumbbells; women should spin wool, "one of the best possible exercises for females.") Both sexes, however, were put through calisthenic paces first thing every morning. The Hygeian Home boasted an "extensive Gymnasium Hall, with abundant apparatus and music," as well as a platform in a riverside grove for the enjoyment of "dancing gymnastics" (a prescient innovation, considering the word "aerobic" had not been applied even to bacteria yet).

Even with dancing, however, the water-cure workout was not particularly strenuous. It was comprised mostly of varied swinging, bending, and thrusting movements of the arms and legs, and jouncing in place in imitation of horseback riding was "considered by many the most important of all" the exertions. The "laughing exercise" was highly regarded as well. Usually the culmination of the session, it involved raising the arms above the head and bringing them down quickly with a forcible expulsion of laughter "till the hall or house rings with the deep, loud and hearty laugh."[26]

Energy for all this activity had to be found in a strictly controlled diet. An officer of the American Vegetarian Society from its founding in 1850, Trall pressed his patients to eat likewise. He did allow the weak-willed small amounts of animal food at the beginning of their stay, but his lectures on proper diet warned them they would never regain full health until they weaned themselves fully from flesh. To assist in the process, he ran a Provision Depot where Graham bread and crackers, oatmeal, hominy, grits, and other farinaceous foods were offered for sale. If the doggerel submitted by one patient is indicative, the depot must have done a brisk business:

> O! dig me a grave, Dig it deeply and wide;
> And a large Graham loaf Lay it snug by my side;
> Tho' I may not want it I'm yet very sure
> There will be in Heaven Dyspeptics to cure.

(In the 1850s *The Water-Cure Journal* even ran what one might call a Graham cracker bake-off, to find the best recipe for this most nourishing of snacks. And as late as the 1890s *The Journal of Hygeio-Therapy* was still singing the praises of "the Graham cracker bold! . . . worth my weight in purest gold/ For I make him well and make him strong/ Who eats me often, and eats me long.")[27]

Graham crackers or no, most hydropathic patients got better. Because it was necessary to travel to water-cures, those with acute or critical conditions were virtually excluded (though many victims of the cholera outbreaks of the late 1840s were treated in urban hydropathy clinics and enjoyed, it was claimed, a much higher survival rate than allopathic patients). As a rule, the sick were victims of relatively mild or chronic complaints, many of which were self-limited, and some of which undoubtedly had been aggravated by the pressures and anxieties of hurried urban lives. "Stress" existed in the nineteenth century, too, and stressed patients surely responded favorably to the early-to-bed-and-early-to-rise hygienic regimen imposed on them at the hydro. As an English nobleman put it, "at the Water-Cure the whole life is one remedy."[28]

Hygeiotherapy and Sexual Hygiene

That remedial life also required sexual restraint, though Trall's teachings on sex deviated somewhat from those of Sylvester Graham. Rather than begrudging God for establishing so sensual a mechanism for procreation, Trall accepted that sexual intercourse was supposed to be pleasurable, was as desirable for recreational as procreational purposes, and was to be enjoyed equally by both partners. He was indignant over male sexual clumsiness, and consequent female sexual frustration, and recognized a serious public need for sex education. His *Sexual Physiology and Hygiene*, one of the most popular works on the subject throughout the latter half of the century, was a clear and patient discussion of human sexual anatomy (complete with unretouched illustrations) and physiology, as close to a eulogy to the joys of sex as a Victorian author might respectably get. The "love embrace," for instance, should be an "at-one-ment" in which "each should almost lose, in the intensity of pleasurable sensation, the consciousness of individual or independent existence." Trall could be as blunt as he was poetic, offering direct exhortations of a sort not often found in nineteenth-century sexual discourse. "Surely, if sexual intercourse is worth doing at all," he exclaimed at the end of one chapter, "it is worth doing well."[29]

Part of doing it well, he further appreciated, was being free of the fear of pregnancy and the threat of early debility or death from too frequent parturition. While most physicians either condemned contraceptive methods or benignly ignored them, Trall forcefully recommended the taking of precautions to avoid unwanted children and clearly explained what ones to take. The primitive diaphragm was one recommendation, but his preferred method was what would one day be called rhythm. Unfortunately, Trall (and many other mid-nineteenth-century doctors who ventured guesses at the female sexual cycle) didn't catch the rhythm quite right. Mistaking menstruation as evidence of the approaching end of the fertile period, he advised that "if intercourse is abstained from until ten or twelve days after the cessation of the menstrual flow, pregnancy will not occur."[30]

Let us hope that the couples who adhered to Trall's schedule had also followed his other rules of clean living so that their offspring at least would be as healthy as they were unexpected. Like Graham, Trall accepted that children inherited the states of health owned by parents at the time of conception, at, in fact, the very hour of conception. Consequently, mother and father (the latter particularly, it seems) could never drop their physiological guard. One tipsy frolic by an otherwise sober parent could result in a half-wit. (How else, Trall asked, could one account for so many clean-living families in which the first child, but not subsequent ones, "was an idiot," if not for "the feastings and dissipations of the wedding occasion?") For the sake of their children and society, if not themselves, therefore, couples had a responsibility to contract only "Sanitary Marriages," committing themselves to lives of physical probity and the rejection of all defiling stimulants.[31]

And since one stimulant was the sexual act itself, intercourse, however delightful an at-one-ment, had to be regulated. Too great frequency equaled too great stimulation and, like alcohol or nicotine, established a morbid craving that drove the indulger to still more frequent activity. Men were especially susceptible to this addiction—and culpable, for since sex involved a partner it was not mere self-abuse. Trall was never more impassioned than when arguing his interpretation of "Woman's Rights," "the right of a woman to her own person." As a potentially injurious access to her person, sex was "under all circumstances, for the female to accept or refuse, and not for the male to dictate or enforce." Many a man did dictate, however; "many a man . . . who would not for his life, much less for the momentary pleasure it afforded, have endangered the health . . . of a well-beloved wife, has destroyed her health, happiness and life (some men several wives successively) by excessive sexual indulgence." (The reason uterine diseases were treated more effectively at water-cures, "or at any other place except home, is because the husband is not continually thwarting what the doctor or Nature is doing for the patient.")[32]

To be sure, women could be culpable, too, if they consented too often. "I have had patients," Trall confided, "who had for years indulged in sexual intercourse as often as once in twenty-four hours, and some who have indulged still oftener. Of course, the result was premature decay, and often permanent invalidism." Once a day, obviously, was too much, but Trall was willing to permit more frequent couplings than Graham. The safe frequency varied according to age, constitution, and state of health, but for the more robust it could be as high as once a week. If that still seemed a bit stingy in view of Trall's urging of people to mate for pleasure instead of procreation, one had to think, apparently, in terms of the distinction between gourmet and gourmand. The epicure found gustatory elation and satisfaction without descending to the gross excess of the glutton. Quality mattered more than quantity; with smaller servings, each bite was more delicious. Less was more in another way, since harboring of sexual energies preserved them. While most people suffered venereal exhaustion by middle age, hygienic livers remained virile through their three score and ten and beyond.[33]

Hygeiotherapy was equally beneficial when it came time for the women in sexually fulfilling marriages to give birth. The ministrations of allopaths, Trall and colleagues charged, were every bit as dangerous when applied to labor and birth as when employed against disease. Under the control of "these Philistines of the apothecary shop," pregnant women were "bled, paregoric'd, magnesia'd, stimulated, mineralized, and poisoned, just as though they were going through a regular course of fever." The experiences of a Mrs. O.C.W. were presented as typical of what ensued when an allopath managed a woman's confinement. "All the 'regular' results followed," Mrs. W. moaned. "A broken breast, sore nipples, O horror! and the like, kept me confined to my bed nearly two months." When this same lady went into labor with her second child, not surprisingly, she dispensed with the allopath and took a sitz bath and a cold water enema instead. The very next morning she was able to get out of bed and eat breakfast (Graham bread and water), and in just a few days she had returned to her usual level of activity.[34]

In the language of more recent times, hygeiotherapy advocated "natural childbirth," as well as "self-help" and "patient empowerment." Being comprised of precisely those life activities over which the individual could exercise control, it was inherently a system of self-treatment. Shew believed that hydropathy was "destined" to transform the public into "their own physicians for the most part," and his *Hydropathic Family Physician* offered more than eight hundred pages of instruction on how to cure virtually anything at home with water. *The Water-Cure Journal* ran regular articles on domestic self-care, and Trall's two-dozen-plus books were all written with an eye toward helping people help themselves. *The Mother's Hygienic Hand-Book* was a clear and informative guide to pregnancy, parturition, and childcare on hydropathic principles, and *Water-Cure for the Million* was exactly the work of democratic domestic medicine its title implied. Even Trall's hefty *Hydropathic Encyclopedia* announced itself first as *A Guide to Families*, and only after as *A Text-Book for Physicians*. Shew declared in 1851 that "there are many times more patients in these United States who are practicing upon themselves at home" than living as inpatients at water-cure institutions.[35]

With a six-foot shelf of the works of Trall (including *The New Hydropathic Cook-Book*, whose recipes would freeze the heart of a bon vivant), one was set to weather all life's storms. One in fact had no choice. To win "physiological salvation," Trall preached, one had to respect the laws of health as divine commandments; what society needed, another water-cure convert suggested, was

> some physiological lore,
> That all may know, that if in sin they go,
> Their organs will all be sore.

"Health reform [this is Trall the hygienic revivalist again] is the veritable corner stone upon which the Christian, the social, the political, as well as the medical reformer must predicate all rational faith in a millenial state of the human family on this earth." Fellow water-curists only said amen to all that. James Jackson, for example, stated that "man's depravity" is rooted not in the soul, as traditionalists believed, but "in his *body*. It dwells there, and if his spirit is also depraved, it has taken it up from sympathy. Look at the vices of society. How large a proportion are the result of ill or wickedly directed *physical* energy. The murders, the burglaries, the arsons, the assaults, the licentiousness, . . . the contempt of religion, the want of patriotism . . . may all, without exception, be ascribed to the ardent spirits, the tea, the coffee, the opium, the tobacco . . . one can add *the drugs which doctors give*." (When Shew passed away shortly before his thirty-ninth birthday, in 1855, Trall diagnosed his demise as the delayed effect of being treated allopathically in his youth and getting "his system badly impregnated with minerals.") Humankind were just as responsible for hygienic sins of omission, furthermore, as commission. It was every bit as immoral not to go into a gymnasium as to go into a tavern. "Physical Puritanism" was an apt term indeed.[36]

Hygeiotherapy and Social Reform

Hygeiotherapy's moral earnestness was the basis of much of its appeal. Its vision of a world freed from mistreatment and exploitation of fellow humans resonated with the politically progressive spirit of the mid-1800s. The last two antebellum decades were among the most reform-minded in the country's history. "Ultras," as political activists were then called, waged war on slavery, capitalism, the oppression of women, Demon Rum, antiquated systems of education, and every other detectable evil. Flaws in the social fabric were numerous, and ultras were kept pretty busy, but not so busy they could overlook the virtues of hydropathy. Like political enthusiasts of any stripe, ultras were given to reflex thinking, to automatic approval or rejection of movements that appeared to share or oppose their own orientation. All systems of irregular medicine were anti-establishment, thus likely to meet with favor; only hydropathy, though, seemed to transcend medicine and commit itself to the furtherance of larger ultra objectives.[37]

To begin with, it had adopted and perpetuated Grahamism, a movement that had aimed ultimately at social perfection. That was the goal also of the temperance crusade, just hitting its full stride in the 1840s. With its exaltation of cold water as the only healthful beverage, the anti-alcohol cause was the most natural reform partner of all for hydropathy. Water-cure periodicals regularly declared support for the temperance campaign, advertised its books and lectures, published its ballads alongside hydropathic hymns, and agreed that water was what "God meant . . . should be our drink."[38]

Water-cure also allied itself with phrenology, the pseudo-science of mind that supposed the human brain encompassed thirty-some distinct organs or regions, each responsible for a specific mental or emotional trait. The prominence of each trait in an individual's personality was directly dependent on the degree of development, the actual size, of its corresponding organ. Philosophers had large organs of causality, thieves large organs of acquisitiveness. The skull, finally, was presumed to reflect the shape of the underlying brain, allowing the expert phrenologist to analyze character by visual and manual examination of the subject's head: the philosopher could be spotted by his prominent forehead, the burglar by his bulging temples. This "bumpology," as detractors called it, was also intended to be a social science. Exercises to strengthen desirable and weaken undesirable mental organs had invaluable applications to psychiatry, education, penology, to everything. Phrenology, one champion babbled, could improve even an oyster.[39]

Hydropaths, at any rate, felt they might benefit from it. America's most renowned practical phrenologists, the Fowler brothers, Orson and Lorenzo, along with a brother-in-law named Wells, ran one of the country's larger publishing firms. Fowlers and Wells turned out a long line of works on phrenology, physiology, temperance, and other reform projects. And when *The Water-Cure Journal* was still languishing three years after its inception, it was the house of Fowlers and Wells that took it over as another reform publication and doubled its circulation in four months. Lorenzo Fowler went on to lecture on mental philosophy at at least two hydropathic schools, and hydropathy was soon clearly linked in the public mind to phrenology.[40]

It was in their feminist leanings, though, that hydropaths most clearly displayed their ultra sympathies. In that matter, they really had little choice. Even had there been no birds-of-a-feather impulse, there was a compelling practical consideration. Female bathers were best handled by female attendants, and those attendants might as well be fully trained practitioners. The Grahamite movement had already instituted the practice of educating women to lecture on delicate topics in hygiene to female audiences. The woman physiology lecturer was an auditorium fixture by the time hydropathy absorbed health reform; the woman water-cure doctor was her offspring. The first class of graduates from the American Hydropathic Institute was composed of eleven men and nine women (one of whom was married to an allopath), and later classes there and at other water-cure colleges were generally from a fourth to a half female. The larger water-cures made it a goal to have at least one woman physician on staff to deal with the more intimate needs of female patients. As a result, the great majority of America's first generation of woman doctors were hydropaths rather than allopaths, which was only to be expected, one water doctoress explained, since hydropathy represented a new, more humane and civilized stage in the evolution of medicine. Women were as far above practicing allopathic medicine as they were above serving as jailers or executioners. Hydropathy, however, good, gentle hydropathy, fostered expression of "the tenderer love, the sublimer devotion, the never to be wearied patience and kindness of woman."[41]

Water-cure wore the trappings of feminist radicalism in a literal sense, too. Its stress on exercise and free breathing clashed with the fashion of heavy dresses and lung-squeezing corsets for females. Feminists outside water-cure institutions were already, by the late 1840s, attacking stylish dress as physically cumbersome and symbolic of woman's social imprisonment, and it was natural for hydropaths to join hands with them. Hygeiotherapist Mary Gove Nichols, for example, gave public lectures in which she denounced fashionable dress as a weapon of men "who wish women to be weak, sickly, and dependent— the pretty slave of man." Women, she decreed, could never advance beyond "small achievement . . . so long as it is the labor of their lives to carry about their clothes."[42]

Female hygeiotherapeutic patients agreed. They had already shown a willingness to wear the "wet dress," a garment designed to allow ladies to walk comfortably while soaking up water. A loose-fitting gown with wide sleeves and a skirt falling over baggy trousers, the wet-dress cut was also ideal for healthy women who wanted comfort and freedom. Soon popularized for general wear by Amelia Bloomer, the wet dress became the Bloomer costume, the quasi-official style of dress of emancipated women. And few publications did more to promote adoption of the new outfit than Trall's *Water-Cure Journal*. While personally denouncing the hoopskirt-and-corset style for rendering women "frivolous and superficial" and dependent, he also ran numerous articles by others explaining the advantages of the Bloomer attire and linking it to female liberation. Trall reserved for himself, though, the most grandiloquent summarization of the significance of the Bloomer crusade, submitting that the freeing of woman from whalebone stays was the first, and an essential, step toward "the reform of the world, the regeneration of society, the full success and final triumph of every Christian and philanthropic enterprise."[43]

His patients often expressed sentiments that differed only in their degree of fervor. The women at the Springfield, Massachusetts, water-cure, for example, celebrated their 1851 donning of Bloomers with formal oratorical exercises concluded by twenty-five different cold water toasts, including one to "The Ladies of the Water-Cure.—The pioneers of reform." A cartoon in the November 1853 issue of the *Water-Cure Journal* placed a robust and earnest looking "Water-Cure Bloomer, who believes in the equal rights of men and women . . . and who thinks it respectable, if not genteel to be well!" next to a pinched and faint-looking "Allopathic Lady . . . who patronizes a fashionable doctor, and considers it decidedly vulgar to enjoy good health."[44]

Health fused with politics in many other areas, for, as Trall announced on the first page of each issue, "It is the appointed and glorious mission of the WATER-CURE JOURNAL to proclaim and hasten the advent of UNIVERSAL HEALTH, VIRTUE AND HAPPINESS." (Hydropathy, an even more sanguine colleague proclaimed, was capable of bringing about the greatest "revolution since the days of Jesus Christ.") His journal took its full title seriously: it was the water-cure journal and *Herald of Reforms*, and its pages had indeed a good word for every reform. Consider, as just one example, its correspondence columns. In the early 1850s Trall established a matrimonial section in the magazine to assist unattached vegetarians in the search for suitable life partners. So many lonely hearts responded, though, he soon had to begin charging an advertising fee of a dollar per hundred words. Letters (and lengthy ones) continued to pour in, each writer begging to be found a worthy connubial candidate. The expectations of prospective mates were in many ways modest: both sexes hoped for healthy partners, the ladies also asking for kind, honest, sober, industrious husbands and denying that wealth mattered. Males ordered independent and open-minded yet congenial helpmates and courteously added that beauty was unimportant. An E.C.W. did specify that "she must not be ugly, nor over thirty years of age," but most were interested in their future spouse's mind rather than her body. Men bragged about the size of their phrenological organs, and some advised ladies not to reply unless they could present evidence of complementary organs from a certified phrenological examination. Millie Maiden asked for a "Christian philanthropist"; Fida wanted a man who "must be a SOCIALIST, a *spiritualist*, and . . . acknowledge the natural right of all to FREEDOM, without regard to sex or color." Agricultor requested a wife "of a decidedly reformatory cast," while Benjamin Radical declared, "My motto, the first love and a natural waist, or no wife." There were many natural waists to choose from, as the women writers nearly all announced themselves as Bloomers—such were Grace Truthful, Fanny Freedom, Abeana Somebody, and Crazy Sabe (who also allowed that "Phrenology and Physiology have always been favorite studies"). A Lover of Truth spoke for all the lovelorn when she concluded her rather desperate plea with an affirmation that she still would "rather live a life of 'single blessedness' than marry any other than a reformer." If she remained in single blessedness, she had only herself to blame, for available to her were Dick Goodenough, a strong temperance man, and Ploughboy, a champion of women's rights, and Honestus, a "progressionist," and Junius, "a friend of all true reforms," and Reformer, Young America, Sobriety, and many, many more, all of them friends of true reform (and more than a few, the reader will be happy to learn, sooner or later withdrew their names from the column, "having found the other half").[45]

Decline of Hygeiotherapy

Because a good reform man in those days was not hard to find, hygeiotherapy enjoyed a considerable following from the mid-1840s into the 1870s. Success was achieved, furthermore, in the face of a volume of criticism from the allopathic profession that was surpassed only by the abuse heaped upon homeopathy. As a physician writing in the late 1840s observed, "hydropathy has become a tabooed subject, being either entirely excluded from medical journals and books, or only admitted into them for the purpose of being ridiculed or utterly denounced." Typical ridicule was the report by a regular doctor of seeing a sick duck in a city park cure itself hydropathically. Wobbling into the lake, the drake first took a foot bath, then floated into a sitz bath, next plunged his head beneath the water for a head bath, and finally threw his head back and flapped his wings as if to shout, "Priessnitz forever," but instead said only, "Quack, quack, quack!"[46]

Even more fun was had at the expense of hydropaths by allopathic cartoonists, who delighted in picturing water-cure patients as swollen with water to the point of exploding or so saturated with water as to require wringing out like a soggy towel. The most that was allowed the water system was that while it was "not very scientific, it is certainly a clever scheme" because many ailing people "require nothing but good air, plain living, rest from their anxious occupations, and agreeable society."[47] As with homeopathy, regulars were convinced, hydropathic patients got better not because their treatments cured them but because the treatments did nothing to hurt them and left nature time to do the job.

Hydropaths counterattacked, comparing allopathy to "sorcery, witchcraft, . . . and many other absurdities." "No age of the world," Trall contended, "presents a medley of medical scribblers in the regular profession more biased and bigoted in their notions, more visionary in their speculations, more puerile in their theories, and more inconsistent in their practices, than is furnished by . . . the medical profession in this country." Worst of all, the puerile physicians were poisoners who "derange and torture" patients with "pharmaceutical filth," the worst component of which was calomel. Trall identified fifty-one distinct "diseases" produced by calomel, including "Stomatitis Mercurialis" ("Mercurial inflammation of the stomach"), "Ostitis Mercurialis" ("Mercurial decay of the bones"), "Paralysis Mercurialis" ("General mercurial palsy"), "Apoplexia Mercurialis," and "Hypochondriasis Mercurialis," which a colleague defined as "a morbid affection of the spirits, . . . terminating often in lunacy or suicide." (Hydropaths also dismissed competing irregular systems, arguing that homoeopathy, for example, was "a chimera" whose effects depended largely on "the workings of the imagination.")[48]

If hygeiotherapy made a big splash in the 1850s, by the end of the 1870s it appeared to be washed up. This was no doubt due in part to the fact that as its novelty wore off, patients came to understand more clearly that the system's emphasis on hygiene meant sacrifice and self-denial for its clients. Most people prefer that doctors cure them directly rather than ask them to heal themselves. "A person sends for a doctor, as a lady sends for a stay-maker," an English MD observed in the 1850s. "If the stay-maker, instead of taking the lady's measure, should begin to discourse concerning the baneful effect of stays upon the frame, and should recommend the lady to acquire an elegant shape by calisthenic exercises, the lady would reject the advice as impertinent, and summon a more submissive stay-maker. . . . So with medical men. They are asked for pills, and not for homilies on temperance; for draughts, and not for dietetics."[49]

More erosive of popular support, however, was a trend toward pessimism during the last third of the century. The horror of civil war disabused American society of its illusions of human perfectibility. A reform spirit that had once seemed dashing came to appear quixotic as ultraism receded. Cynicism, then the vulgar materialism of the Gilded Age of the 1880s and '90s, came to dominate the national mood, making optimistic hygeiotherapy appear hopelessly naive at best, and socially disruptive at worst, and depriving the water-cure of the idealistic young who had constituted so much of its patronage.[50] By the end of the century, only a handful of water-cures remained in business. Nevertheless, hygeiotherapy was on the verge of revival and would soon get to enjoy a second life in the form of naturopathy. That revival will be considered in Chapter 9.

5

Magnetism and Mind: From Mesmerism to Christian Science

T he power which a man's imagination has over his body to heal it or make it sick," Mark Twain remarked, "is a force which none of us is born without." Yet if left to his own devices, he believed, "a man is most likely to use only the mischievous half of the force—the half which invents imaginary ailments for him and cultivates them"—and is "quite likely to scoff at the beneficent half of the force and deny its existence." To help such a person, then, "*two* imaginations are required: his own and some outsider's. The outsider, B, must imagine that *his* incantations are the healing-power that is curing A, and A must imagine that this is so" as well, when in fact the outsider is doing no more than the engineer who drives a locomotive. He "turns on the steam," but "the actual power is lodged exclusively in the engine. . . . If the engine were left alone it would never start of itself."[1]

Turning on the steam in the sick person's mind and getting it to start up was an activity that engaged many alternative practitioners in the nineteenth century. Homeopathy and hygeiotherapy both recognized that mental state influenced physical functioning, but neither elevated the mind to the position of primacy in healing. A primarily mental approach to cure did develop contemporaneously with those systems, however, flowering in several forms from seeds planted by an eighteenth-century Austrian physician, Franz Anton Mesmer (1734–1815; Fig. 5.1).

Mesmerism and the Origins of Magnetic Healing

Mesmer was a well-established Vienna practitioner who in the 1770s began to test a theory he had developed in his medical school dissertation. Believing

103

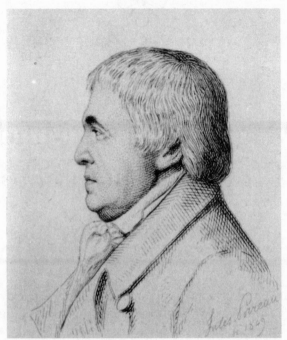

Figure 5-1. Franz Anton Mesmer [Courtesy of the
National Library of Medicine]

that the gravitational pull of the sun, moon, and planets created tides in the
earth's atmosphere, and that this aerial ebb and flow could affect the nervous
fluid within the human body, he hypothesized that illness might be cured with
magnets since they, like celestial bodies, could influence other physical entities
without being in direct contact. Accordingly, toward the end of July 1774, he
began treating a woman suffering from recurrent attacks of hysteria by placing
one magnet on her stomach and another on each of her legs soon after an
episode had begun. There was a nearly instantaneous reaction, his patient
declaring she felt "painful currents of a subtle material" moving within. Her
seizure gradually subsided, and she was well for several hours. When the
attack was renewed the next day, Mesmer reapplied the magnets with the same
success, and over the course of the next two weeks the woman was restored
to complete health. ("She married and had some children," he was pleased to
relate.)[2]

Mesmer thus was the exception to the irregular rule of empiricism.
Whereas others discovered treatments from clinical trials and then postulated
theories to rationalize the methods, he began with a theoretical framework
from which he deduced his therapeutic innovation and then tested it empirically. More experimentation followed, other patients were found to benefit,

and eventually Mesmer discovered that wooden and other non-magnetic articles achieved the same results—but only if wielded by him. Clearly, if nervous fluid could be altered by virtually any object, the effect must not be one of ordinary mineral magnetism but instead be a manifestation of the healer's own vital influence. Still "magnetic" by virtue of its power to attract and impart movement to the nervous fluid, it was "animal magnetism."[3]

The revised theory that now took form in Mesmer's mind centered on a kind of magnetic ether, "a universally distributed and continuous fluid ... of an incomparably rarefied nature," that he supposed to be the medium for transmission of influence from celestial bodies to the earth and into the human nervous apparatus. This animal magnetism, his clinical experience had indicated, could be "communicated to other animate and inanimate bodies" and directed toward the ill so as to cure sickness. In sum, Mesmer proposed, his newly discovered form of magnetism could replace traditional therapeutics and "the art of healing will thus reach its final stage of perfection." He resolved "to dedicate my remaining life [to] the preservation of my fellow creatures" both from disease and from "the incalculable hazards of the application of drugs."[4]

The next stage through which Mesmer carried his art was the wholesale "magnetization" of the patient environment. (Magnetism, remember, could be communicated to inanimate bodies; he supposed it could be reflected by mirrors as well.) He handled and thereby infused with his personal magnetism every item in the clinic precinct of his stately home. The patients he attracted awoke between magnetized sheets, bathed with magnetized water, took breakfast from magnetized china and silver, and strolled the estate's grounds in magnetized clothing. In the evenings, they gathered in the garden to immerse their feet in the magnetized fountain, clinging to metal cables attached to magnetized trees while the master soothed any remaining nervous agitation with music from the magnetized glass harmonica on which he was a virtuoso.[5]

Mesmer's unorthodox methods brought him into conflict with his medical confreres, however, so early in 1778, desperate to secure "the relaxation I so much needed," he moved to Paris. Initially, at least, his reception there was more congenial. Patients flocked to him, and the cures performed in his rooms in Place Vendôme were soon the talk of *tout Paris*. There was the case of "vaporous melancholia with spasmodic vomiting"; another of "decay of the organs of perspiration"; several of "longstanding stoppages in the spleen, lining and mesentery"; and the unprecedented restoration of a patient suffering from "paralysis with trembling ... the result of frost-bite ... aggravated by the effects of a putrid and malignant fever ... contracted six years before in America."[6]

Mesmer's success in Paris owed much to his perfection of magnetic instrumentation, the *baquet*. The prosaically named device (*baquet* simply means tub) was a condensed and modernized version of the magnetized fountain of Vienna. Four to five feet in diameter and a foot or so deep, the circular (sometimes oval) oaken tub held bottles of magnetized water arranged concentrically above a bottom layer of pieces of magnetized glass and iron. Through the cover of the *baquet* there protruded narrow iron bars long and flexible enough to be applied to any ailing part of a patient's anatomy. Numerous patients could congregate about the tub; by holding hands and winding themselves in a cord attached to the *baquet*, they could form a human conducting chain. (His clinic was actually equipped with four *baquets*, three for paying clients and one for the poor.) Music, tranquil or martial according to the patients' needs, issued from the piano in the corner, to which accompaniment Mesmer entered in flowing lilac robes, walking with majestic pace from patient to patient, gazing into each with his commanding eyes, and touching or stroking each with his energy-filled fingers and magnetic baton. As he introduced his powerful magnetic current into a client, the subject's own sluggish fluid was stirred into a movement that quickly built to a crescendo of nervous agitation. "When I pointed my wand at him," Mesmer reported of one patient, it "caused him to tremble wildly; his face became flushed; he appeared to suffocate; he perspired profusely"; finally, "he fainted and fell back on the sofa unconscious." A Mlle. Belancourt "staggered and fell to the floor in violent convulsions" when the wand was directed at her.[7]

Whether brought about instantaneously or gradually, convulsion was Mesmer's goal. Supposing illness to be a sign of a greatly depressed or even arrested flow of animal magnetism through an individual's nerves, he believed the inert fluid must be temporarily pushed to an equally extreme velocity to reactivate body parts and reestablish normal function. Hence the need for *une crise* as a proof of cure. "A disease cannot be cured without a crisis," he declared. "The crisis is an effort of nature against the disease, tending, by an increase of movement, tone and intension, through the action of the magnetic fluid, to disperse the obstacles which impede circulation, to dissolve and evacuate the molecules which form such obstructions, and to reestablish harmony and equilibrium within all parts of the body."[8]

Undeterred by the violence of the crisis, throngs filled the salons of Mesmer and his disciple Charles Deslon, likewise an erstwhile orthodox practitioner. In the single year of 1784, the pair treated an estimated eight thousand patients, the majority from the higher social strata, and those who were not treated at least talked of mesmerism. In examining the broad range of French popular literature of the 1780s, Robert Darnton has determined that mesmerism "probably inspired more interest than any other topic of fashion" until the approaching revolution turned all eyes toward politics at the end of the decade. Subject of poetry and pamphlet, play and burlesque, cartoon and café debate, mesmerism for a while constituted a veritable "frenzy": "Everyone is occupied with mesmerism. One is dazzled with its marvels, and if one admits doubts about its powers . . . at least one dares no longer deny its existence."[9]

In truth, one group did deny mesmerism. In 1784 Louis XVI appointed a commission of eminent scientists to investigate the claims of magnetic healing. Directed by Benjamin Franklin, the international authority on electricity (at the time serving as American ambassador to France), and including Antoine Lavoisier, the pioneer of modern chemistry, and Joseph de Guillotin, a physician who had greater fame lying ahead, the commission carried out experiments with mesmerized patients that convinced them that Mesmer's magnetic fluid did not exist and that the healing crises were the result solely of suggestion from the magnetizer and the imagination of the patients. "Imagination without magnetism produces convulsions," their report concluded, but "magnetism without imagination produces nothing." The implicit possibility that imagination and suggestion might be harnessed to the work of healing was left unexplored, for the investigation had focused on Mesmer's fluid, and that had been found to be "non-existent" and therefore "without utility."[10]

Imagination was not, however, without danger, and the potential evil results were itemized in titillating detail in a second, secret report from the commission. Most of Mesmer's patients were women, it had been noted, and women patients experienced crisis much more frequently and with more violence than male ones. ("Women are weaker, more delicate, more impressionable than men," a nineteenth-century mesmerist would explain, "which signifies [that] the nervous system in them is the predominant system"; they were also particularly susceptible because "dependence" was "one of the prominent traits of their organism and habits.") All of Mesmer's practitioners and assistants were men, the latter in fact being carefully selected from among "*les plus beaux, les plus jeunes et les plus robustes*" of men. As therapy involved close proximity—treatment commonly began with the doctor enclosing the seated patient's knees between his own and progressed by touching and stroking of the patient's body, particularly the abdomen—female crisis might easily imitate orgasm. The woman's "face becomes flushed by degrees," it was observed; "the eye becomes ardent, . . . respiration is short and spasmodic; and the breast rises and falls tumultuously; tremors begin along with precipitate and brusque movements of the limbs or the entire body. . . . The end . . . is often a bodily spasm. Langour and quiescence follow this stage." Even Mesmer's supporters admitted that it would be an easy matter to "outrage" a patient in such a state, and repeated denials that liberties were ever taken only cranked the rumor mill faster. Bawdy songs congratulated Mesmer for conquering "many a female" and having "old ones, young ones, ugly ones, beautiful ones" all in love with and faithful to him. Others joked that what Newton had done for physics, the magnetizer "has done for love."[11]

Rise of Hypnosis

Gossip failed to drive Mesmer away, but with the storming of the Bastille, the city turned inhospitable for a man who had made a fortune catering to the *ancien régime*. Mesmer fled, eventually settling in Switzerland, where he died in 1815. By then followers had refined his technique in such ways as to avoid producing the violent crisis, bringing about in its stead a peaceful state of "sleep" at first called somnambulism and eventually (in the 1840s) termed hypnosis (from Greek *hypnos*, sleep). Theory had been altered as well by some practitioners, somnambulism being explained as a mental effect produced by the mesmerist's willpower rather than a material fluid transmitted from his body. Mesmerism would remain split into two theoretical camps through the middle of the nineteenth century, with the fluidists outnumbering the animists (proponents of psychic influence) until the end of that period.[12]

Extraordinary phenomena were reported from both sides as experimentation with hypnotic response spread into new areas. For a time, the mesmeric trance was employed by a few practitioners to obviate the pain of surgical operations. (There were no pharmaceutical anesthetic agents available until 1846, when ether was introduced.) A painless mastectomy was reported from France as early as 1829, and from the late 1830s into the '40s a well-placed London surgeon gave a number of demonstrations that dramatized the power of hypnosis to make patients insensible to pain. A handful of other surgeons in Britain and America also utilized hypnosis for anesthesia. Most noteworthy was James Esdaile, an Englishman practicing in India, who in the 1840s reported dozens of painless operations, including such procedures as mastectomy, amputation of limbs, and "toe nails cut out by the roots." Mesmerism also came to be employed for the relief of labor pains and to comfort the dying. (In recent years, it has come back into vogue for painless childbirth; there is even a Hypnobirthing Institute in New Hampshire.)[13]

For the great majority of the medical profession, however, the mesmeric fluid still smacked of the occult; it was one of the "mock sciences," an English physician scoffed, bearing the same relation to physics "as astrology does to astronomy." Mesmeric surgery was surely some sort of "imposture," most physicians concluded; a Georgia doctor who actually witnessed a magnetic operation without evidence of pain concluded that it "is not a reality; . . . that the phenomena ascribed to it, are firstly due to the imagination and excited feelings." "No more shall we hear the afflicted complain," a British poet-physician chuckled,

> Operations will give more of pleasure than pain;
> And ladies will smile in their mesmerised trance
> As the pains of their uterine efforts advance.
> Then shut up the schools, burn the Pharmacopoeia,
> Let us carry out all Dr. Mesmer's idea:
> And whilst skeptics their agonized vigils are keeping
> His disciples will through their afflictions be sleeping.

In short, most physicians reacted, "mesmerism is too gross a humbug to admit of any further serious notice. We regard its abettors as quacks [who] ought to be hooted out of professional society." So strong was professional opinion against the apparent humbug of mesmeric surgery that James Elliotson, the London physician who introduced hypnosis for surgery into Britain and theretofore a gentleman highly respected by colleagues, was in fact hooted out of the hospital position he had held for years in 1838.[14]

If there were to be an acceptable anesthetic agent, it had to be a scientific one, and there is reason to believe that ether owes its discovery and acceptance in part at least to mesmerism. It was mesmerist surgeons who raised the possibility of operating without pain, and surgical experimentation with ether, a substance previously used only as an intoxicant, followed hard on the heels of demonstrations of mesmeric surgery. When Robert Liston completed the first amputation in Britain using ether, two months after its introduction in America, his first words to his audience were "This Yankee dodge, gentlemen, beats mesmerism hollow"; that evening, he wrote a friend, "HURRAH! Rejoice! Mesmerism, and its professors, have met with a 'heavy blow, and great discouragement.' " (Liston's operation was performed, ironically, in the same hospital from which Elliotson had been banished.) An American journal echoed the sentiment, declaring that ether "is based on scientific principles and is solely in the hands of gentlemen of high professional attainment," which was not the case, it was noted, with "the farce and trickery of mesmerism." Ether, along with chloroform, an agent discovered in 1847, steadily displaced mesmerism in surgery over the next ten years because, in spite of the dangers of chemical anesthetics, they worked on everyone; many patients were resistant to the deep mesmerization required for painless surgery.[15]

Mesmerism in America

Mesmerists were not particularly dismayed by ether's ascendance, because they believed the chief value of their science to be not for surgical anesthesia but for the cure of disease. That application of magnetic healing was introduced to America by Charles Poyen in 1835. (Lafayette, one of Mesmer's most fervent followers, had beseeched George Washington to try the new method of healing as early as the 1780s, but his plea came to nought.) A Parisian whose treatment by a mesmerist included the advice to go to the New World for his health, Poyen settled in Lowell, Massachusetts, intending to teach French. As he discovered Americans' ignorance of magnetism, though, he was motivated to offer a course of public lectures on animal magnetism. The lectures were an extraordinary success, largely because of the demonstrations of clairvoyance Poyen gave with an assistant who was able to read the thoughts of audience members and the contents of sealed containers while in the mesmeric trance.[16]

Yet while some welcomed mesmerism as a "Gift of God . . . mercifully vouchsafed by the beneficent Creator for the mitigation of human misery," for others the revelation of these mysterious and previously unsuspected powers was highly disquieting. For those of an anxious disposition, the mesmeric trance was, in the mid-1800s, what radioactivity would be in the mid-1900s, a dark and uncontrollable force that might bring about inconceivable horrors. There was an opinion, apparently widely shared, "that Mesmerism is a mysterious and unholy power, from the exercise of which good men and Christians ought to keep aloof." At the least it might well undermine religious faith, for mesmeric cures were so similar in appearance to the healings performed in the New Testament that one might be led to the conclusion that "the reputed miracles of Scripture were but the result of strong Mesmeric power," that "Christ only raised the dead by Mesmerism."[17] Indeed, more than one magnetic healer would conclude exactly that.

Mesmerism, the public was cautioned, was "so fearful a power," a force "so pregnant with mischief," that "no one can answer for what may happen"— though if anyone could answer, it was Edgar Allan Poe. His answer, of course, was not pretty. In "The Facts in the Case of M. Valdemar," he told the tale of an ailing man who has himself mesmerized to escape his imminent death, only to die wretchedly anyway when "awakened" months later: "His whole frame at once—within the space of a single minute, or even less, shrunk— crumbled, absolutely *rotted* away beneath my hands. Upon the bed . . . there lay a nearly liquid mass of loathsome—of detestable putridity."[18]

Nor could one overlook the possibility of sexual exploitation of mesmerized females by their entrancers. There were already reports from Europe of mesmeric seducers who were constantly in search of "fresh food [for their] libidinous propensities," of a Paris mesmerist who had disgraced himself "by a series of orgies which only occur amongst licentious enthusiasts," and of young Russian men studying mesmerism in London for the purpose of using it "on unsuspecting females" on return to their own country. "What father of a family," a London physician asked, "would admit even the shadow of a mesmeriser within his threshold? . . . Should we not shun such pretenders more than lepers?" That seemed more than ever necessary after the publication of an American-written *Confessions of a Magnetizer* in which the understandably anonymous author boasted of regularly taking pleasure with his more comely patients after placing them under his hypnotic power. Respectable mesmerists admitted that there were indeed practitioners who were motivated only by a "degrading and wretched concupiscence" but insisted that their numbers were few and that honest hypnotists took pains to "avoid whatever may wound the most scrupulous modesty, or cause the least embarrassment" when treating ladies; they also ensured that a family member or female friend was present throughout the session. Even so, there seemed good reason for a Liverpool minister's sermon denouncing mesmerism as a "Satanic Agency."[19]

Uneasiness with the moral implications of mesmerism faded, however, as its healing potential was made manifest. Poyen often treated people who attended his lectures and claimed to have accomplished cures of rheumatism, liver disease, and other ailments. Thanks to his medical triumphs he was able, barely a year and a half after launching his lecture campaign, to announce that "Animal Magnetism has sprung from a complete state of obscurity and neglect into general notice, and become the object of lively interest throughout the country." So lively an interest developed that even the faculty of Harvard Medical School extended Poyen an invitation to speak, though by and large medical opinion of the new practice was, as in England, anything but complimentary. Animal magnetism, one Boston-area physician expostulated, was "of a piece with fortune-telling, juggling, necromancy, astrology, magic, augury, [and] Scottish second-sight." Were it actually as effective as devotees claimed it to be, the medical profession was obsolete: "Doctors must shut up shop, burn and bury their medicaments, take a last, long, lingering look at their anatomical preparations, and betake themselves to some other employment—to whaling, perhaps"; coffin makers and gravediggers were about to be thrown out of work, too. Ridicule was no retardant, however. "A mighty host" of magnetic healers "sprung up in a trice," the *Boston Medical and Surgical Journal* reported, and promptly "swarmed throughout the length and breadth of the northern States, like locusts." By the 1840s even the South was infested, Alabama being "not more thoroughly overrun with the disciples of *doctor* Thomson than those of Dr. Mesmer."[20]

Mesmeric practitioners were a diversified lot. They differed one to the next in the methods used to induce somnambulism. They differed to some extent in the ways they operated upon the entranced patient to manipulate her magnetic fluid or stimulate her willpower. They commonly made "passes" over the patient's body with their hands, but where some maintained physical contact with the body, others moved their hands through the air near the body's surface (either way, "the magnetized person perceive[d] a heat escaping from the ends of your fingers" or experienced tingling or some other evidence of magnetism entering her body). A few even employed a magnetized iron wand, à la Mesmer, taking care to keep it to themselves "and not lend it to any person, lest it should be charged with different fluids." They called their method any number of names: mesmerism, animal magnetism, electro-biology, electrical psychology, etherology, mental electricity, neurology, neurohypnology, pathetism, psycheism, psychodunamy, therapeutic sarcognomy, and still other things. Under whatever name, and whatever the presumed mechanism of action, it was understood by all practitioners to be "the power that man possesses of materially acting upon man, independently of touch."[21]

Nowhere is diversity more in evidence than in the theories spun by mesmerizers to rationalize their abilities. Fluidists played nearly infinite variations on *magneto-*, *electro-*, *galvano-*, *ethero-*, *neuro-*, and similar prefixes in describing their supposed health-adjusting fluid. Some even dragged in phrenology. Joseph Buchanan, perhaps the reigning phreno-magnetist, believed in the nervaura, a blend of electricity, heat, and willpower emanating from the individual phrenological organs in the brain, each of which regulated a specific organ of the body. By putting the patient into a nervauric trance, Buchanan healed any diseased part by concentrating his galvanic power on the associated phrenological faculty. Laroy Sunderland had a comparable theory, pathetism, which allowed for twice the usual number of phrenological organs.[22]

John Bovee Dods

Mesmerism's profligacy in theory is perhaps best demonstrated in the work of John Bovee Dods, father of electrical psychology. A Universalist minister, Dods was attracted to magnetic healing by Poyen's lectures and eventually converted. In the early 1840s he resigned his pastorship and took up a new ministry, preaching the wonders of electrical psychology, "the highest and most sublime science in the whole realm of nature." He was, it would appear, no ordinary preacher. No other magnetist, at any rate, was invited to speak by both the Massachusetts state legislature and the United States Senate. (The invitation from the latter was signed by Henry Clay, Daniel Webster, and Sam Houston.) For six consecutive evenings in 1843, more than two thousand people jammed Boston's Marlboro Chapel to hear him speak ("chained in the most profound silence"), while "multitudes" were turned away. (Such numbers "congregated together, night after night," seemed "almost incredible" to the editors of the *Boston Medical and Surgical Journal;* it was "with deep mortification" that they watched their city, the Athens of the New World, being "disgraced with a class of exhibitions so low and so contemptible.") Three thousand published copies of the Boston lectures were sold within a month, and a British edition of Dods's works on mesmerism was issued as late as 1886, well over a decade after his death.[23]

The reason for all the fuss was that in the span of six lectures Dods explained the universe and the meaning of life, and in oratory so thundering as to allow no doubt: he ventured to throw "the light of truth on rolling worlds . . . to step back beyond the threshold of creation—to lift the dark curtains of primeval night, and muse upon that original, eternal material, that slumbered in the deep bosom of chaos, and out of which all the tangible substances we see and admire were made. That eternal substance is *electricity*." From that beginning Dods flew off into mystical transports of wonderment at the vastness of space and time, the continuing creation and destruction of worlds throughout the universe, the minuteness of the human race and yet its greatness for being a manifestation, however ephemeral, of the primal substance and energy of creation, and so forth.[24]

But eventually he came back down to earth, to the human body and particularly the brain, the source of the electricity responsible for all vital function: "*Electricity* is the connecting *link* between MIND and MATTER." Using that link was the key to restoring the matter of the body to health. One had first to understand, however, the nature of the body's electrical fluid. It was not, according to Dods, some magical substance or force that transcended the laws of ordinary nature. The reason mesmerism had not won an even greater following, he held, was that other lecturers left it shrouded in mystery, as if its phenomena were impossible to explain. The main thrust of his theorizing, therefore, was to show that magnetism was as natural, as scientific, as physics and chemistry—it *was* physics and chemistry. As atmospheric air is taken into the lungs, he conjectured, oxygen and electricity are extracted from it and absorbed into the blood. The iron of the blood is at once made magnetic by the electricity, while the serum is made acidic by the oxygen, so that by a process still more vague the altered, energized blood is "propelled to the extremities." Then, as it courses through the arteries, the friction of the vessel walls causes the electrical power to escape into the nervous system and pass to the brain, from which it is secreted as "nervo-vital fluid." That fluid is stirred by the will with every desire for movement and causes the voluntary nerves to vibrate, which contracts the associated muscles.[25]

Nervo-vital fluid was essential to health in other ways, too, so clearly any disharmony or diminution in that fluid must bring on sickness: "There is but one grand cause of disease," Dods proclaimed, "*which is the electricity of the system thrown out of balance.*" For once Dods failed to elaborate, merely citing certain causes of nervo-vital disruption—eating, drinking, physical impressions from outside, and anxiety or other psychic upset. Causes were relatively unimportant, though, for therapy was the same in all cases. Dods held the patient's hand in his, pressed one or another nerve in the hand for half a minute or so, asked the subject to close his eyes, and lightly brushed the lids with his fingertips several times; if susceptible, the patient would be mesmerized and ready to have his fluid reserves raised. "Now let a person whose brain is fully charged come in contact with one whose brain is greatly wanting in its due measure of this fluid," Dods instructed, "and let the person possessing the full brain gently and unchangeably hold his mind upon the other, and by the action of the WILL the fluid will pass from the full brain to the other, until the equilibrium between the fluids in the two brains is attained. . . . This is MAGNETISM; and it is in perfect accordance with all the principles of philosophy in the known realms of nature."[26]

The fully charged brain in the foregoing passage was, one might guess, Dods's, but proud as he was of his skill as a magnetizer, he gave final credit to nature: he supplied nervo-vital fluid to the patient; the body did the rest. "The healing principle is in man," he lectured, a principle that "must equalize the electricity . . . and call it to the proper spot." (Plants likewise healed themselves, through an electro-vegetative fluid that "moves and equalizes the sap.") Further, his method was safe, unlike allopathic therapy, "because its pharmacy is of God and rests on the bosom of nature." As the gift of God, naturally, it was capable of miracles. Should a person break his arm, he need only have the arm (not the whole person, just the arm) mesmerized, then set, and if the limb were kept magnetized it would heal rapidly and painlessly. If a limb were badly mangled and required amputation, the surgery could be performed without pain under mesmerism. Lucy Ann Allen, of Lynchburg, Virginia, had not walked a step for eighteen years, but after a fifty-minute exposure to Dods's nervo-vital fluid she regained the use of her legs. Well could Dods inform the Senate that his science "must stand when the pillars of strength and beauty that support our Capitol shall fall and be crumbled to dust."[27]

Electrical psychology was immortal. Dods directed the whole of his last lecture in the Marlboro Chapel series to an exposition of mesmerism as the method of healing used by Christ and the Apostles and suggested that those seeming miracles outstripped any achieved by more recent magnetizers solely because of the greater goodness and stronger faith of Jesus and the disciples. "But let us bring up our children in the faith as we ought," he proposed, "and they will learn to mesmerize as naturally as they learn to walk."[28]

In the long run, that was the purpose of electrical psychology—to teach people to bring up their children, and themselves, as they ought. To understand electricity was to know God, for everything "that transpires amidst the immensity of his works, from rolling globes down to the falling leaf . . . is performed, through electricity as his agent." "Psychology" meant, literally, the science of soul. Hence electrical psychology, while curing the ills of the body, opened the doors to the soul, allowing one to expand her understanding of herself and her Creator, and her place in the creation. It was a science of mental and spiritual well-being, of secular salvation. With an exalted awareness of its place, humankind would act in accord with divine intention. Electrical psychology bound with the gospel, Dods concluded his lectures to the Senate, "is destined to renovate the world and usher in the millenial morn."[29]

In the meantime, even Dods was perturbed by the ignoble uses to which the mesmeric art was being put by opportunists. "Very many ignorant individuals," he complained, "have gone into the field as lecturers on Animal Magnetism, and by making it a mere puppet show, have brought it into degradation in the public mind." He referred here to the numerous popular exhibitions (put on by "one traveling mountebank after another," physicians jeered, to amuse "their silly admirers") in which hypnotized subjects played dominos while blindfolded, tasted foods through their fingertips, and apparently read audience members' minds. Its exploitation as vulgar entertainment only further discredited mesmerism with the medical community, who delighted in fabricating the most outrageous spoofs of the clairvoyant powers of the *mesmerizée*. "Animal magnetism will be of inestimable benefit to morals," mused a Massachusetts physican of *nom de plume* Mesmer; "the profligate son may always be under the inspection of his father, into whatever company he goes," he explained, "and the jealous wife may always have an eye upon her unfaithful husband." And just think, if the Secretary of War were to magnetize all his clerks, they would be able "to point out every swamp, cave, or hollow tree, in which a single Indian is concealed"; if only that had been done before, the Florida campaign against the Seminoles would have been brought to a close "in three months, instead of three years."[30]

Phineas Quimby and Mind Cure

Exactly such clairvoyant capabilities were in fact claimed by more than one magnetic healer, who enabled their mesmerized subjects to see every swamp and hollow of disease inside a person's body and thus to point out to the practitioner precisely where to focus his magnetic energies. One such collaborator with clairvoyants was a clockmaker from Belfast, Maine, Phineas Parkhurst Quimby (1802–1866), who turned mesmerist at age thirty-six after attending one of Poyen's demonstrations. Flattered by the lecturer's assurances that he possessed exceptional magnetic powers (and indeed he was described by others as having "piercing black eyes" and a "power of concentration surpassing anything we have ever witnessed"), Quimby began experimenting to learn how to exercise his abilities. In time he became adept at putting subjects into trance, and by 1840 he was treating people for illness, believing he healed them by impelling from his own brain into the sufferer's body a subtle fluid and that "electricity had more or less to do with it." "Quimby has been doing miracles," it was soon reported; "he has cured a man that couldn't walk nor speak" and another who had not been able to lift his arm for two years. In addition, on at least one occasion he employed his electrical fluid to anesthetize a patient for a surgical procedure performed by a regular physician.[31]

What brought Quimby to public attention, however, was a third variation of medical magnetism. Soon after perfecting his skills, he was fortunate enough to meet a boy in his late teens who under hypnosis exhibited "astonishing mesmeric powers." Lucius Burkmar could read others' minds, astounding audiences with his ability to minutely describe people and places he had never seen but that were being thought of by audience members. He also could read others' bodies, penetrating into their viscera to uncover evidence of disease. At the time they met, in fact, Quimby was certain that his lungs and kidneys were being destroyed by "consumption" (for which "I had taken so much calomel that my system was . . . poisoned with it; and I lost many of my teeth"), and Burkmar confirmed it: "Asleep, he described the pains I felt in my back [and] told me that my kidneys were in a very bad state."[32]

Burkmar was equally adept at suggesting remedies for the ailments he saw in others, and for four years, between 1843 and 1847, Quimby employed him to diagnose and prescribe while in the mesmeric trance. (Burkmar strayed away for part of that period, incidentally, being enticed to work in the same capacity for John Bovee Dods.) But although the two of them became celebrated throughout the Northeast for their successful practice, eventually Quimby dispensed with Burkmar's services, realizing they were unnecessary. Relating just one disillusioning experience, Quimby remembered that "I put him to sleep to examine a lady, expecting that he would go on in his old way." His old way was to recommend one herb or another, but this time "he wrote a long prescription in Latin" instead. Quimby awakened his subject and asked him to translate the prescription, but the unlettered Burkmar was unable to read Latin while unhypnotized, so the prescription was taken to an apothecary, who said the indicated drugs would cost twenty dollars. "This was impossible for the lady to pay. So I returned and put him to sleep again; and he gave me his usual prescription of some little herb, and [the patient] got well." Thus, Quimby concluded, "any medicine would cure if he ordered it," because "the cure is not in the medicine, but in the confidence of the doctor."[33]

Healing worked through the mind, Quimby now realized, and did not require clairvoyance or magnetism. A practical-minded man, he commented often on the "absurdity" of Burkmar's diagnoses and remedies. When his protégé had told him his kidneys were in a bad state, for instance, he had elaborated by saying one of the organs "was half-consumed, and a piece three inches long had separated from it, and was only connected by a slender thread." He then proceeded to effect a cure by placing "his hands upon me, and said he united the pieces so they would grow. The next day he said they had grown together." He proposed equally implausible things to other patients, such as the man who was told that "his lungs looked like a honeycomb, and his liver was covered with ulcers." When such a supposedly disease-corroded patient recovered after taking "some simple herb tea," it seemed undeniable that a mental rather than physical effect had been induced. In the case of his own kidneys, "I discovered that I had been deceived into a belief that made me sick," and with other patients, he decided, Burkmar had not seen into their bodies at all but into their minds, there perceiving what they already believed to be wrong. Cure, therefore, should be simply a matter of identifying and correcting a patient's negative beliefs; with a positive state of mind, the body would be freed to function properly and overcome its pathology.[34]

Quimby thus parted ways with magnetism and electrical fluids, eventually denouncing mesmerism as "one of the greatest humbugs of the age." The true explanation of disease, what he had learned through his therapeutic experiences, was that people are comprised of both an "outward man," the body, and an "inward man," the mind and soul, and that illness can exist only "when these are at variance or out of tune." "Disease is what follows the disturbance of the mind," he taught; if the inward man were to be agitated by some mental or emotional shock, "this disturbance . . . produces a chemical change in the fluids of the system." Further, when the body's fluids fell into a "distressed state," the inward man or mind/soul was upset by the change "and the soul stands apart from the disturbed part and grieves over it," compounding the mental distress. But grief was unnecessary, he insisted, as the part could be restored by giving the inward self a positive outlook that lifted the mental blockade preventing the body from healing itself. "Come with me [mentally] to where the trouble is," Quimby directed one patient, "and you will find . . . it is kept hot and disturbed [only] by your mind being misrepresented."[35]

The method Quimby thus came to employ was not to hypnotize anyone; hypnosis he now thought of as a charade designed to dazzle patients and onlookers, a performance one would resort to only if he "had no other aim than dollars and cents." Rather, "I retained my own consciousness and at the same time took the feelings of my patient," mentally connecting to both the inner and outer person and working "as a mediator between these two principles of soul and body" so as to bring the one "back to harmonize with" the other. When he came to the side of a sick person, Quimby claimed, he saw a "vapor" or "cloud" enveloping the patient's body, a vapor that "contains the identity of the person." Engaging the spiritual identity in the cloud, he bade it "carry me spiritually to the place where their trouble commenced." Then began the task of conversion of the victim's spirit from a state of belief in being sick to one of faith in recovery: "The cure of your limb depends on your faith," he exhorted a Mrs. Norcross; "your faith is what you receive from me."[36]

Quimby instilled faith in his clients, convinced them they were in fact healthy, by talking them through all the negative thoughts that kept them sick and convincing them the thoughts were in error. Consider the case of Mr. Robinson, a man who had been confined to his bed for four years until Quimby visited him "and sat down, and commenced explaining to Mr. R. his feelings, telling him his symptoms nearer than Mr. R. could tell them himself." He explained as well "how his mind acted upon his body," and when the patient voiced some doubt, "Mr. Quimby commenced taking up his feelings, one by one, like a lawyer examining witnesses, analyzing them and showing him that he [had] put false constructions on all his feelings." Steadily Robinson was won over, his healer's arguments being "so plain that it was impossible not to understand," even though they were unlike "any that I ever heard before from any physician." By the end of the session, Robinson "felt like a man who had been confined in a prison for life" and then been granted "a pardon and . . . set at liberty." By the next day, he "felt as well as ever. . . . I had no desire to take to my bed, and have felt well ever since."[37]

So profound was Quimby's ability to merge his inward man with his patient's that he frequently practiced "absent treatment," curing people at a distance through letters in which he professed to be present in spirit, talking with the sufferer. (His in-person practice was in Portland, Maine.) "I will sit by you a short time," he wrote a New Hampshire patient, "and relieve the pain in your stomach and carry it off. You can sit down, when you receive this letter, and listen to my story and I think you will feel better. Sit up straight," he commanded, for "I am now rubbing the back part of your head. . . . I do not know as you feel my hand . . . but it will make you feel better. When you read this, I shall be with you," Quimby assured. "I am in this letter, so remember and look at me, and see if I do not mean just as I say." He closed with a "Good evening" and a wish the recipient would "let me know how you get along."[38]

As Quimby pondered this phenomenon of spiritual communion over great distances, it gradually dawned on him that all souls were parcels of the divine wisdom that had created and still filled the universe and that the healing power of spiritual intercourse was nowhere more fully demonstrated than in the New Testament, "in Christ's teachings and works." As one of his patients put it, "his formula of faith is confessedly that of the Saviour," but he did not think of scriptural or his own healings as miracles. They were entirely natural events, he believed, the result of interactions between agencies that were as comprehensible and subject to science as any physico-chemical forces. His, however, was the highest science, a "Science of Health" that bestowed wholeness by reuniting the error-prone human mind with the unfailing divine spirit that had manifested itself most powerfully through Christ. "Christ," in fact, was interpreted by Quimby to mean the divine spiritual counterpart to Jesus the physical man. The "Christ" was eternal Truth and eternal Wisdom; every person possessed a "Christ within," and it was with that inner Christ that Quimby established rapport when he healed. In Quimby's mind, Christ and science were synonymous; his method of healing he thus called the Science of Christ and even, toward the close of his life, "Christian Science."[39]

Mary Baker Patterson and the Development of Christian Science

By the 1860s Quimby's fame had spread throughout the country. "His patients come from the four winds of heaven," one admirer marveled, then corrected himself to note that southerners need not apply: "The Doctor is a strong Union man; and would as soon cure a sick rattlesnake as a sick rebel." One Yankee he helped, though never fully cured, was a forty-one-year-old woman named Mary Baker Patterson, who arrived in Portland in October 1862 in so gravely debilitated a state her friends feared for her life. They needn't have, as invalidism was by then second nature to her. Although she had descended from hardy New Hampshire pioneer stock, Mary Baker (1821–1910) was sickly from early childhood, low in energy, unstable emotionally, and subject to recurrent spells of pain along her spine. The Baker family doctor diagnosed her as a case of "hysteria mingled with bad temper," and her condition only worsened with age and motherhood. Homeopathy was tried, as were Grahamism and hydropathy, yet mesmerism alone could bring ease when one of her paroxysms of pain and emotion struck. It was perfectly reasonable, then, that as she reached an all-time physical low in the early 1860s her second husband, Daniel Patterson, would turn for help to the man renowned throughout New England for taking healing to the next step beyond mesmerism.[40]

While Quimby was known in his own right during his lifetime, he is remembered today only because of his association with Mary Patterson, who would become internationally celebrated under the name of her next husband as Mary Baker Eddy, founder of Christian Science (Fig. 5-2). There is a long-running controversy between defenders of Quimby and representatives of the Christian Science Church over the question of Patterson's debt to Quimby, the former asserting she borrowed freely but without attribution from

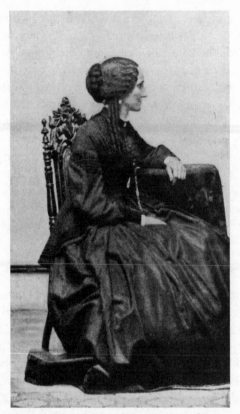

Figure 5-2. Mary Baker Patterson [Georgine Milmine, Mary Baker G. Eddy, *Mc-Clure's Magazine* (1906–7) 28:610]

Quimby's teachings and unpublished writings, the latter maintaining she received inspiration from no one but God. The details of the conflict are tangential to present purposes, except to observe that it is beyond dispute that Mary Patterson benefited from treatment from Quimby for several years and was profoundly influenced by him whether she plagiarized or not. After his death, she first disavowed any debt to her mentor, then made so bold as to denounce his views as mere "scribblings" that "commingled error with truth"; she even claimed that she was in fact the author of the manuscripts attributed to him and that she had perfected Quimbyism with ideas "far in advance of his."[41]

According to Eddy, it was in the year 1866, only two weeks after Quimby passed away, that "I discovered the Christ Science." In February she suffered a concussion and other injuries when she fell on an icy street. On the third day after, however, her pain suddenly subsided while she was poring over biblical passages describing Christ's healing ministry: "As she read, the presence and power of God seemed to flood her whole being, and she rose, healed." She "named my discovery Christian Science," ignoring the fact that Quimby had sometimes used "Christian Science" to identify the method he thought of as *his* discovery. He had, of course, more often used the term "the Science of Health," and *Science and Health*, perhaps coincidentally, was the title chosen by Mary Patterson for the 1875 book she wrote to enlighten the world about the approach to healing she had developed. That publication was nevertheless not to be mistaken as Quimby's book but rather had to be recognized as "God's book." Over time, Patterson convinced herself that she had received her insights into eternal truth by divine revelation. She would "blush," she wrote, for people to think that the book was "of human origin," for she could not have written it alone, "apart from God."[42]

By the date of the volume's publication, incidentally, the author's name was once again Glover, the surname of her deceased first husband. (Second spouse Patterson had left her shortly after the famous fall, presumably in search of "the fleshpots" that, in his wife's opinion, he "craved"; she finally obtained a divorce from the debauchee in 1873.) In its original version, *Science and Health* was 450 pages of repetitious obscurantism (more than 600 in subsequent editions) and so baffling as to convince Mark Twain that among "all the strange and frantic and incomprehensible and uninterpretable books which the imagination of man has created," *Science and Health* was "the prize sample."[43]

The book's originality was fundamentally epistemological. Whereas Quimby had arrived at his interpretations of disease and healing empirically, through clinical experience leavened with intuition, Glover relied on logic, constructing nothing less than a new reality through syllogistic reasoning that provided "immortal proof" of her contentions. Further, she bound her analysis much more tightly to religion than had Quimby; her book's full title was *Science and Health With Key to the Scriptures*, and it so embellished Quimby's basic insights with scriptural interpretations as to create a new theological sect. Glover erected her argument on what seemed to her unshakeable premises about the nature of God. Scripture, she observed, reveals both that "God is All" and that "God is Spirit." From those statements it followed that "all is Spirit and spiritual," that "Mind is All-in-all." Quimby had hinted at something of the sort, but while he removed sickness from the body and placed it in the mind, he still supposed that there existed a corporeal body to be injured by mind. Yet the way Glover would have it was that since mind was all, matter was therefore nothing and the material body did not exist. What people thought of as the body was in fact only a misguided belief; the notion of the "body" was a product of what she called the "mortal mind," a mental "per-version," a "carnal" mentality that afflicted humankind and inhibited them from communing with "divine Mind." In theory, at least, "a man could live just as well after his lungs had been removed as before, if he but thought he could."[44]

Even if there had been a body, it would have been of no consequence with regard to health, for by the Glover analysis there was no such thing as disease, either. Another of her premises was that "God is good," and since God is also all, all is good and evil cannot be. "Evil is but an illusion," she taught; "evil is a false belief." Disease, of course, is evil by definition, so "what is termed disease does not exist." Illness, like the body, was a wrong idea: "The soil of disease is mortal mind." The nonexistence of disease not-withstanding, however, people believed themselves and their nonexistent bod-ies to be sick, and they called for help. "The remedy," Glover taught, "consists in probing the trouble to the bottom, in finding and casting out by denial the error of belief which produces a mortal disorder." So in the end, all religion and metaphysics aside, she did what Quimby had done: she educated her clients to see disease as the consequence of wrong thinking and convinced them to cast the devil of erroneous belief from the mind; "the discords of corporeal sense must yield to the harmony of spiritual sense, even as the science of music corrects false tones and gives sweet concord to sound." (Spiritual sense also accounted for the apparent efficacy of homeopathy, Glover suggested, as "the highest attenuation of homeopathy . . . rises above matter into mind.")[45]

Such was the method of healing Glover practiced and taught for seven years before publishing her book. As early as 1868 she began taking on stu-dents with the promise she would instruct them how to heal "with a success far beyond any of the present modes," and do so in only twelve lessons. At first charging a hundred dollars for the course, she soon raised her rates to three hundred, "a startling sum for tuition lasting barely three weeks," she acknowledged, but a fee to which "God impelled me." The incompatibility of demanding dollars while preaching that money and the things it buys do not exist seems to have been overlooked, however, for over the years Glover passed several thousand students through her program. (Many graduated as Doctors of Christian Science from her Massachusetts Metaphysical College, which operated between 1881 and 1889.) One of these was Gilbert Eddy, a man who had sold sewing machines until a reversal of health in the mid-1870s impelled him to seek for aid in Christian Science. He found more than he sought, for not only did he complete the class and regain his health, he so endeared himself to the teacher that the two were wed on the first day of 1877.[46]

Growth of Christian Science

In 1879 Mrs. Eddy founded the Church of Christ (Scientist). During the first three years, church membership did not advance beyond fifty, but by 1890 it approached nine thousand and would surpass forty thousand in the early 1900s. Between 1900 and 1925 Christian Science was far the fastest-growing denomination in the United States, reaching a membership of more than two hundred thousand by the end of that period. (Many of the new members were converts from other Protestant denominations, particularly the Congregational and Methodist churches; members came overwhelmingly from the middle classes, and nearly two-thirds were women.) In the interim, numerous editions of *Science and Health* were issued, along with other works by Eddy; a *Journal of Christian Science* was launched (1883); many local churches and instructional institutes were opened; and several thousand Christian Science healers (more than 80 percent of them women) set up practice throughout the country. Eddy meanwhile ruled the church first from Boston, where she relocated in 1882, then from Concord, New Hampshire, where she retired in 1889 to live the life of a well-off recluse on the very considerable income from her teaching and publishing endeavors. Eddy, Mark Twain joked, had turned Quimby's "sawdust mine" into "a Klondike"; others referred to her as "the 'Profitess' of Christian Science." When she died in 1910, Eddy left more than two million dollars to the church (her son contested the will, but lost).[47]

The rapid growth of Christian Science was achieved in the face of competition from more than a few other mental healing groups. Followers of Warren Felt Evans, himself an erstwhile patient of Quimby's, practiced the Primitive Mind Cure, while the devotees of Anetta and Julius Dresser (the latter also a successfully treated Quimby client) employed the techniques of Mind Cure Science. These and like-minded bands of healers constituted what came to be called the New Thought movement in late nineteenth-century America and freely acknowledged Quimby as their founder. The advantage enjoyed by Christian Science was that, in contrast to the New Thought mélange that diluted Judeo-Christian traditions with Transcendentalism, spiritualism, mysticism, and Asian philosophy, Eddyism was unadulterated *Christian* Science, a method of healing derived wholly from the tenets of the faith of the masses and one that by denying the reality of evil promised to eradicate sin even as it drove out sickness. At a time when American Protestants were feeling uneasy with liberalizing trends in theology, Christian Science appeared to herald a return to the pristine church, an institution that had put healing at the head of its mission. "The first day I read from its sacred pages," one convert said of *Science and Health*, "I was convinced its teachings were the same truths as Jesus Christ had taught"; "I entered a Christian Science church," another related, and "loved Christian Science from the very start." Eddy repeatedly attacked all forms of mind cure associated with New Thought because they relied on the action of one human mind upon another instead of operating through divine Mind.[48]

Christian Science practitioners healed as Eddy had taught them, by "demonstrating over false claims," talking to the patient so as to convince her or him that sickness and pain were illusions allowed to thrive only by the individual's inadequate acceptance of the truth that all is good. Human error being as deeply entrenched as it is, repeated treatments, or demonstrations, were often needed to destroy the illusion of suffering ("years of prayer and regeneration of character" were sometimes required), but ultimately Christian Science practitioners laid claim to an impressive record of cures. "Testimonies" of healing became a monthly feature in the *Christian Science Journal* and other church periodicals, piling up until their numbers were in the thousands. People testified to being cured of cancer, blindness, gunshot wounds to the chest, and dental injuries sustained from calomel. Even a few MDs admitted to being able to regain their health only through Christian Science prayer, as did a number of celebrities. There was, for example, the operatic prima donna whose "delicate little nose" was dealt "a staggering blow" when the stage curtain descended upon her head; yet before the curtain was raised for the next day's performance, her grotesquely swollen nose and badly bruised eyes had regained their accustomed beauty.[49]

Many victims of false belief did not bother to summon a practitioner but cured themselves directly simply by reading *Science and Health*. (Eddyites were expected, in fact, to attempt to cure themselves first.) Among the cases whose afflictions vanished with a single reading of the book were the Seattle woman relieved of "constipation of thirty years' standing," the South Dakota man broken of his addictions to tobacco, alcohol, and profanity, and the Los Angeles child whose rickety bones "grew perfectly straight" after his mother read Eddy to him. A New York woman whose entire body was covered with liver spots saw them disappear before her eyes while only halfway through *Science and Health*, and a Salt Lake City woman needed only ten minutes of reading for her arm, broken in a fall from her bicycle, to mend itself. (There were as well many reports of pets and livestock cured by Christian Science of everything from overeating to snake bites.) It is no surprise, then, that souls were healed by Eddy's book too, more than one doubter experiencing the transformation "from a worldly, godless agnostic to a God-loving Christian." Indeed, the disappearance of external illness was significant primarily as evidence of inward spiritual grace. Ultimately what was healed was the alienation between the mortal mind and God; in that sense, the bodily healing was an act of worship. (In contrast to all the claims of the healing power of Christian

Science, incidentally, more than one twentieth-century study of longevity has found the church's members to be more short-lived than the general population.)[50]

Medical Opposition to Christian Science

Orthodox physicians, need it be said, were not often to be found among the worshippers. The tenets of "the new theologico-philosophic therapeutics" seemed to them even more asinine than those of homeopathy. Homeopaths at least accepted the existence of matter, even if they diluted it beyond perceptibility before administering it. Yet while Christian Scientists denied matter altogether in theory, when theory came to be translated into action they often spoke and behaved contradictorily. Mrs. Eddy herself, for example, proudly reported using *Science and Health* to save the life of a woman experiencing a difficult labor and to deliver her of a healthy twelve-pound infant. "Considering there was no body to this bouncing offspring," a Chicago physician laughed, "and not an ounce of matter in it, but only a round, plump convolution of spirit . . . twelve pounds on the scales was a very satisfactory result." Then there was the case of the Christian Science healer called to attend to an acutely sick heifer. The cow "so completely recovered that she chased the 'Scientist' twice around the barnyard, and he was only rescued by a hired man with a pitch-fork." Why did the practitioner run, a regular doctor wondered; apparently "the line of the non-existence of matter has to be drawn at enraged animals." A Detroit doctor questioned whether the line could be drawn at all, proposing an experiment in which Christian Scientist volunteers would be injected with drugs whose material effects were well documented and then asked to negate those effects through faith; no volunteers came forward.[51]

"That such a farrago of nonsense is taken seriously by people of education and intelligence," one physician shook his head, "almost makes us despair of human progress." Yet it had to be acknowledged that the most absurd logic could still result in effective practical applications, that true healing might be accomplished in spite of a nonsensical rationale. In fact, argued Harvard Medical School's Richard Cabot, "most" of the cures claimed by Christian Scientists "are probably genuine." Their genuineness derived, however, entirely from the application of the power of suggestion and placebo to functional complaints. Carefully examining one hundred cures reported in the *Christian Science Journal*, Cabot determined that at least three-quarters were functional or emotional ailments, conditions famously susceptible to mental influence. "The complication is in the patient's mind," he concluded, not in the body (Eddy would have agreed); "chronic nervous (that is, mental) disease is the Christian Scientist's stock in trade." Physicians generally concurred that the only people helped by Christian Science were "hysterical patients, the morbidly introspective, the worriers, the *malades imaginaires*." "In every county," famed clinician William Osler remarked, "there were dyspeptics and neurasthenics in sufficient numbers to demonstrate the efficacy of the new gospel," hypochondriacs so "unquiet in a drug-soaked body" that they "rose with joy at a new Evangel." MDs concurred as well with Cabot's contention that Christian Science "cures" of such things as broken bones and cancer could not be taken seriously, because of practitioners' ignorance of medical diagnosis; as one cynic observed, "it is undoubtedly as easy to imagine a fictitious illness as to deny the existence of a real one."[52]

Yet if Christian Science ofttimes "worked" despite the "logical bankruptcy" of its "weak-kneed theory," it also all too often failed and thereby constituted a threat to the public health. Physicians voiced no objection to Eddy's practitioners helping the nervous and hypochondriacal, as one could do little damage to people who were not really sick. But when those who truly did have a malignancy or heart disease or smallpox were told it was all in their mind, tragic consequences could follow. He was "awful sick," a doctor-in-disguise wrote a Christian Science healer in Illinois, sick with what a physician had diagnosed as "appendix-bogusitis and say I got to be cut open to let it out." Describing repeated attacks of abdominal pain and vomiting, he begged, "If you can treat me by what they call absent treatment, I wish you would." Absent treatment was immediately promised, at a dollar a session. "Here," the doctor objected, "was a presumably dangerous condition calling for surgical intervention, which [he] was willing to treat by sitting in his office, probably mumbling over some formula. Is this not a return to medieval exorcism?" In a similar vein, the health commissioner of Colorado in 1900 only half-jokingly predicted that the mortality rate in Denver, hitherto the lowest in the country, would soon "increase in an alarming ratio" now that Christian Science had established a foothold in the state.[53]

In the medical profession's estimation, mortality had already increased nationwide. Once Eddy's movement assumed national prominence in the 1890s, "Death Under Christian Science," "Victims of Christian Science," and like titles began to appear regularly in medical journals over notices of deaths from appendicitis, diphtheria, cancer, mushroom poisoning, and every other acute ailment that Christian Science's "homicidal pretenders" treated with their "fatal inactivity" (one woman was "kept in torture for a year" while a Christian Science healer prayed over her tumor). A fifteen-year-old girl who was treated for deafness by an Eddy practitioner not only failed to recover her hearing but over the course of her ten treatments acquired an "acute religious mania" that left her "violently insane." A Baltimore man sued two Christian Science practitioners for twenty thousand dollars for "ill treatment," complaining that one kept him confined to his room for three and a half months so as to insulate him against the influence of mortal mind, and "in the meanwhile he suffered excrutiating pain, his limbs and body swelling and gangrene affecting both limbs." When a second practitioner was appointed to replace the first, his condition only worsened until, near death, he summoned an MD, "under whose care he has greatly improved."[54]

Whether in the end he survived or won his suit is unclear, but Christian Science healers were occasionally charged with manslaughter in the movement's early years; such was the case, for example, in the death of the prominent English author and journalist Harold Frederic in 1898. As a rule, practitioners were acquitted on the grounds that their patients were freely exercising their religious beliefs, and physicians eventually came to accept that however "depressing [an] exhibition of folly and cruelty" such lethal treatments might be, "if some adults think they can get any benefit from Christian Science [they] have a right to risk their lives." For non-adults, however, the situation was different. "Small children should be protected from the ignorance" of Christian Science healers," physicians protested; "to subject a helpless infant" to their control "is so obviously criminal" as not to be disputed. Medical journals reported more than a few cases of children dying who might have been saved by standard medical care, enough so that one critic could charge that Christian Scientists "are Molochs to infants." (There was a bright side to be found in the carnage: the hard-nosed realist H. L. Mencken asked where was the harm ultimately if a Christian Scientist treated his child "with Mrs. Eddy's rubbish, and so sacrifices its life. What if he does? It is *his* child, and if it lived it would simply grow up into another Christian Scientist.")[55]

Christian Scientists were seen not only as Molochs to infants but also as "pestilential perils to communities." Eddy's "miserable compound of . . . fantastic vagaries, grotesque nonsense, imbecile contradictions, anarchy and infidelity" would not be worthy of notice by doctors, one physician wrote, "were it not for its possible influence on the spread of infectious disease." By the late nineteenth century, public health policy required physicians to report cases of communicable disease so that authorities could institute measures to contain the pestilence. But how could Christian Science healers report diseases they couldn't diagnose? Would they sign a smallpox victim's death certificate with the statement that "the late departed believed herself dead so strongly that they had to bury her?"[56]

Eddy did not believe in communicable disease, of course, but for purposes of avoiding legal conflict and negative publicity, she came around to recommending "that Christian Scientists decline to doctor infectious or contagious diseases." For the same reasons, church members agreed to accept medical treatment for seriously ill children, as well as vaccination of children.

Cooperation with the medical establishment, however, was not entirely a matter of public relations. In many instances, Christian Scientists found they were unable to cope with disease otherwise. To consider only the example of the church's leader, in her later years Eddy used eyeglasses and a dental plate, and when in the early 1900s she began to suffer from gallstones she readily accepted a physician's prescription of morphine; she in fact resorted to the drug repeatedly for the rest of her life. Mrs. Eddy also had her grandchildren vaccinated and paid for a mastectomy for her sister-in-law. Her justification for yielding to the errors of mortal mind, a rationalization subsequently adopted as church policy, was that the world had not yet advanced to the state of enlightenment whereby union with the divine Mind was always easily achieved. Sometimes healing would be stalled by the inadequacy of the patient's faith and understanding of Truth, and in those instances it was permissible to call for medical assistance. "Until the advancing age admits the efficacy and supremacy of Mind," she taught, "it is better for Christian Scientists to leave surgery and the adjustment of broken bones . . . to the fingers of a surgeon."[57]

Failures of Christian Science healing were also attributed to a darker force, the operations of the evil power that Eddy ominously called MAM. Malicious Animal Magnetism was her version of the early nineteenth-century fear of mesmerism as an occult work of Satan. For Eddy, MAM was the agency utilized by rivals and enemies to undermine her benevolent mission of healing. "The author's own observations of the workings of animal magnetism," she wrote in *Science and Health*, "convince her that it is not a remedial agent, and that its effects upon those who practise it, and upon their subjects who do not resist it, lead to moral and to physical death." Quimby had been a mesmerist, she recalled of the man she had once adored, and the words of tribute she had offered him had been involuntarily composed while she was under mesmeric influence. Worse, the methods he had perfected lived on after him to be employed by others against her and her church and even her family. When Eddy's husband passed away in 1882, she announced in the *Boston Post* that his death "was caused by malicious mesmerism," even though the autopsy she had requested showed that he had been stricken by heart disease. Whenever attempts at healing through Christian Science failed, it was due to someone subverting the process with MAM. Whenever her church was criticized in medical journals or popular magazines, or whenever she suffered a financial reverse, or whenever she was challenged in any way, animal magnetism was presumed to be at work: "You're so full of malicious animal magnetism," she chastised a defiant student, "your eyes stick out like a boiled codfish's." She brought lawsuits against those she suspected of using magnetism against her, and there was no doubt that her health problems, especially her gallstones, were the treachery of spiteful magnetizers. Even as she lay dying she insisted that MAM was the cause. Her warning in *Science and Health* had been prophetic: from "animal magnetism . . . comes all evil."[58]

Fear of MAM so permeated Eddy's writings that her followers obsessed over it nearly as much as she did. "Suppose Mrs. Eddy should commit a crime," a skeptic asked a Christian Scientist close to the church's leader. "Suppose certain reputable persons . . . President Roosevelt, the Archbishop of Canterbury, and the Pope of Rome—saw her rob the bank. Suppose they all went upon the witness-stand and swore that they saw her do this—would you believe their testimony?" "No" was the answer, and the explanation given was that malicious mesmerism must have been used to "lead astray the senses of all these high-minded witnesses and force them to bear false testimony." Thus "the real secret of the horrors" of the Spanish-American War, a physician suggested in 1899, was "not explosive bullets, asphyxiating gases, or missiles . . . but malicious thoughts, which are far more deadly." American troops henceforth should be trained not to shoot but to make faces at the enemy.[59]

Even without the silliness of MAM, Christian Science was a rich source of material for non-medical humorists. Eddyism was superior to both allopathy and homeopathy, Ambrose Bierce pointed out in his *Devil's Dictionary*, because it "will cure imaginary diseases, and they cannot." It could even restore amputated limbs, Finley Peter Dunne suggested. Just meditate on the lost leg, his Irish character Mr. Dooley proposed, "an' afther awhile a leg comes peepin' out with a complete set iv tootsies, an' by th' time th' las' thought is expinded, ye have a set iv as well-matched gambs as ye iver wore to a picnic. But ye mustn't stop thinkin' or ye'er wife or th' Christyan Scientist. If wan iv ye laves go th' rope, th' leg'll get discouraged an' quit growin'. Manny a man's sprouted a limb on'y to have it stop between th' ankle an' th' shin because th' Christyan Scientist was called away to see what ailed th' baby."[60]

The best, if not the last, word was had by Mark Twain, who told a tale of falling over a cliff in the Alps and incurring a "series of compound fractures extending from . . . scalp-lock to . . . heels." The only medical assistance available was a Christian Science practitioner vacationing in a nearby village. "It hurts," he told her when she arrived. "It doesn't," she replied; "pain is unreal." She then administered treatment, first present, then absent, and Twain's bones soon "were gradually retreating inward and disappearing from view. . . . Every minute or two I heard a dull click inside and knew that the two ends of a fracture had been successfully joined. This muffled clicking and gritting and grinding and rasping continued during the next three hours, and then stopped—the connections had all been made." The next day the practitioner "brought in an itemized bill for a crate of broken bones mended in two hundred and thirty-four places—one dollar per fracture." "Nothing exists but Mind?" the patient asked. " 'Nothing,' she answered. 'All else is substanceless, all else is imaginary.' I gave her an imaginary check," Twain related, "and now she is suing me for substantial dollars. It looks inconsistent."[61]

PART II

The Early Twentieth Century: Drugless Healing

"I've given him pills," said old Doc. Squills, "And he's taken a gross, I guess;
And jalap and rhubarb and ipecac—But it's puzzlin', I confess.
I've given him wine and syrup of pine, and iron and calomel;
And he takes it mild as a little child; But he don't seem to get well!
I blistered his back at the first attack And I greased his chest with lard;
And I looked at his tongue and sounded his lung When I found him breathing hard.
If I've written him one he's had a ton Of my prescriptions, I think.
He's had every kind of drug, by jing! That a mortal can eat or drink. . . .
He's had morphine when his pain was keen And plenty of aconite;
And digitalis whenever 'twas seen That his heart wasn't working right.
He's had his skin full of medicine Sence at least six weeks ago,
Swallered and hypo'd and some rubbed in; But he gets well awful slow!
So I'm just about clean plumb run out Of drugs and idees too;
And everything's been done, by jing! That a mortal man can do.
And I can't tell if he's going to get well, If he's going to live or die;
But when it's done I don't want none To say, 'Doc. Squills didn't try.' "

"The Doctor at Bay" (1919)

6

The Licensing Question: The Campaign for Medical Freedom

Before early twentieth-century alternative medicine can be examined with respect to individual systems of practice, it is necessary to consider an issue that was of paramount importance to all, that of the revival of medical licensing laws. No matter was more disturbing to irregulars, no threat provoked so much outraged—yet reasoned—criticism of the regular profession, than the attempts of the medical establishment to bar non-approved healers from practice. Since every system responded to the threat with much the same objections and actions, it is more efficient to address the subject of opposition to medical licensing in a short chapter that serves as a foreword to the twentieth century than to take it up individually for each school of practice.

As was discussed in Chapter 2, the first wave of medical practice laws had been enacted from the late 1700s into the early 1800s, only to encounter the Thomsonian political offensive of the 1830s and '40s that triumphed in the repeal of nearly all licensing legislation by mid-century. From then until the later 1800s, the majority profession relied on the American Medical Association's "consultation clause" discussed in Chapter 3 to suppress medical heresy. By the 1890s, however, the clause was falling into abeyance because it was backfiring. First, in trying to isolate irregulars as incompetents undeserving of public confidence, the AMA instead made its own members appear petty and more attentive to personal image than patient need. In the 1870s, for example, a Connecticut woman died in labor after orthodox physicians refused to respond to her homeopath's call for assistance. But would any allopath have been able to save her? After all, proposed a skeptic reacting to the profession's opposition to the appointment of homeopaths to public hospital positions, "there is only one thing that is harder to get out of a hospital than an allopathic doctor, and that of course is his patient."[1]

Enforcement of the consultation clause, furthermore, made regular doctors look like ill-tempered bullies brutally hazing the innocent and weaker new kids in the neighborhood. To be sure, that image might have been acceptable to regulars had the new kids been frightened off. But their attacks only strengthened their victims' resolve. As Oliver Wendell Holmes had pointed out as early as the mid-1800s, irregular practitioners actually "welcome every cuff of criticism." Every disparaging remark directed their way is "a gratuitous advertisement," he warned, another bit "of exposure which enables them to climb up where they can be seen." Denunciation and ridicule only make them "grow turgid with delight," for however ignorant of medicine they might be, "they understand the hydrostatic paradox of controversy: that it raises the meanest disputant to a seeming level with his antagonist." Thus by 1900 there were in the United States, the only Western nation imposing ethical sanctions against intercourse with homeopaths, an estimated "88% of all [homeopaths] in the world." With approximately 110,000 mainstream practitioners in America, there were "no fewer than 9,369 persons" calling themselves homeopaths (nearly 10 percent of the number of allopaths, in other words), "all fat, all thriving, and all fervently hoping that our *good old prohibitory clause* would long continue." (There were an estimated ten thousand practitioners of other alternative schools of therapy combined at the time as well.) "The one thing that makes organized medicine grind its teeth in rage," a naturopath laughed in the early 1900s, "is to have the drugless practitioner invite martyrdom. There is no better way to incur public sympathy than through persecution."[2]

Largely because of the beneficial publicity that the consultation clause gave irregulars, but also because of the harmful consequences it could have for patients, regular practitioners subjected the clause to increasing scrutiny and reconsideration over the course of the last two decades of the nineteenth century. During that same period, moreover, it became increasingly evident to the majority profession that those fat and thriving homeopaths, the heretics for whom the consultation clause had been chiefly intended, were not deserving of such ostracism. However strange their beliefs and practices, homeopaths were well-intentioned practitioners, "a body of educated men," as one MD acknowledged in the early 1900s, "men of good professional character, correct morals, and much esteemed by those who know them best." Ultimately, the AMA abandoned the old code of ethics in 1903, replacing it with an "advisory document" that disparaged medical practices "based on an exclusive dogma" but with regard to consultation enjoined physicians to follow the promptings of conscience, putting patient welfare first. "The broadest dictates of humanity," the document counseled, "should be obeyed by physicians whenever and wherever their services are needed to meet the emergencies of disease or accident." "Our profession," regulars proclaimed, "has changed the tomahawk for the olive branch."[3]

Nevertheless, the profession still believed irregulars to be misguided and dangerous, so the appearance of the olive branch hardly signaled the end of hostilities. To the contrary, the battle had grown hotter than ever by the opening of the twentieth century. Between 1875 and 1900, licensing statutes were reinstituted by virtually every state in the country in response to the dramatic advances in medical science and practice (particularly surgery) that grew out of the germ theory of disease. Certain steps taken by the medical profession to raise standards in its schools also influenced state legislators to lend a sympathetic ear to the allopathic appeal to enact licensure requirements. The resurrection of licensing did not, however, drive irregulars from the field, for by the last quarter of the century two unorthodox groups—homeopathy and eclecticism—were too well established, attracting too many patients, to be outlawed. The regular profession's victory in reviving licensing restrictions, in short, was a Pyrrhic one, obtainable only by accepting that homeopaths and eclectics be granted their own licensure acts too.[4]

The extension of licensing to those old-school irregulars did not, of course, carry over to new systems still struggling to get themselves established. As osteopathy, chiropractic, naturopathy, and other newcomers appeared, their practitioners found themselves in the same position as homeopaths and Thomsonians had been in the 1830s, guilty of practicing medicine without a license. Actually, their position was worse, as the licensing laws of the early nineteenth century had not been vigorously enforced, and punishment had usually been nothing more than denial of the right to sue patients who neglected to pay their bills. Late nineteenth-century laws were applied more seriously, however, and the penalties for violation were more severe: fines and time in jail.

Among the newly established unconventional practitioners, only Christian Scientists were able to evade restrictions. This was not due to their being overlooked by physicians, for they were in fact among the most abominated of irregulars. "Steps should be taken to restrain the rabid utterances and the irrational practices of such ignorant and irresponsible persons," a commentator on "the immorality of Christian Science" opined in the 1890s; "liberty is one thing, and license another, and the crime of even suggesting such obviously false doctrines and immoral practices should be prevented by severe punishment." But while Christian Science practitioners were occasionally arrested for practicing medicine without a license, their defense that they were practicing religion, not medicine, was generally accepted by the courts, which granted them their constitutional right to freedom of religion. Physicians found

it "a wild absurdity," as the *Journal of the American Medical Association* editorialized in 1898, to allow "that any . . . shrewd and conscienceless exploiter
of human credulity, can defy the law and practice the rites of any cult, no
matter how degrading, vicious or dangerous, provided . . . the knave takes the
precaution to call the cult a 'religion.'" In the few states that refused to
concede that Christian Science was not the practice of medicine, practitioners
got around the law by not charging for their services, as licensing statutes did
not interfere with free medical assistance. (Practitioners did, of course, make
it known to clients that they were willing to accept voluntary expressions of
gratitude, even though in theory—or theology—money was non-existent.)[5]

Otherwise, the new legislative environment provoked an angry political
backlash, both from individual members of the various healing schools and
from national organizations formed expressly to fight for "medical freedom":
such were the American Medical Liberty League, the Constitutional Liberty
League of America, and the National League for Medical Freedom. The case
made for medical freedom was based primarily on the need to protect constitutional liberties. These included first of all the liberty of citizens to choose
the treatments they thought best for their own bodies. Americans were guar-
anteed the right to elect representatives in government according to their
political beliefs and the right to choose a religious faith according to their
spiritual beliefs. Why then, it was often asked, should they not have the right
to choose physicians according to their medical beliefs? "Medical legalized
monopoly ruthlessly tramples upon the most sacred private domain," a writer
in the popular current affairs periodical *The Arena* objected in 1893. "It is
moral robbery, masquerading as humane legalism." The allopathic profession
did not have "any more moral right to impose its peculiar therapeutic methods
upon an unwilling individual than a Baptist majority in any state would have
to require universal immersion."[6]

Orthodoxy's answer, of course, was that lay people did not have the
scientific knowledge to distinguish between effective physicians and incompetents, so the choice had to be made for them and for their own good. (Few
shared the sentiments of Mencken, who believed there was "evil, indeed, in
every effort to relieve the stupid of the biological consequences of their stupidity. If the sort of yokels who now dose themselves with Swamp Root were
deprived of it by law, and forced to consult the faculty of the Harvard Medical
School when they were ill, what advantage would there be in being too intelligent to take Swamp Root?")[7]

The response to medical paternalism—in echo of Thomson—was that
intellectual sophistication was hardly required to choose a physician, since
anyone with a modicum of common sense could tell if she was being helped
or harmed by a doctor. "We demand the right," a physical culturist wrote,

"to patronize any practitioner whose principles of cure and methods of procedure appeal to our reason and conscience." If the patient's reason determined the practitioner to be inept, she would vote with her feet, and the marketplace would shortly eliminate the pretender and all others of his kind. Further, even if the lay person was incapable of making wise medical judgments, there was a more fundamental principle at stake. No less an intellect than Mark Twain raised the point when testifying in favor of the licensing of osteopaths in New York State. "What I contend is that my body is my own," he protested; "at least I have always so regarded it. If I do harm through my experimenting with it, it is I who suffer, not the State."[8]

The second constitutional liberty being challenged was that of the freedom of every person to choose a career or follow a calling. "I don't know that I cared much about these osteopaths," Twain continued in his testimony to the New York legislature, "until I heard you were going to drive them out of the State; but since I heard this I haven't been able to sleep." No one who treasured freedom should be able to sleep, alternative practitioners argued, as long as there was a profession that behaved as if it were the "National Established Church of Medicine" empowered "to weed out dissent" through "harsh and vindictive measures." There was considerable popular sympathy at the turn of the twentieth century for the charge that "medical orthodoxy has always been as intolerant and bigoted as religious orthodoxy, and about as ready to torture and destroy."[9]

Irregular doctors milked that sympathy to the last drop. Drugless healers "are treated as common criminals and outlaws and are relentlessly persecuted at the behest of intolerant official medicine, by means of the most pernicious laws and regulations that disgrace our statute books." Those statutes "are the only remnants of monarchical intolerance and despotism legalized, in 'the country of the free.'" Instituted and enforced by "medical bigots that are no better . . . than the religious bigots of olden times who burned the followers of another faith at the stake," they should "be abolished and medical freedom established in the interest of humanity, progress and science." Those words of a naturopath provide just a taste of the passion with which he and irregular comrades carried out their crusade against "The Most Evil of All Monopolies . . . the Medical Trust." (That Trust was understood to be embodied in the American Medical Association, a "juggernaut" of "a political machine," an osteopath asserted, "second not even to Tammany Hall.") Their goal, however, was not to abolish allopathic laws, as their nineteenth-century forbears had done, but to establish licensing provisions for themselves. The solution in a free society was to institute licensing requirements for every system of care, with competence to practice being demonstrated by examination in the applicant's special field: "We must grant social justice and equity to all duly qualified practitioners of every approved healing method. That's the meaning of Medical Freedom in America."[10]

The orthodox profession found this interpretation of medical freedom even more offensive than the argument that the licensing of MDs should be abolished, for it necessitated far greater political exertion, and expense, to turn back the irregular legislative onslaught. Bills to legalize alternative schools of practice were nothing but "mush legislation," an Illinois physician objected in 1921. "Nearly every year some new group of imaginary healers with little or no education attempt [sic] to be recognized by State legislatures and to be made by law the equals of medical men who have given years of study to qualify themselves to treat the sick. The growing enslavement of the medical profession has reached an acute stage," he grumbled, and it was time to call a halt to "the everlasting meddling by politicians and derailed menopausics with the practice of medicine." To New York's commissioner of public health, the licensing of "cults" was "a hydra-headed monster. You destroy one and others rise up against you. It is a preposterous spectacle," he complained in 1927, "to see the medical profession always on the aggressive to prevent a host of these persons from jimmying their way into the realm of medicine."[11]

The real reason allopaths were upset, irregular doctors countered, was that they were frightened. Medical democracy meant fair and square competition, but MDs were afraid to play fair. A chiropractor suggested in 1915 that the reason regular physicians attacked his profession so viciously was that they were desperately "protecting themselves against the competition of a strong and meritorious science." Behind all their scheming, he maintained, "is a recognition and a fear on their part that chiropractic is another step in the logical evolution of the healing art, and that this new step has carried that art beyond the scope of the old school." The old school of practice was coming to "apprehend that unless they stamp [chiropractic] out in its infancy they will have to give way before its vigorous young manhood." That was an article of faith shared throughout irregular ranks. Only give "the drugless physician . . . a fair chance with the allopath," a naturopath pled, "and he will soon make his brother of the older school take a back seat in the healing art." Certainly "if orthodox medicine has any merits worth preserving," another drugless physician reminded, "it should not need special state protection from honest, heterodox competitors."[12]

MDs sought state protection, it was charged, not for their professed purpose of guarding public welfare but out of economic self-interest: as a chiropractor would put it later in the century, "the ermine glove of altruism frequently conceals the brass knuckles of greed." Medical monopoly paid much better than open competition. With more doctors on the scene offering to heal without recourse to drugs or the knife, an osteopath joked, "the undertaker has ceased to be the only man to whom [allopaths] must relinquish their patients." The economic benefits of monopoly to the regulars, furthermore, equated to economic exploitation of the masses. In the words of the president of the National Association of Drugless Practitioners in 1921, "the government would levy a tax on over 30,000,000 good people, who want drugless therapy, and then spend this money to deprive these same people of their right to have drugless therapy." The restriction of medical licensing to allopaths was taxation without representation, it was objected, and "a meaner conception than this was never born in the brain of man."[13]

Finally, obtaining their own licensing statutes was perceived by alternative practitioners as a critical measure for purging incompetence and quackery from their own ranks. "Where there is no official recognition and regulation," the founder of naturopathy, Benedict Lust, maintained, "you will find the plotters, the thieves, the charlatans. . . . [The] riff-raff opportunists bring the whole art into disrepute." By the time Lust said this, shortly before his death in 1945, frustrating experience had demonstrated that "that is the fate of any science—any profession—which the unjust laws have placed beyond the pale."[14] In following the evolution of alternative medicine over the first third of the twentieth century, it is essential to keep in mind that constant battle of each system to bring itself within the pale.

7

The Rule of the Artery: Osteopathy

A t first glance, Andrew Taylor Still (1828–1917; Fig. 7-1), the founder of osteopathy, appears to be the South's answer to Samuel Thomson. Born in a log cabin in Virginia, he too was largely self-taught in matters medical, acquiring mastery of anatomy while still a boy by studying the bones of animals he brought down with his rifle and of Native Americans he pulled up from burial grounds ("Indian after Indian was exhumed and dissected, and still I was not satisfied"). Rough-hewn in manner, haphazardly schooled, and intensely practical-minded, he was every bit as proud to be plebeian as Thomson had been.[1]

Yet there is no hint in his life or writings of the peevishness and acerbity that made Thomson so insufferable, and only a touch of the botanic's air of self-importance. His autobiography, so different from Thomson's saga of deprivation and persecution, is a savoring of the challenge and adventure, the downright fun, of frontier boyhood. It brims with hard-won practical knowledge—the fine points of shooting a flintlock and selecting a coon dog, the fight and grit in a rattlesnake. Even the eighteen-by-twenty dirt-floored cabin in Missouri that his family moved to when he was nine is described with a fond remembrance of the opening left in the wall to admit enough light to allow him to work on his reading and writing. Still, in short, was irregular medicine's answer to Abe Lincoln, an emancipator with a puckish sense of humor and down-home eloquence. So like Honest Abe was he that in young manhood, in the 1850s in bleeding Kansas no less, he took a firm stand against slavery and fought on the side of the Union in the War Between the States. (In later years he was given to telling people that he "helped to free the colored man from slavery and am now engaged freeing the white man from slavery—the slavery of drugs.")[2]

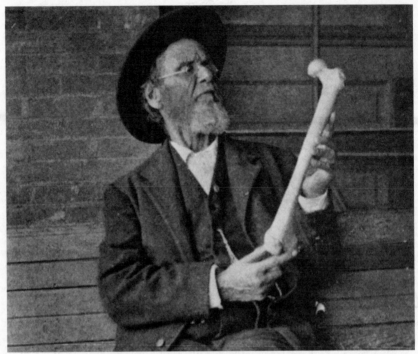

Figure 7-1. Andrew Taylor Still [George Webster, editor, *Concerning Osteopathy*, 2d edition (Norwood, MA: Plimpton, 1921), 221]

Origins of Osteopathy

Still's father, Abram, was a Methodist preacher who, like many another frontier reverend, dabbled in medicine, ministering to the bodies as well as the souls of his flock. Young Andrew studied healing with his father, supplementing his practical training by reading medical texts and perfecting his knowledge of human skeletal structure by identifying bones while blindfolded; through this tactile training in anatomy "I became as familiar with every bone as I was with the words 'father' and 'mother.'" He then moved on to the careful study of muscles, ligaments, and the vascular system, acquiring all the while a conviction that intimate knowledge of anatomy was the key to practicing medicine. (When half a century later a would-be student of osteopathy asked Still what he might read in preparation for medical school, he was told, "*Gray's Anatomy*, and nothing else.")[3]

Still began practicing regular medicine on his own in 1854; it will be recalled that at this time medical licensing laws were all but extinct, so there was no barrier to his entrance into the profession. The outbreak of civil war interrupted his medical career (although he served briefly as an army hospital steward), but in 1864 he returned to practice in Kansas. Almost immediately his confidence in medicine was shaken. An outbreak of spinal meningitis struck down three of his children despite the best efforts of several MD colleagues. Still already felt some misgivings about standard remedies, having lost several teeth to calomel during his teenage years. His children's deaths were a far more affecting demonstration of the uselessness of drugs, however, moving him to a realization that hit-or-miss prescribing of toxic pharmaceuticals could not be nature's way of healing. The rough-and-ready frontiersman who prided himself on being "as independent as a wolf when he knows the dog got the strychnine" was set on a course of rebellion against orthodox medicine.[4]

Still had received a hint of nature's way while yet a child. At the age of ten, he found himself suffering one day with a headache. Instinctively seeking relief by applying pressure to the back of his head, he made a "swinging pillow" by wrapping a blanket around a rope swing lowered to about ten inches above the ground. He lay down with his head resting on the blanket and soon "went to sleep, [then] got up in a little while with headache all gone." (Ever after that, if he felt a headache coming on, he would "swing my neck," as he called it.) That "first lesson in osteopathy" was succeeded by a similar experience when, bothered with diarrhea, he lay on the ground with his lower back across a small log "and made a few twisting motions." That movement "restored the misplaced bones to their normal position," he decided, "and that was the last of the flux."[5]

Experiences such as those came back to mind when, as an adult, Still began to suspect that drugs could not cure. Although he continued to employ drugs in his practice on into the 1870s, he used them less and less as time went by, relying more on various manual techniques for alleviating pain that he gradually developed over the 1860s and '70s. These seem to have been arrived at through empirical trial-and-error testing guided by intuition and his expert's familiarity with human anatomy. To illustrate: one day while strolling through town Still noticed a line of blood spots along the sidewalk. Following the trail to a young boy walking with his mother, Still realized the child was affected with bloody diarrhea and asked if he could do an examination. "Beginning at the base of the child's brain, I found rigid and loose places in the muscles and ligaments of the whole spine, while the lumbar portion was very much congested and rigid." Then, "like a flash," Still said, a thought occurred to him, "that there might be a strain or some partial dislocation of the bones of the spine or ribs, and that by pressure I could adjust the bones and set free the nerve and blood supply to the bowels." He did so, and by the next day the child was well. There happened to be a good bit of the bloody flux in town at the time, and as word of Still's method got around, the sick flocked to him and he "cured them all."[6]

To be sure, physical manipulation of the body was hardly a new procedure. Massage had been employed in Europe since Hippocratic times or earlier, and massage therapy experienced a resurgence of medical interest in the early nineteenth century. At that same time, there appeared an offshoot of massage in the form of the system of "medical gymnastics" developed by Swedish fencing master Per Henrik Ling. Making its way to America in the mid-1800s as the Swedish movement cure, Ling's program involved both active exercises performed by the patient and passive musculoskeletal flexions and extensions carried out by a therapist. Touching and stroking of the ailing person's body, and particularly the spinal column, had also been a common practice among mesmerists; Still in fact briefly advertised himself as a magnetic healer in the 1870s.[7]

Finally, there was a long history of so-called natural bonesetting practiced by people who claimed an instinctive knowledge of skeletal structure and an intuitive ability to remedy not just fractures, dislocations, and sprains but virtually all other ailments as well by pushing or pulling one or another misplaced bone back into alignment. In America, several generations of the Sweet family of Rhode Island had won renown for their skill at bonesetting, the family patriarch Job having treated the daughter of Aaron Burr. (Orthodox medical opinion of natural bonesetters is evident in a mid-nineteenth-century physician's characterization of them as "Natural Fools.")[8]

Still devised his own bonesetting procedures but was no less subject to being rejected as a natural fool. When in 1874 he announced that he was severing all ties to regular therapies (at ten A.M., June 22, "I flung to the breeze the banner of Osteopathy"), he was denounced by doctors, ministers, and neighbors and effectively run out of his Kansas hometown. He relocated to Kirksville, Missouri, where the "show me" people were less hostile but hard to impress nonetheless—at least at first. Unable to drum up enough business, Still became a medical circuit rider who scratched out a living traveling from town to town while his wife and remaining children stayed behind in Kirksville. The medical vagabond met with skepticism everywhere, being heckled as a "hoodle-dooer" and a "hypnotist." ("Yes, madam," Still responded to the latter attack, "I set seventeen hips in one day.") At most towns, "he did not tarry long," and even those who employed him requested he make his call at the back door.[9]

Before long, however, the "lightning bonesetter," as Still styled himself, was being welcomed properly. This was partly a matter of personal charisma. A bearded, tobacco-chewing eccentric in a dowdy felt hat and wrinkled suit, baggy pants stuffed into his boots, one hand holding a long wooden walking stick and the other a bagful of bones slung over his shoulder, Still looked every inch the convention-flouting prophet. He impressed more than one person as having a sort of medical clairvoyancy, an ability to "see" into people's bodies and know just what bone to set. Still also had a gift for baffling metaphoric language (his autobiography is largely parable and allegory, at times verging on speaking in tongues) that captured people's attention and even spellbound some. "Dr. Still would come to my store and the store would fill up with a crowd and stay as long as he staid," one patient recalled. "He would often come in in the evening and talk Osteopathy till ten o'clock or after; all would stay to listen to him."[10]

More persuasive, however, must have been Still's ability to minister to the sick. By more than one account, lightning bonesetting often truly was as startling and powerful as a bolt from the blue. An Irish woman came to him for relief of shoulder pain; he found some upper vertebrae out of place, "set" these and several ribs, and sent her home. A month later she returned to report that not only was the pain gone from her shoulder, but "divil the bit of asthma [a problem she had not mentioned before] have I felt since you trated me first." Still rid a heavy-drinking blacksmith of his taste for whiskey by realigning his ribs, and at the state insane asylum he adjusted the upper spine of a woman who three years before had lost her mind while playing the piano. In a flash she became rational and aware of her surroundings, asking, "Where is my piano and music?" In whatever town the itinerant healer set up shop in his wagon, "people came from great distances to see him," according to his son. "It looked to me just like the old-fashioned camp-meeting, as everybody who was treated went off happy and shouting," leaving behind the "plaster paris casts, crutches, and all classes of surgical appliances" with which they had previously been encumbered.[11]

Finally, "the old doctor," as Still came to be known, "was generous hearted. If he thought it hurt a man to pay," one of his satisfied patients reported, "he would not take it. He cured me of a headache. I sent him a check; he sent it back." "The poor," another observed, "always got their treatment free." Thus it was inevitable that even Kirksville would sooner or later be won over by the old doctor. The victory there was clinched by the miracle cure of the daughter of a town minister. The child had lost her ability to walk and defied the skills of all the local doctors. Her father refused to let Still try his hand, but when business called the minister away from town, his wife called the hoodle-dooer in. A quick spinal manipulation was administered, and when the father returned home, his little girl walked down the stairs to welcome him. Kirksville society now eagerly opened its front door, and Still was able to give up his life as a medical itinerant. In 1887 he situated permanently in Kirksville, soon opening an infirmary to which patients traveled to see him. Kirksville was fast becoming "the great Mecca for invalids" seeking cures that were "marvelous even unto the miraculous."[12]

The town was also the birthplace of "osteopathy." By the time he settled there, Still realized his method of healing was superior to natural—or even lightning—bonesetting. It needed a distinctive, more dignified name, "so I began to think over names, such as Allopathy, Hydropathy, Homeopathy, and . . . concluded I would start out with the word os (bone) and the word pathology, and press them into one word—Osteopathy." Taken literally, that meant "bone disease," though Still, stung by allopathic ridicule of his invention, insisted the word could mean "bone usage." His true feeling about the matter, though, so typical of the stubborn frontiersman, was "I wanted to call my science osteopathy, and I did not care what Greek scholars said about it."[13]

Early Osteopathic Theory

That science of his was really religion to a good degree. Its practical half was derived from observation and experiment, to be sure, but the theory was straight out of what the nineteenth century referred to as "natural theology." How, a proponent of natural theology would ask, could the natural world have so complicated yet harmonious an order unless it had been designed by an omniscient and omnipotent divine architect? Nature proved the existence of God. Still, the son of a preacher, agreed. One morning while strolling through a dew-covered meadow, for example, "my spirit was o'erwhelmed with the unmeasurable magnitude of the Deific plan on which the universe is constructed." The same awe engulfed him when he contemplated the human body, which he saw as an astonishingly intricate piece of machinery, complete with all the "drivewheels, pinions, cups, arms and shafts" needed to distribute all the substances required for the maintenance of life. It followed that those substances must be provided in adequate amounts by infinite intelligence, and if the body was chemically self-sufficient, the doctor who operated as a chemist, adding drugs or chemical substances to the body, was wasting his time and poisoning his patient. The doctor, rather, should be an engineer. Still built osteopathy "upon this principle: that man is a machine, needing, when diseased, an expert mechanical engineer to adjust its machinery." To be a true healer, one had to recognize that function depends on structure and to use his knowledge of divinely designed structure to remove physical (not chemical!) impediments to right functioning: "An Osteopath is only a human engineer."[14]

Still was particularly o'erwhelmed by the thought of blood corpuscles. Those conveyors of fuel, lubricants, and reparative materials for the body machine had to be instilled with divine wisdom. "Every corpuscle goes like a man in the army," Still imagined, "with full instructions where to go, and with unerring precision it does its work—whether it be in the formation of a hair or the throwing of a spot of delicate tinting at certain distances on a peacock's back. God . . . simply endows the corpuscles with mind, and in obedience to His law each one of these soldiers of life goes like a man in the army, with full instructions as to the duty he is to perform." Corpuscles "go forth to fulfill their appointed mission in unswerving obedience."[15]

That explained why drugs were unavailing to the sick. All-wise and complete, the soldier corpuscles had no need of reinforcement with external substances. Still was confident that "the brain of man was God's drug-store and had in it all liquids, drugs, lubricating oils, opiates, acids, and anti-acids, and every quality of drugs that the wisdom of God thought necessary for human happiness and health." Surely "the Architect of the universe was wise enough to construct man so he could travel from the Maine of birth to the California of the grave unaided by drugs"; to suppose anything else would be "accusing God of incapacity." This crude, faith-grounded hypothesis of blood as a curative medium would by the early twentieth century be asserted by some overzealous osteopaths to constitute the founding of the science of immunology. That overestimates Still's scientific acumen and originality by a considerable margin, yet osteopathy's founder did appreciate the dependence of the health of all tissues on a full supply of blood. Imagine, he instructed with one of his many parables, that a community of people in California were "depending upon your coming in person with a load of produce to keep them from starving. You load your car with everything necessary to sustain life and start off in the right direction. So far so good. But in case you are side-tracked somewhere, and so long in reaching the desired point, your stock of provisions is spoiled; if complete starvation is not the result, at least your friends will be but poorly nourished." The moral was that if the body's blood were side-tracked somewhere, and its stock of provisions delayed, the organ depending on that stream of blood to nourish it would suffer. "So if the supply channels of the body be obstructed, and the life-giving currents do not reach their destination full freighted, then disease sets in."[16]

What could produce such obstruction? What else but the abnormality treated by bonesetters for centuries—a bone out of place and exerting enough pressure on a vessel to divert its life-giving current? Just as the whole person might bleed to death if badly wounded, an individual organ might bleed to death in a sense if there were a loss of the blood supplied to it. The organ would show the effects, the pain and other symptoms, but the cause, the true seat of the disease, would be back at the point of vascular obstruction, at the "osteopathic lesion." Whether produced by strain, fatigue, or any other stressing of the skeletal system, osteopathic lesions were not as a rule large-scale displacements of bones. "When there is the least particle of abnormality of position of spinal structure or when there is a change in the relation of bones, ligaments and muscles," one of Still's protégés explained, "these conditions constitute lesions."[17]

Still spoke as if he could account for all disease with osteopathic lesions. "A goitre is no mystery to a mechanic," he confided, explaining that swelling of the thyroid was caused by dorsal vertebrae, ribs, or clavicles pressuring the blood vessels of the neck. Gout, which he found most frequently in merchants and clerks, was occasioned by lumbar displacements resulting from the workers stretching to place goods on high shelves. A dislocated femur, on the other hand, precipitated rheumatism and might even cause tuberculosis. The most sensational event in the development of medical bacteriology, the 1882 discovery of the tuberculosis bacillus, elicited nothing more than a snort from Still. As far as he was concerned, tuberculosis, and any other so-called infection for that matter, could be accounted for by stagnation and fermentation of fluids detained from their appointed rounds by an osteopathic lesion. "Bacteria do not cause disease," Still maintained; they were merely "the 'Turkey Buzzards' of the body," scavengers that "live on dead cells" generated by an osteopathic lesion. Germs, in other words, were an effect of disease, invading the body only to get at the carrion of impure blood. (Yet if he didn't believe in germs or some sort of contagious pathogens, why did Still order his students to tell patients worried about gonorrhea "to keep their pants buttoned as they should and keep out of that mess"?)[18]

Unbuttoned breeches aside, what sustained health in Still's interpretation was not avoidance of germs but "the rule of the artery," the freedom of arteries and all other vessels from flow-inhibiting pressures. "The artery," Still preached, "is the father of the rivers of life, health and ease, and its muddy or impure water is first in all disease." "The rule of the artery," he declaimed elsewhere, "must be absolute, universal, and unobstructed. . . . Interfere with that current of blood, and you steam down the river of life and land in the ocean of death." The rule of the nerve had to be unobstructed as well. Still stood in wonder before the nervous system, too, that almost impossibly complex network of "the telegraphy of life." He confessed he had no idea what electricity was, but the brain was apparently an "electric battery," the "dynamo" that drove the body by its discharges of electric vital energy. As the conduits of that energy, nerves had a primal power that gave them authority even over the artery. The intuitive Still was "sure that the artery takes blood from the heart for the purpose of depositing it into the womb-like cells of the nervous system in which atoms of living flesh are formed by nerve processes that act to give life, motion and form to organs, muscles and all parts of the body." In his opinion, "the laboratory of the nerves is the place in which the arterial blood goes through the final process and the atoms become qualified to make muscle or flesh of any kind."[19]

Interference with nerve functioning thus also constituted an osteopathic lesion, indirectly by its suppression of the perfecting of arterial blood, and directly by its retardation of the flow of nervous power to connecting organs. The rope swing had cured his childhood headache, Still determined, because the pressure of the rope against his neck had "suspended the action of the great occipital nerves, [giving] harmony to the flow of the arterial blood to and through the veins." Any misplaced or malaligned bone could harmfully impinge, but the spinal column, the bony center of the nervous system, seemed especially prone to the formation of osteopathic lesions, given all the jars, twists, and falls to which most people's backbones were subjected. Consequently most "bony lesions" occurred around the vertebrae and attached ribs.[20]

Osteopathic Practice

It should be apparent that the original theory of osteopathy was a highly speculative creation inspired by Still's mechanical orientation and spiritual beliefs and only flimsily based on any medical science other than anatomy. But what mattered ultimately was practice, not theory, the administration of empirically derived techniques of correction of skeletal abnormalities. First the lesion had to be located. This was done by palpation, of course, the practitioner feeling the patient's body in search of abnormalities. But it was also accomplished by the standard patient history, measurements (blood pressure), and laboratory tests (urinanalysis); taken together, these allowed the osteopath to diagnose the affected organ and from that to deduce what vessels and/or nerves must be inhibited. The manipulative corrections that followed are less easily described, as techniques were "exceedingly complex and difficult of proper execution, requiring . . . a highly sensitive touch." They were best taught, in other words, through demonstration and repetition in the clinic, not in books. Still offered some attempt at written instruction nonetheless, generalizing that bones had to be used "as fulcrums and levers" and giving more detailed explanations for specific common problems. To set a shoulder, for example, "after a thorough loosening at the articulation, use but little force to push the elbow towards the contracted muscles at the shoulder then rotate the humerus into its socket." The "soft hand" and the "gentle touch" got the best results, and the dramatic "popping" sounds the public had come to associate with the operations of crude bonesetters were not necessary. The popular view that the treatment must be "strenuous, rough and painful," a trial "that only the strong can withstand," something that left "the patient hanging on for dear life and wondering which way the tornado had gone," was in error.[21]

Nor did Still have need of tables or other specialized appliances to carry out his manipulations. He simply pressed the patient against a chair or a door jamb or any other immovable object that might be handy whenever sturdy body support was needed. Typical was the case of "an old darky woman with a crooked neck and a stitch in the muscles" whom Still came upon "at the old Wabash crossing." Setting one foot against a fence railing, "and with the old lady resting against his knee," Still "placed one hand on the neck and the other on the head and gave it such a twist that he corrected the lesion at once." As this suggests, none of his operations, contrary to cynics' assumptions, were massage. He did not knead or rub, Still asserted, he manipulated bones and surrounding cartilage, ligaments, tendons, muscles, and fascia.[22]

The lesion removed, the body recovered its health automatically, under the direction of the *vis medicatrix*. The ancient inner force of healing was given a new, mechanical dimension by Still, however. Dependent on the structural integrity of the body, the *vis* would be effectively extinguished by anatomical derangement and would be able to act only when the mechanical impediment was eliminated. "The Osteopathic physician removes the obstruction," Still explained, "and lets Nature's remedy—Arterial blood—be the doctor." Nature could repair almost anything "if you know how to line up the parts." But only if. The creed of the osteopath therefore was simple: "Find it, fix it, and leave it alone." That was in essence the creed of the hydropath, the homeopath, and other natural healers as well. But while all irregulars boasted of utilizing natural methods, none was so tenacious as Still in his claim to be nature's spokesman, nor were any so outspoken about their system bearing the stamp of approval of the Author of nature. "God or Nature is the only doctor whom man should respect," and clearly osteopathy, Still took every opportunity to propose, was God's own medicine. Manipulation was "a prescription written by the hand of the Infinite," which he had discovered at "the University of Deity." The life-affirming corpuscles of the free-flowing artery had been "prepared and proportioned" on "the balance-scales of the Infinite," and Still had always been able "to find all remedies in plain view on the front shelves of the store of the Infinite." He "stood in the courts of God as an attorney," and when people asked him how old his science was, he replied, "Give me the age of God and I will give you the age of Osteopathy." "Osteopathy is God's law" and, Still might as well have added, "I am his prophet." (Indeed, he did report experiencing more than one "vision" revealing osteopathic truths to his mind.) A hint of his estimation of his place in the cosmic medical scheme was dropped in his suggestion that "when Christ restored the withered arm, He knew how to articulate the clavicle with the acromian process, freeing the subclavian artery and veins to perform their functions."[23]

Growth of Osteopathy

Like that predecessor, Still eventually took on disciples to spread his teachings. About the time he settled permanently in Kirksville (1887), he began informally teaching his son Harry to diagnose and treat osteopathic lesions. In short order, his three other sons were initiated into practice, and by 1889 Still was able to open an osteopathic infirmary that drew patients to town by the trainload. Three years later, a school—the American School of Osteopathy— was opened in Kirksville; students earned the DO degree (Doctor of Osteopathy) by attending two five-month terms of training in manipulation, as demonstrated by Still on infirmary patients, and classroom instruction in anatomy. Taught by Scottish MD William Smith, a new convert to osteopathy, the anatomy course had to make do with limited resources its first decade. There was only one cadaver (stolen from an Illinois graveyard by Smith), and it, a regular physician found, "had been rendered so hard by the process of embalming that nothing but a cold-chisel could make an impression on it. A painted wooden Indian used for a cigar store sign would answer the purpose for demonstrating anatomy just as well." Not until 1903 did the state of Missouri grant the American School of Osteopathy legal rights to cadavers.[24]

Meanwhile, enrollment at the school had grown from a mere eighteen students in the first class to several hundred, and the faculty expanded to half a dozen or more, depending on the session. A considerable number of the trailblazing students, moreover, were female, a reflection of Still's position as a staunch supporter of women's rights. (One of his graduates related that the emancipation of women was a "passion" with him, so much so that he often proposed that the federal constitution needed an equal rights amendment.) Women seemed particularly desirable recruits for osteopathy for the purpose of improving obstetrical care. Like earlier developers of irregular systems, Still deplored allopathic obstetrical practice. The MD's routine use of "the brutal forceps of death," he believed, often left women lacerated and "ruined for life" and was "the cause of so many fools and idiots among children to-day." Still performed osteopathic deliveries himself, using manipulations to make labor brief and painless, but he felt women could practice "nature's system of midwifery" even more effectively. Having deeper empathy for their own sex, he supposed, they would work harder to master obstetrical techniques. Apparently they (as well as male osteopaths) did. A woman DO writing in 1921 justified the statement that "equal suffrage and Osteopathy" were the greatest boons for women to occur over the past century by pointing out that thanks to osteopathic obstetrics "the unspeakable wretchedness" of morning sickness had been banished, "the hours of labor ... much shortened, and the pains greatly lessened." When one threw in the consideration that osteopathically delivered mothers regained their strength more quickly "and were able to preserve good figures," there could be no question but that osteopathy had been "a wonderful emancipation for half of the race."[25]

The osteopathic educational system expanded quickly. In 1895 a school was opened in Baxter Springs, Kansas, and over the next five years institutions were founded in Anaheim, Minneapolis, Denver, San Francisco, Milwaukee, Boston, Des Moines, Wilkes-Barre, Philadelphia, and Chicago. By the early twentieth century, graduates of these schools had set up practice throughout the United States and as far afield as Canada, Mexico, the Caribbean, England, Ireland, and China[26]

Unfortunately, not all early osteopaths graduated from serious programs. The sudden expansion of the new system naturally drew entrepreneurs into the game, and get-rich-quick educational schemes flourished from the outset. Conscientious osteopaths of the time were greatly upset by the "many incompetents" who launched schools "without capital, equipment, brains, experience, or purpose, except to make money." There were correspondence schools that "blatantly forced themselves upon the attention of the people by advertising" and individual practitioners who, "with 'an itching palm,' took pupils and professed to teach them all about Osteopathy in a few lessons. Others claimed to give Osteopathy by teaching a few 'movements,' and even issued books with cuts purporting to represent movements." William Smith, the anatomy professor at Kirksville, told of visiting the director of a bogus institution in Kansas City: "I introduced myself as a Dr. Stuart, told him fairy tales, told him straight out that I wanted to buy a diploma and secured it." Still, friends reported, was "moved to tears on more than one occasion" when he heard stories of osteopathic charlatans who "faked the people and virtually robbed them of honest money." He raged at such "drunken scoundrels," such "trash . . . no more fit [to practice osteopathy] than a donkey is to go in a jewelry shop," but was most concerned that "the impressions they have left have proven injurious to Osteopathy" overall.[27]

Medical Opposition

Even had the new therapeutic system not been tarnished by educational hucksterism, early osteopaths would have met with biting criticism from allopathic rivals. (One may as well approach "Satan for information about Christianity," Mark Twain joked, as "ask a doctor's opinion of osteopathy.") Regular practitioners looked down upon even the graduates of Kirksville as poorly educated in the medical sciences and blindly subservient to a leader who was "particularly vague, windy, and pompous" and "a master dispenser of hokum," to a profession that was "Still born," to professional literature that was "hyperbolic" and "ill-written," to a rationale that was more mysticism than science ("an absurd and impossible theory"), and to a practice that was nothing more than "a rather rude massage": "It hurts [the osteopath's] feelings to call the proceedings massage, and it is indeed rather hard—on massage; but that is what it is." Osteopaths, it was agreed, were guilty of "claiming impossible things and doing harmful ones," and when perchance any good did come to one of their patients it was due purely to "mental suggestion" and the relaxing effects of massage. To claim anything more for osteopathy was "the *ne plus ultra* of absurdity," as it was a system "encumbered with endless falsities." To one MD, osteopathy was "a complete system of charlatanism, empiricism and quackery calculated and designed to impose on the credulous, superstitious and ignorant, and fraught with danger to the health, limbs and lives of the citizens"; to another, it was "a disgrace to this century."[28]

Such a disgrace had to be put down—by law. The first osteopath to feel the hand of the law was Still's own son Charles, who moved to a small town in Minnesota in 1893 and at once found himself in the middle of a diphtheria epidemic. Treating victims with manipulations of the head and neck, he enjoyed enough success to come to the attention of state health authorities, who had him arrested as an unlicensed practitioner. By the time the case came to court, though, Still's public support had grown to such a degree (so many patients sought him out, he complained, he had no time left for fishing or hunting) that the charge was dropped. Nevertheless, many other arrested osteopaths were taken to trial in the 1890s. Fortunately, a common judicial attitude was the one expressed by an Illinois judge who pardoned the defendant after deciding "the people seemed to want to try this new humbug."[29]

The central issue in these early legal battles was whether or not the new humbug was actually a form of practicing medicine. Did "medicine" mean any and all measures employed to treat disease, or only drugs and surgery? If the former, osteopaths clearly were in violation of the law when they performed their manipulations. Most courts, however, sided with the latter definition, allowing osteopaths to practice so long as they used no pharmaceutical or surgical measures. Counting long-term on the goodwill of the judiciary, however, was a gamble, especially when allopaths were campaigning throughout the country to have osteopathy prohibited as dangerous. The brunt of the regulars' attack rested on the sweeping objection that could be made to any ineffective therapy of whatever system: it injures by not doing any good, occupying the patient with harmless but useless procedures when she could genuinely benefit from orthodox drugs or surgery. But direct injury was often charged as well. In 1915, for example, the *Journal of the American Medical Association* reported the case of a football player who incurred a spinal injury, was stabilized by an allopathic surgeon, but then at the family's insistence was attended by "an arrogant, boastful osteopath" whose treatment resulted in "renewed shock, a scream and . . . death . . . two hours later." MDs insisted, moreover, that osteopathic manipulations were likely to worsen infections, not just injuries; adjustment of the cervical vertebrae of a diphtheria case, for example, "would invariably kill the patient." Consider the orthodox opinions expressed in merely one court case, that of a Kentucky osteopath who was denied the right to practice in 1900: "The doctrines and practices of osteopathy are utterly preposterous and . . . would do no good on earth, but on the contrary would do harm, and in many cases likely kill its victims"; "the osteopathic treatment of diseases is positively and highly dangerous"; "the practice of osteopathy is not only dangerous to the limbs and lives of the public, but in many instances is inhuman and barbarous." "It is singular, indeed," the judge in this case concluded, "that in an enlightened age like this such humbug schools and ignorant pretenders could find recognition by the laws of any state." The only way to protect themselves, the first generation of osteopaths recognized, was to obtain licensing statutes specific to their type of practice; otherwise, it was predicted, "our ancient foe will work us woe."[30]

Professionalization of Osteopathy

DOs thus plunged into the business of exploiting popular distrust of medical monopoly, depicting the AMA as "the great allopathic octopus, seeking to grasp and strangle to death every system of healing" but its own, and denouncing the medical trust's denial of the right to practice as "the most dangerous, the most impudent infringement of personal rights ever sought to be foisted upon the people of an enlightened country." Osteopaths, furthermore, showed formidable tenacity in lobbying state legislators for their rights. "What they lacked in numbers and logic," a spokesman for regular medicine observed, "the osteopaths made up in energy." (Some even provided gratis treatments to legislators.) As early as 1895, in fact, a state legislature approved a bill providing for the licensure of osteopaths. The state, of course, was Missouri, though the act was promptly vetoed by the governor with the objection that graduates of the American School of Osteopathy had not received a thorough medical education. Indeed, with just anatomy and osteopathic theory and technique in its curriculum, the school did provide only the most narrow scientific basis for practicing the healing art. Still himself conceded the point, responding to the veto by expanding his course of study to include physiology, pathology, histology, chemistry, midwifery, and even surgery, spread out over four terms of five months each. (This necessitated the hiring of additional faculty, nearly all of whom held MD or PhD degrees.) Essentially the only thing missing from the revised curriculum was drug therapeutics. At the sitting of the next legislature, in 1897, a new osteopathic bill was submitted; it quickly passed, and was signed into law by a new governor. Kirksville celebrated: "Bells rang and whistles blew. Anything that would make a big noise went," and ASO students paraded through the streets chanting:

> Rah! Rah! Rah!
> Missouri passed the bill
> for A. T. Still
> Goodbye Pill
> We are the people
> of Kirksville.[31]

In the meantime, Missouri had been edged out as the first state to license osteopaths by Vermont, which enacted its law in 1896 after an osteopathic practitioner successfully treated the state's lieutenant governor and several legislators; shortly after, North Dakota passed a law, leaving Missouri to become the third state where osteopaths could lawfully practice. By 1901 fifteen states had admitted osteopathy to legal standing, and by the early 1910s the total had reached forty. (Not until Mississippi's law of 1973, however, did osteopathy win legal support in every state.) That steady advance of legalization was, of course, a major stimulus to the growth in numbers of osteopathic schools and students. At the same time, the licensure process was furthered by continued polishing of osteopathy's professional image. In 1894 a *Journal of Osteopathy* was begun, and three years later the American Association for the Advancement of Osteopathy (renamed the American Osteopathic Association in 1901) was founded, not just to fight for legal protection of practice but also to raise educational standards, encourage research, and wage war on quackish imitations of osteopathy. Over the next two decades, the curriculum at osteopathic colleges was expanded and strengthened, though it still lagged well behind the orthodox standard.[32]

Research was pursued at osteopathic schools as well as at the A. T. Still Research Institute, the chief object being to "prove the lesion." There were experiments, for example, in which slight skeletal displacements were performed on anesthetized laboratory animals; when the animals were sacrificed some days or weeks later, "the nerves showed congestion and inflammation at the site of the lesion, and the organs they supplied gave evidence of congestion, inflammation and disordered functions." Similar observations were made of human tissues during autopsies, and X-ray studies were also reported to verify the osteopathic lesion. But the strongest proof, to osteopaths' minds, was the superior cure rate they believed they obtained by adjusting lesions:

"The osteopathic tide," they boasted, had swept "tens of thousands of cases pronounced hopeless" by allopaths "into the ranks of perfectly healthy men, women and children."[33]

Expansion of Osteopathic Practice Into Surgery and Drugs

Just beneath that smooth and yearly brighter surface, however, was a widening rift caused by disagreement over the scope of therapy permissible to an osteopath. From the profession's earliest days there were practitioners who doubted that manipulation could be a cure-all and who wanted to buttress it with other—allopathic—treatments. The first area of osteopathic expansion was to be surgery, a realm of treatment about which Still felt more than a little ambivalence. On one hand he was repulsed by contemporary MDs' eagerness to resort to the knife. Modern aseptic technique in the operating room was developed from the 1860s through the '80s and revolutionized surgery, making it possible to invade all the major body cavities with much less fear of the acute infection of wounds that had so restricted surgeons before. Understandably, physicians were suddenly as determined to use surgery as they had been to avoid it, and epidemics of appendectomies and hysterectomies swept the land. ("In memory of our father!" a newspaper's fictional epitaph ran. "Gone to join his appendix, his tonsils, his olfactory nerve, his kidney, his ear-drum, and a leg, prematurely removed by a hospital surgeon.") In truth, surgical hysteria was not quite so out of hand as to justify Still's remark that surgical patients were "slashed up as if you had had a fight in Russia with three wild boars" or his estimate that nearly half the country's women "bear a knife-mark," but he was correct in asserting that many operations were "unwarranted." Still believed that osteopathic treatments could cure many conditions commonly submitted to surgery ("The osteopath uses the knife of blood to keep out the knife of steel"), but if osteopathic methods failed he was willing to cut as a last resort.[34]

The fact that others resorted to the knife so much more readily was not the fault of surgery, of course, but of the surgeon, and Still had no difficulty rationalizing surgical interventions when no alternative was left. An operation, after all, was a kind of manipulation of body structure, much like osteopathy, though performed internally with instruments. As Still put it, "osteopathy is surgery from a physiological standpoint," and in the right cases surgery became "but a branch of osteopathy." By 1897 surgery had been introduced into the Kirksville curriculum, taught by two faculty with orthodox surgical training. Soon after, advertisements for Still's infirmary began to tout the institution's surgical service, promising patients "that they will in no case be subjected to unnecessary surgical operations" but at the same time assuring them that if going under the knife were necessary they could expect "the highest order of skilled surgery [performed by] a corps of the very best surgeons in the United States."[35]

The highest order of surgery was thought of as a specifically osteopathic surgery, an approach to cutting that minimized the use of drugs (mercifully anesthetics and antiseptics were allowed) and employed manipulative treatments to supplement operative procedures. If, for example, the patient's vitality were elevated by pre-operative manipulations, no stimulants would be needed during surgery, osteopathic surgeons maintained. Manipulations post-surgically were believed to increase the body's resistance to infection, and osteopaths reported a virtual elimination of pneumonia and pleurisy, with mortality "wonderfully decreased"; even the vomiting caused by anesthesia became a rarity in osteopathic hands. It was possible, then, to think of surgery as "the complement of Osteopathy," but a complement reserved for use only when manipulative methods were of no avail. The primary reason for teaching surgery to the osteopathic student was "so that he shall thoroughly understand when *not* to operate." Where restraint was exercised, one might envision a future golden age when "Osteopathy and surgery (rationalized and changed much from its average status of today) will align themselves against the fallacies of medicine." Indeed, Still's own son predicted such a course was "inevitable." The inevitable nevertheless got off to a slow start; relatively few osteopaths attempted more serious procedures than setting fractures or closing wounds before the 1920s. Their original licensing laws did not permit them to do surgery, and until those laws were expanded and more opportunities for advanced surgical training developed, osteopathic surgery was as much dream as reality.[36]

Initially, the dream that "a new system of surgery may be devised" was inspired by one essential, inviolable principle. "Let us call our surgery Drugless Surgery," one advocate proposed; "then it can be truly said that osteopathy is a complete system of healing and is drugless." For Still and his followers, drugs were a far more invidious attack on nature than surgical interventions. They were, after all, the defining characteristic of allopathic practice. The difference between his medicine and that of the regular doctors, Still proposed, was that "osteopathy does not look on a man as a criminal before God to be puked [and] purged"; "take strong medicine," he added in disgust, "and die like rats." (In his autobiography "the greatest snake fight I ever had" was recounted to teach the lesson that since the snake represents poison and all drugs are poisons, the fight was the first clash between osteopathy and allopathy.) It was "the reckless use of drugs . . . which gave rise to osteopathy," and just as irregulars of the mid-1800s had piled scorn on "mineral doctors," early osteopaths sneered at "drug doctors": they were "fetich-worshipers" obsessed with "blind searching for panaceas"; they were deluded practitioners of a "futile alchemy—worse than the attempts at transmutation of lead to gold in the olden time!"[37]

In truth, the public of the late nineteenth century, though largely liberated from calomel, was anxious about the reckless use of other drugs. Morphine and cocaine, both compounds popularized as medications by mainstream physicians, were just then being recognized as addictive substances that had already wrecked hundreds of lives and threatened to undermine the economic and moral foundations of society. (One of Still's own brothers was numbered among the hundreds of thousands of "morphine sots" created by allopathic doctors.) A parallel recent development had been the rise of the mass-production pharmaceutical industry to displace the lone apothecary compounding remedies in his street-corner shop. These big businesses advertised their products aggressively to the medical profession, encouraging doctors, critics feared, to prescribe even more drugs. A popular magazine article decrying this trend in 1904 represented society's growing unease with large-scale drug manufacture. Speaking of Detroit, the center of the pharmaceutical industry, the author pointed out that if the city's "annual pill harvest . . . was strung on thread like Christmas popcorn, the rope of pills would reach twice around the earth, with enough over to tie in a bow knot. If this string of pills was cut in pieces each of the 36,000,000 women and girls in America could have a different necklace of pills for every day in the year, with an extra long one for each Sunday." In 1901 the governor of the state of Washington, himself a former pharmacist, vetoed a bill passed by the legislature to outlaw osteopathy with the observation that osteopathy was harmless but "the contents of the drugstore are perhaps more dangerous to the future well-being of the race than those of the saloon." Allopaths, he submitted, "are guilty of poisoning the springs of life."[38]

Original osteopaths objected to drugs not just as poisons but also as an insult to the wisdom of the creator. An assumption of Still's medical theology, remember, was that God had placed all materials necessary for life in the blood: "The body has its own chemical laboratory, and man cannot improve it"; "the blood has a hundred drugs of its own of which the doctor knows nothing"; "God did not make man's stomach to be a slop-pail for any dopes or pills." Fellow osteopaths at first agreed, pointing to the allopathic assumption that God placed medicaments outside the body, in the environment, as "the point of departure between Osteopathy and medicine." To look to the mineral and botanical kingdoms to repair God's noblest creation was illogical; "as well say, twice two is a pot of beans." In osteopathy's palmy youth, drugs had no place. Still's greatest contribution, admirers believed, was not that he introduced skeletal manipulation but—"and this is a huger fact"—that he "was the originator of drugless medicine." This was perceived as "perhaps the only forward step that medicine has taken since the time of the ancients."[39]

As will be seen in subsequent chapters, "drugless medicine" and "drug-less healing" were appellations used by several alternative systems of practice in the early twentieth century, not just osteopathy. There clearly was a deep reservoir of public uneasiness about the effects of drugs that could be freely tapped. Praising Still as the originator of drugless medicine, however, not only overlooked the founders of hydropathy, mesmerism, and still other non-pharmaceutical systems of the nineteenth century, it also failed to foresee that osteopathy would not remain drugless medicine for long.

It was the adoption of surgery that opened the door that let drugs into osteopathic practice, for—given Still's anti-drug philosophy—the employment of anesthesia and antiseptics had to be rationalized in accord with professional principles. In doing this, osteopaths followed the lead of the old doctor, who had himself administered antidotes in cases of poisoning on the grounds that snake venom and rabid dog's saliva were external toxins against which the body had not been supplied with internal neutralizers. Consequently, osteopathic surgeons apologized for surgical antiseptics with the argument that they "remove a destructive element from the cell environment,"—that is, they restored the molecular integrity of the bloodstream, the rule of the artery, the same as an antidote for snakebite. Anesthetics were then excused along similar lines. The agony of surgery without anesthesia was an extreme disturbance of bodily equilibrium that surely weakened nature's normally sufficient efforts to sustain health: eradicating pain gave "the nervous system rest and an apportunity [sic] to co-ordinate disturbed forces in order that the processes of repair may operate."[40]

Thus, through the process of explaining how the drugs used in surgery could be understood as "natural" interventions, osteopaths stepped onto a slippery slope that led down to acceptance of agents that Still had considered the very antithesis of natural healing. After all, if it is deemed "osteopathic" to relieve surgical pain with ether, then what objection can be made to relieving severe non-surgical pain with morphine or some other analgesic? That, too, will give the nervous system rest and a chance to regroup its disturbed forces. And, that step taken, how does one resist the proposition that if destructive elements can be removed from the cell environment of the surgical patient with antiseptics, the destructive elements of infectious disease can be removed from non-surgical patients with other drugs? Still's contempt for bacteriology notwithstanding, most osteopaths by the early twentieth century had accepted the overwhelming experimental evidence that germs cause disease. To be sure, at first they interpreted the germ theory from a Still-like perspective by emphasizing individual immunity over bacterial virulence:

germs could obtain an infection-producing foothold only in tissues that had already been weakened by an osteopathic lesion. And even then, it was maintained, osteopathic manipulation of the lesion would overcome the infection by stimulating the production of more antibodies. "Osteopathic treatment," in fact, "aborts infection by increasing the natural resistance of the body faster than is the rule with Nature when it is left alone"; beyond just freeing nature to work, it stimulated nature to a higher level of activity in its manufacture of blood, and "healthful blood [is] nature's best germicide."[41]

In the first decade of the twentieth century, however, it was laboratory germicides that were generating excitement within the regular profession and capturing the attention of the general public. The discovery of germs as infectious agents had sparked an all-out research campaign to synthesize organic compounds that might operate as "magic bullets" (that now hackneyed term came into use during the early 1900s), striking down bacteria while sparing the body's cells. In 1910 the first of the new era's magic bullets was brought into clinical practice in the form of Salvarsan, an organic arsenical that cured syphilis. It was anticipated that drug cures for many other infections would shortly follow, and though the process of discovery took somewhat longer than expected (the next breakthrough was not until the 1930s, with the sulfa drugs), there was ample reason for liberal-minded osteopaths to suppose that allopathic medicine might at last be onto something good and that pharmaceuticals might be a useful (and "natural") adjunct to manipulation.[42] The idea struck other osteopaths as blasphemy, of course, and the resulting debate over the admissibility of drugs into osteopathic education and practice quickly became the profession's hottest intramural contest during the 1910s.

As indicated, osteopaths' descent into the acceptance of drugs was a stepwise process. It began with the establishment by osteopathic schools of courses intended to help students get to know the enemy better so they could more effectively resist it. At Kirksville, for example, there was introduced early in the century a class in "Comparative Therapeutics" in which the properties and effects of drugs were studied for the purpose of demonstrating that "as a rule, whatever desirable results might be obtained from a drug can be obtained by drugless methods." But other considerations soon intruded to give such courses a different bent. First, there was political pressure. State legislatures generally resisted osteopaths' appeals to expand licensure provisions to include the practice of surgery with the objection that if they wished to move in the direction of allopathic practice they should be required to study all the subjects in the allopathic curriculum, including drug therapy. That pressure, which osteopathic schools yielded to, was compounded by osteopaths' conviction that they were losing patients because the public did not think of their practice as "a complete system." People were "absolutely convinced" of the merits of medications, one DO argued, and looked upon osteopaths as "more or less fanatics" for denying it. The result was that even those who sought osteopathic treatment thought of it as limited in scope: they "regard us as qualified to use a 'method' of cure useful for 'some things' only" and "still patronize the medical man" for everything else.[43]

Internal Dissension

Finally, many osteopaths themselves came to feel that it was more or less fanatical to condemn drugs altogether. "There is a wide difference between sanity and fanaticism," one of the profession's leaders observed in 1908; "we can not serve our cause . . . by being blind to other consistent supplementary measures." He was hardly alone in fearing that Still's opinions were acting as blinders on DOs. "Is the osteopathic profession to be developed as a creed," another asked, "or is it to be developed as a complete system or science of the healing art?" Bridling at Still's continuing hold on the profession, thinking of him as the *old* doctor in the sense of a set-in-his-ways codger out of touch with progress, advocates of pharmaceuticals wondered how their system could be complete "when its development is hampered by previous opinions, beliefs and traditions? . . . [and] we refuse to accept truth in any form." Truth was the recurring theme. The reflex dosing with calomel that had turned the young Still so irrevocably against drugs was a delusion of the distant past. The truth of the present was that effective drugs were being developed, and if osteopaths wanted to render their patients the best care available, they would have to integrate drugs into their practice. (One reformer estimated that 90 percent osteopathy and surgery and 10 percent drug therapy was about the right balance for creating "the greatest physicians in the world.") "Why cannot our osteopathic colleges teach the best known things to do for sick folks under all conditions and circumstances?" a Minnesota practitioner wondered in 1916; why could they not evolve "unfettered by anybody's theory about disease?" He confessed that initially he had shared Still's opinion of drugs, but events had forced him to change his mind, and he was "now convinced that it is the duty of the profession to adopt the truth."[44]

One DO's truth was another's heresy, of course. "Are We Falling From Grace?" one defender of the original faith asked editorially in 1915. The "great and masterful fundamental principle" of osteopathy, he warned, "is being frozen to death" by those practitioners who had pursued "the 'broader' training." Such men were "spineless practicians," so unsure of their osteopathic roots that "in a crisis" they would at once "throw up their hands and turn to drugs." The profession had gone "seriously wrong," he concluded, "and unless it is righted, osteopathy will cease to exist as a distinct system." Indeed, osteopathy had fragmented into two systems. On the one side was the system of "straight" or "bony lesion" practitioners who adhered faithfully to Still's belief in manipulation (manual or surgical) as virtual cure-all. On the other stood the system of "mixed," "broad," "liberal," or "unrestricted" osteopaths who buttressed manipulation and surgery with not just drugs but "mechanical devices, vibrators, electrical apparatus, [and] hot air appliances" as well. Drugs were the crux of the conflict, however, as evidenced by straight practitioners' use of the labels "ten-fingered osteopaths" and "three-fingered osteopaths" to distinguish the two camps. Ten-fingered doctors relied on both their hands to effect cures by manipulating osteopathic lesions; three-fingered men used the thumb and adjacent fingers of one hand to inject hypodermic syringes filled with drugs.[45]

By the 1910s osteopathy was suffering considerable pain and dysfunction from its own "professional lesion." Broad osteopaths believed their obligation to be the provision of all effective therapies; their purist brethren saw theirs to be the preservation and elevation of a unique therapeutic method (manipulation) and fundamental medical philosophy: trust in nature. Wasn't it necessary, they asked, for osteopathy to shun pharmaceuticals if the price of using them was to impress the public "that this system is becoming more like medical treatment and those who demand a strictly non-drug system must go to some other?" At a time when people were becoming ever more reliant on drugs when they fell ill, "is it not one of our duties . . . to restore to mankind confidence in the ability of their bodies to right their functions under proper conditions?" If an osteopath actually believed some drug might benefit a patient, should he not refer the person to an allopath? Osteopaths who answered no to such questions had "sold out for a mess of pottage," they were told; drug prescribers were "run[ning] after strange gods" and "pollut[ing] with unholy unions," they were "impudent and thieving impostors" who had taken the noble tree planted by Dr. Still and "grafted on thorns and thistles until it no longer bears the true fruit." It was even reported that wholesale drug houses on the West Coast sold greater quantities of certain drugs to osteopaths than to allopaths.[46]

No one felt those thorns and thistles more painfully than old Dr. Still himself. In 1915 a Pennsylvania DO told of having recently "sat at [Still's] feet, and his face gave me the impression of one who was filled with infinite sadness." He was in mourning for the future of osteopathy, worried that it would soon die as a distinctive medical system because its practitioners could not "be trusted to perpetuate this great truth unsullied and undiluted." Yet that same year, Still sent a poignant letter to the president of the American Osteopathic Association, for publication in its journal, attempting to rally "all Simon Pure D.O.'s who are willing to go on the fighting line" for a last stand against the invasion of their profession by drugs. In his late eighties by then, he was physically incapable "to take the generalship." Nevertheless, "as the Father of osteopathy . . . I make this appeal to my children. . . . Hold up the pure and unadulterated osteopathic flag. Do not allow it to be trampled in the mud by the feet of our enemy. . . . Offer no compromise unless it be the golden truth. D.O. means Dig On."[47]

Two years later, the old doctor passed away following a stroke. At the time of his death, there were in the United States an estimated six thousand osteopaths and eight schools of osteopathy. Practitioners momentarily united in an extraordinary outpouring of affection for their profession's founder. Still seems truly to have been held in the regard expressed in the oration delivered at his funeral: "Daddy, dearest of daddies, to your thousands of children who love you so dearly." Before long, however, the children were fighting again; angry exchanges between straights and broads continued through the 1920s. A lasting truce was imposed only in 1929, when the American Osteopathic Association approved a resolution calling on all schools to include instruction in drug therapy. Outnumbered though they were, the three-fingers had beaten the ten-fingers, and as state after state granted them permission to prescribe drugs, osteopaths became, as straights had feared, more and more like allopaths. By 1937 twenty-six states had extended osteopaths the same practice privileges enjoyed by MDs, and DOs had in the process further alienated regulars and irregulars alike. Osteopathy, a prominent allopath asserted in 1925, "is essentially an attempt to get into the practice of medicine by the back door"; osteopathy, a naturopath charged in 1922, "has been medicalized and made sterile. We cannot treat it as a real member of the Drugless profession."[48]

The subsequent evolution of osteopathy into osteopathic medicine is a development better saved for a later chapter. For the moment, attention will be directed to the one thing that straight and mixed osteopaths could agree on as therapeutic error: osteopaths of both schools utterly despised the adherents of a second system of skeletal manipulation, those "fakeopaths" who practiced "chiroquacktic" and "quackopractic," the chiropractors.[49]

8

Innate Intelligence: Chiropractic

I f there was anything the first generation of osteopaths hated as much as allopathy, it was chiropractic. That rival method of musculoskeletal manipulation was simply "pseudo-osteopathy," they believed, a "violent imitation" of osteopathy carried on by "fakers" whose "theft" had debased Still's methods into "a cheap and inferior grade of osteopathy"; chiropractors were "plagiarists" notable "only for their utter ignorance." Whether any plagiarism was involved or not, the charge of ignorance is unquestionably true, at least when applied to chiropractic in its formative stages. Even one of the most sympathetic historians of chiropractic acknowledges that in its early decades the system was "infected with faddism and quackery." Furthermore, since the first impression that chiropractic made upon conventional medicine was such a lasting one, coloring relations between the two sides down to the end of the twentieth century and largely shaping the medical profession's attitudes toward all unorthodox systems, this chapter will concentrate on the negative facets of chiropractic during the first three decades of the twentieth century. The positive changes made by the profession since the 1930s will be addressed in a later chapter; for now, the task is to illustrate why Morris Fishbein, the editor of the *Journal of the American Medical Association* and the man who charged osteopaths with trying to sneak into medicine by the back door, asserted chiropractors were even worse, as they were trying to crawl in "through the cellar." Further, he reminded, "the man who applies at the back door at least makes himself presentable. The one who comes through the cellar is besmirched with dust and grime; he carries a crowbar and he may wear a mask!"[1]

Origins of Chiropractic

The alternative medical principle that effective therapeutic procedures can be developed purely through empirical trials without the guidance of sophisticated

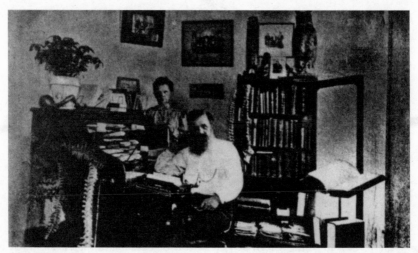

Figure 8-1. D. D. Palmer (with his last wife, Mary) [D. D. Palmer, *The Chiropractor's Adjuster: Text-Book of the Science, Art, and Philosophy of Chiropractic* (Portland, OR: Portland Printing House, 1910), 153]

scientific theory has no stronger proof than the evolution of chiropractic. The founder of the system was D. D. Palmer, "the Discoverer," as he was fond of calling himself, "of this, the grandest and greatest science the world has ever known." As "the Fountain Head of Chiropractic," he declared with characteristic humility, he was "one of the few great thinkers," an "equal" to Edison; indeed, he had actually "solved one of the most profound and perplexing problems of the age, namely, what is life?"[2]

D. D. was born Daniel David Palmer (1845–1913; Fig. 8-1) in the backwoods east of Toronto. He obtained some brief schooling under a rod-happy master, but family financial reverses made education a luxury. Then, when employment in a local match factory proved too seasonal, the twenty-year-old Palmer set out for America. He settled first in Muscatine County, Iowa, an area so in need of a schoolteacher it was willing to hire a young immigrant who advocated hanging disobedient pupils by their thumbs. Five years of teaching and disciplining students in several jurisdictions followed, until in 1871 Palmer attempted to sink roots by taking his first wife (there would be five) and purchasing a plot of land in Illinois where he tried his hand as an orchardist and apiarist. He seems to have made a success of horticulture until the thirty-below temperatures of the winter of '81 killed all his bees, moving him to return to Iowa and become a grocer. He turned to doctoring at last in 1885, when his fancy was captured by magnetic healing.[3]

Medical magnetism had passed its heyday by the time Palmer took it up, but there was still sufficient public interest in the method for him to attract patients when he began to advertise himself as a "Vital Healer." By 1887, in fact, he was managing quite well practicing in the big city, Davenport, where the city directory listed him as "D. D. Palmer, Cures Without Medicine." Upwards of a hundred patients a day thronged to his offices, lured by the liberally circulated advertisments brimming with case histories of invalids restored by magnetism: Ella Post cured of malaria with a single treatment, Jane Wilson of a ten-year-long sore throat in a single visit also, and seventy-five-year-old Mrs. E. M. Hoxie "raised from death unto life" after six treatments. Where, the ads asked rhetorically, "can you get cured quicker or for less money, and without making a drug store of yourself?"[4]

Palmer's life-renewing powers were probably as much a manifestation of personal style as of magnetic substance. Though a short five foot four (and sensitive about it), D. D. had a stocky build, a beard just unkempt enough to be intimidating, and intense, penetrating eyes. His presence was enlarged further by a domineering manner. Even at the memorial service following his death, eulogists were unable to forget how he "loved a wordy quarrel," was "too combative and aggressive and too much set in his own way," and had "squelched us at times with bitter sarcasm." So feisty and self-assured was Palmer that some years after discovering chiropractic he would be able to invade a Kansas City allopathic medical society meeting, gain the floor for a lecture on his method, and actually demonstrate the technique on the back of the society's president to the applause of its members; "chiropractic," D. D. wrote to a colleague, "captured the meeting."[5]

D. D.'s hands were as strong as his personality. His grandson remembered them as having "tremendous warmth," with "large and extremely sensitive" fingers. When healing magnetically, he recalled, Palmer "would develop a sense of being positive within his own body; sickness being negative. He would draw his hands over the area of the pain and with a sweeping motion stand aside, shaking his hands and fingers vigorously, taking away the pain as if it were drops of water." Those movements were intended to allay anxiety and mental turmoil as well. While yet a magnetizer, D. D. jotted down in his journals such holistic maxims as "the mind must be cured as well as body," and "thots [sic] are real substance and modify all they toutch [sic]." Business grew apace, forcing Palmer to lease more and more space, until by 1891 his original suite of three rooms had expanded to forty-two and was decorated with "the finest collection of mounted heads of animals in the west" as well as a glass enclosure holding four live alligators. "His increase in business shows what can be done in Davenport even by a quack," the local paper sniffed, but the editor, and the regulars who scouted D. D. as a "mountebank" huckster of "gold-brick devices," hadn't seen anything yet.[6]

Throughout the nine years he was a magnetic healer, Palmer later claimed, he had slowly acquired an awareness of the relation of physiological function to physical structure. That such an orientation was an advance beyond magnetism nevertheless went unappreciated until September 18, 1895, and an encounter with the janitor in his office building, Harvey Lillard. In D. D.'s telling, Lillard had been extremely hard of hearing for nearly twenty years, ever since a day "when he was exerting himself in a cramped, stooping position [and] felt something give way in his back and immediately became deaf." Palmer examined the man's back and found "a vertebra racked from its normal position. I reasoned that if that vertebra was replaced, the man's hearing should be restored." Lillard agreed to let him have a try, and Palmer "racked it into position by using the spinous process as a lever and soon the man could hear as before."[7]

For the record, Lillard remembered the incident differently, relating that on the fateful day he had been swapping jokes with a friend in the hall outside Palmer's office. D. D. couldn't help overhearing a conversation loud enough for Harvey's ears, so he came out to join the group and was so amused by one story's punch line that he slapped the janitor on the back with a book he was carrying. A few days later, Lillard told Palmer he believed his hearing had improved, and it was then that Palmer began his experimentation with manipulative procedures. Whatever the exact course of events, Palmer's allegiance quickly shifted from magnetism to manipulation. Soon after Lillard's cure, a patient with heart disease was found to have a racked vertebra, too, and similarly she was returned to health by restoration of the bone to its normal position. Palmer then "began to reason if two diseases, so dissimilar as deafness and heart trouble" were produced by displaced vertebrae, "were not other diseases due to a similar cause?" The answer, experience proved, was yes. Undertaking "a systematic investigation for the cause of all diseases" Palmer discovered that "instead of . . . a few rare cases of vertebra [sic] which had been wrenched from their natural position, I found them very common"; indeed, they were virtually universal among the sick.[8]

Among the early successes with the new method was the Reverend Samuel Weed, a Davenport-area minister who had at first assumed D. D. to be a quack. That opinion changed in 1893, when magnetist Palmer cured the reverend's daughter "of a sprained ankle that threatened her life." After one treatment, she walked home, "carrying her crutches in her hands." The next year her father sought magnetic relief for a poorly functioning spleen, but Palmer had by then changed methods and relieved the patient with manipulative therapy instead. Part of Weed's payment for these services was to assist the unlettered Palmer in finding a dignified name for the new healing. Palmer particularly wanted a Greek name, and Weed, something of a classical scholar, proposed "chiropractic," denoting "done by hand." In January 1896 the new method of healing was launched under that name.[9]

Chiropractic Theory

The method had been discovered empirically, and, following the norm, a theoretical rationale followed quickly. Unfortunately, to arrive at an understanding of the theory, one has to read Palmer's 1910 *The Chiropractor's Adjuster*, a text that, the author promises, provides "much new thot [sic] for thinkers." Unearthing those thots, however, requires one to clear away a mountain of rubble—fatuities and redundancies, petty polemics and garbled grammar—only to learn after 985 baffling pages that life and health can be reduced to a proclamation that was made on the book's title page: "FOUNDED ON TONE." That was it. "Life is the expression of tone," and tone is just the "normal degree of vigor, tension, activity, [and] strength" of the body's tissues, particularly the nerves. Disease, consequently, must result from fluctuations of tone above or below that ideal level; in lay language, "nerves too tense or too slack." (Palmer arrived at his conclusions in part, it should be acknowledged, through extensive reading of orthodox texts in anatomy, physiology, and pathology; many of his references were outdated, however, and he regularly misinterpreted even the recent ones.)[10]

How did nerves become too tense or slack? Palmer's experience showed that every case of illness involved a skeletal subluxation of some sort and that alleviation of the subluxation invariably cured the patient. (A subluxation is a minor dislocation, one in which some degree of contact is preserved between the bones in a joint; in a full luxation, the displacement is so extreme as to remove all contact between joint surfaces.) Most subluxations, he had found, occurred in the spine, and it was there that the central nerve channels of the body originated and branched out through openings between the vertebrae (the intervertebral foramina). It followed, for Palmer, that a spinal subluxation would cause a narrowing of the adjacent intervertebral foramen. The narrowed passage would in turn impose upon the nerve passing through it a pressure that would make it "sensitive, enlarged, contracted, tense, rigid." (The nerve was not, Palmer stressed, "pinched," which would mean squeezed between two bones, but impinged, pressured by a single bone.)[11]

All would agree, of course, that if a nerve actually were impinged, functioning in some part of the body likely would suffer. But Palmer's interpretation of how dysfunction would come about was unique to chiropractic. It was, in the discoverer's own words, "The New Theology" of healing, an integration of physical health with "the Intelligent Life-Force of Creation . . .

God." The vital force of the human body, Palmer explained, was "a segment of that Intelligence that fills the universe," a power that "is eternal, always was and always will be." An "inborn intelligence in every living being," even "in every plant that grows," it was properly called "Innate Intelligence," or simply, as Palmer preferred, "Innate." Innate was that which "never sleeps nor tires, recognizes neither darkness nor distance, and is not subject to material laws or conditions." Innate "continues to care for and direct the functions of the body as long as the soul holds body and spirit together," but because it circulates through the nerves, an impingement caused by a subluxation could disrupt its governance and cause illness to result.[12]

The rule of Life-Force was not, Palmer protested, a mechanical regulation of the sort accomplished by Still's divinely directed corpuscles. He considered the machine analogy, with its connotations of unimpassioned automatism, to be an insulting image for the self-conscious and individualized spirit of Innate. His elaboration of how Innate actually sustained vital functioning nevertheless calls to mind no adjective so readily as "mechanical." All the phenomena of life, according to Palmer, were activated by impulses of Innate transmitted through the nervous system. These impulses were of the form of a vibratory wave occurring at a frequency of two hundred vibrations per minute in health. (The clever Palmer determined the frequency by counting every other one of his own vibrations, then multiplying the total by two; exactly how he—or anyone else—detected nerve vibrations so as to count them was left unexplained except for the clue that he was able to succeed only after "a little practice.") In any event, "nerves too tense or too slack" meant nerves vibrating at too high or too low frequencies, nerves impaired by "too much or not enough functionating."[13]

What produced subluxations? Minor trauma from bending, lifting, and "sudden movements [during sleep] superinduced by dreams" was an obvious answer, and with some occasional toe-stubbing and other everyday skeletal mishaps thrown in, physical accidents might easily have been stretched to accommodate all subluxations. Observant clinician that he was, however, Palmer recognized that illness was often preceded by chemical insults so he devised a poison category of subluxations to balance the physical one. Chemical irritants in the blood, he divined, affected nerves in such a way as to force vertebrae out of position. The nicotine of cigarettes, for instance, "affects sensory nerves which in turn contract motor nerves, drawing bones to which they are attached, out of alignment" and leading to "pain, misery, paralysis, abnormal physical desires and mental aberrations." Every other form of pain and misery that human flesh had to endure also stemmed from subluxations, as did afflictions of the mind: "So far as my experience goes," Palmer reported, "all insanity is caused by displaced vertebrae." Even so, harmful subluxations did not always occur in the spinal column. Palmer somehow determined that only "95 per cent of diseases were caused by subluxated vertebrae; the remaining 5 per cent by slightly displaced joints other than those of the backbone." These other joints were usually the fingers and toes, with bunions, corns, and ingrown toenails being the consequence. But whether beginning in backbone or big toe, some injury or toxin had "set the ball rolling, that eventually made the subluxation which caused the impingement, which produced the irritation, which modified the animal temperature, which augmented or decreased the force of the impulse that changed normal functions to abnormal" in the house of theory that D. D. built.[14]

There was no room in that house, of course, for bacteriology. Perhaps the one question on which Palmer agreed with Still was the role of germs in illness. Where Still used the analogy of buzzards and carrion, or of flies and dead dogs, Palmer compared microbes to "the mold found in decaying cheese"; both meant that the decay of disease supported bacteria, not vice versa. The theory of chiropractic subluxation, Palmer predicted, "will in time, knock the bacterial origin of fever into oblivion. It is difficult—impossible—to mix medical etiology and the causation of disease as known by Chiropractors." A causal role for bacteria did in fact come to be accepted by chiropractors by the 1920s, but through an interpretation similar to that of early osteopaths: germs caused sickness only in those already weakened by a subluxation. ("Would you, as a chiropractor, put a gonorrheal germ in your eye?" a lawyer asked a witness in 1921. "I would not be afraid to do so as long as my spine is normal.") Looked at that way, "bacteriology . . . would be of no more use" to a chiropractor, a Utah practitioner announced in 1916, than "a smokestack to an aeroplane."[15]

Chiropractic Technique

As with other alternative systems, though, the proof of chiropractic was found not in theory but in practice. "Chiropractic," after all, meant accomplished by hand, not by mind; theory merely made rational what had been demonstrated in clinical experience. The art of the chiropractic clinician began, just as it did for the MD, with diagnosis, the determination from the patient's history and symptoms of the site of disease. For the chiropractor, though, the irregular heart and enlarged spleen were only secondary sites of illness, remote manifestations of a central disturbance. Having identified the affected organ, Palmer instructed, one should consider the nerve connected to the organ, the part of the spine from which the nerve emanates, and finally, by touch, confirm that a subluxation does indeed exist in that section of the spine. There would be found, Palmer affirmed, only one impingement per disease, and a constant relation between specific ailments and individual vertebrae. Smallpox was connected to the fifth cervical, for example, heart disease to the fourth dorsal, heartburn to the fifth dorsal, and gonorrhea to the second lumbar. At the first lumbar was to be found an allopathic paradox, the source of both syphilis and impotence.[16]

The last patient could be restored to either sexual purity or licentiousness by removal of the single impingement at fault. Indeed, any patient whatever, whether a victim of bunions, hallucinations, diphtheria, tuberculosis, stroke, or ear wax (a small sampling of the conditions Palmer claimed to cure), could be set to rights with an adjustment. Osteopaths often used the word "adjustment" to describe their manipulations, too, but for chiropractic that was the official professional term for removal of a subluxation. As with osteopathic manipulations, adjustments were not easily explained in words but had to be learned through experience and acquisition of "knack," as Palmer called it. Consequently he made only a nominal effort to describe the adjustment process in detail in print. Near the end of his textbook, referring to photographs of his own operations on an Asian gentleman, he explained how "the Jap getting a back-set" was done. (The subject in those photographs was Shegataro Morikubo, a chiropractor himself, and one of the first to be arrested for practicing medicine without a license.) The patient, whatever his nationality, should be made to lie face down on the adjusting table, a bench with an open section in its middle, the subluxated portion of his body above the open space. The chiropractor should then stand on the side of the body toward which the vertebra had been displaced, grip his right wrist with his left hand, place the heel of the right hand against the vertebra so as to use its projections as levers, "then follow with such force as experience has taught us to be capable to move the vertebra as desired."[17]

Great force generally was not needed, at least not for Palmer. He complained of frequently seeing chiropractors lift the hand up and down several times before thrusting, as though "trying to get a good swing," and some, he reported, would even "jump up and down several times before giving a thrust." Palmer described one case in which the adjustment he gave a "twisting [and] screaming" accident victim produced "a crashing sensation that could be felt and heard," but normally he used as little force as possible and found that speed could be substituted for power, a quick movement accomplishing as much as the hefty shove. His reader is left with the impression that the Discoverer's adjustments were free of the discomfort, even pain, of those given by his followers (although his first patients, in pre-adjusting-table days, had had to lie face down on the floor, and "not a few left the office with a telltale red handkerchief held to their noses"). At least adjustments were over with quickly, it would seem, as Palmer treated upwards of a hundred patients some afternoons; chiropractic treatments could be dispensed, he stated, "at the rate of one a minute."[18]

Nothing more was required for healing than a resetting of the subluxated vertebra. That accomplished, the body restored itself through Innate ("the Allopath's Vis Medicatrix Naturae"): "The Chiropractor removes the obstacles to nature's healing processes." As one of Palmer's several poetry-writing admirers elaborated,

> The spinal column holds, we know, a most important place.
> When normal, it is beauteous, a form of wondrous grace.
> But when distorted, it becomes the seat of many ills,
> Which are, frequently, mistreated with ineffective pills.
> Adjust the subluxations till crooked spines grow straight.
> Take off from nerves the pressure which induce [*sic*] an evil state.
> Thus many ailments vanish and health appears for all
> Who, wisely, on Dame Nature for real assistance call. . . .
> Away with drugs which poison and instruments that kill.
> Let us use, in wisdom's way, of mental, manual skill.
> The hands, by mind directed, can drive our ills away
> And bring us advantageous health for which we all shall pray.[19]

Palmer himself anticipated that a good bit more than advantageous health would be generated by chiropractic. By his lights, adjustments were not just the culmination of medical progress but the dawning of the golden age to which human history had always pointed but so slowly ascended. The cosmic questions—"What is life, disease, death and immortality?"—had long been asked, he observed, but had "remained unanswered until the advent of Chiropractic." It was only with the appearance of that "science" that the world was given the "knowledge for which humanity has been hungering since the dawn of civilization" and that "in time [will] do much to relieve poverty and crime, for they are largely diseased conditions. It will in time empty our jails and penitentiaries," he promised, and "give us a conscious connection with that unseen life which is believed in by all nations. . . . Then death, instead of being feared, will be welcomed because the life beyond the veil will be comprehended and known to us as we now know and comprehend this." One will not be surprised to learn that both Palmer and his son, who would eventually assume leadership of the profession, gave serious thought to declaring chiropractic a religion instead of a system of medicine.[20]

It went without saying that a therapy so profoundly revolutionary was far superior to osteopathy, but Palmer delighted in saying so anyway. Bothered by the public's confusion of the two superficially similar systems, as well as mistreatment by jealous osteopaths ("slander and misrepresentation" were but two of the indignities he had to endure from their hands), Palmer seized every opportunity to show how the two systems "are as different as day is from night." His own brighter science was at once simpler and more refined. It cured disease with a single quick adjustment instead of protracted multiple manipulations. Whereas Still's "bloody delusion" supposed the artery was the regulator of health, chiropractic saw the nerve as the source of vitality for arteries and all other body tissues, and appreciated its power to be spiritual rather than material. Palmer interpreted Still's mechanical orientation to physiology to mean a denial of immaterial vital force, of Innate Intelligence. Hence the man who had presented osteopathy as a divine revelation and himself as a prophet was treated by Palmer as an ignorant blasphemer: "Osteopathic treatment and chiropractic adjustment," Palmer ruled, "have nothing in common."[21]

Development of Chiropractic

Palmer was so fiercely proud of his theory and methods, and so swollen with self-importance as the Discoverer, that one is at first amazed to hear he kept his discovery secret for two whole years. But he was above all a practical man, and his new method was "so simple he was afraid someone would see how it was done," his grandson admitted, "and become a competitor in Davenport. He wanted to keep the discovery for himself." From 1895 to 1897 D. D. confided his therapeutic secret to no one but Reverend Weed. It took a brush with death in a train accident to elevate the altruist above the businessman. Had he been "snatched from earth-life it might have been a long time before the same combination of circumstances, combined with the same make-up of an individual, would evolve a science such as I saw in Chiropractic."[22]

Thus, even though suffering from injuries that were "serious in nature," Palmer took on an apprentice, a young Illinois man, and taught him enough of the new science to heal its discoverer's wounds. That tutorial system was soon replaced, however, with a more formal program conducted within Palmer's offices in Davenport. In 1897 the doors of the Chiropractic School and Cure were thrown open, and one short year later the first class, a homeopath named William Seeley, entered and soon graduated. (Palmer's original program consisted of only three weeks of coursework in anatomy, physiology, pathology, symptomatology, diagnosis, chiropractic philosophy, and techniques of adjustment, for five hundred dollars.) The following year, enrollment tripled, to three, and by 1901 it had risen to five. Fully a third of the students in those first classes were MDs looking to expand their horizons, and three (20 percent) were women. Although he once was reminded by a younger brother that the first rule of success is "do not be deceived by women, three times have they been a curse morally, physically and financially," Palmer seems to have welcomed women interested in studying chiropractic. In later years his school would offer discount rates to ladies who matriculated jointly with their husbands. The tolerance of later chiropractors extended only so far, however; Harvey Lillard, the janitor through whom chiropractic was discovered, was a black man, yet the catalogue of the Palmer School in the early 1920s, after Palmer's death, specified that members of all races were welcome, "with one exception." The gatekeepers at other schools were similarly discriminating.[23]

And there were other schools, many others. The second was an American School of Chiropractic, opened in 1902 or '03 in Cedar Rapids, Iowa, by two of Palmer's first graduates; two of the American School's first graduates then opened schools in Minnesota, while Palmer, meanwhile, founded a school in Portland, Oregon, in 1903. He left the Portland College of Chiropractic in a matter of months, however, and moved on to Oklahoma City, where there already existed a thriving Carver-Denny Kiropractic College, to start up two more schools over the next two years. By the 1910s chiropractic colleges had sprung up throughout the country ("like wild flowers following a spring rain on a meadow," by one educator's simile), conferring upon their graduates the degree of DC, Doctor of Chiropractic. Schools were especially numerous in the Midwest and along the West Coast, though, like Palmer's institutions, many were short-lived; of the 392 chiropractic schools known to have been opened, fewer than half survived beyond their first year. (One chiropractor testified to the U.S. Senate that "we had at one time 200 schools in the state of Michigan. They would start up with anything, in a back parlor for instance. We had a man over on East Capitol Street a few years ago who was advertising to teach chiropractic in 30 days for $10.") To their credit, chiropractic's leaders regularly acknowledged problems with their educational system ("fraudulent schools and unscrupulous practitioners," "diploma mills . . . releasing a horde of incompetents whose chief ambition was to get rich quickly") and called for steps to eliminate the abuses.[24]

Professional journals and associations followed in short order behind educational expansion. *Backbone*, issued by the leader of the Cedar Rapids school, was the first journal of chiropractic, initiated in 1903. The following year, Palmer began publishing *The Chiropractor*. Cedar Rapids was also the center of the first would-be national organization, the American Chiropractic Association, founded in 1905 primarily to bring together school alumni. The next year, Palmer's son B. J. started the Universal Chiropractors Association, an organization whose name was not quite as hyperbolic as it might seem; chiropractic was far from universal, but it would soon be international, entering into Great Britain around 1908 and reaching the Continent by the early

1920s; by 1930 chiropractors could be found on every continent but Antarctica. Finally, during the 1910s chiropractic infirmaries and hospitals began to appear, growing to as many as one hundred inpatient facilities in the United States during the 1920s and '30s. (Chiropractic infirmaries decreased dramatically after World War II, as hospital costs rose and no federal funding assistance was available.)[25]

Criticism From MDs and DOs

As the list of schools, journals, and associations might suggest, there were endless disagreements among early chiropractors, regarding adjustment techniques, equipment (many were strongly opposed to the X-ray machine at first), and anything else they could find to wrangle over. But to the allopathic profession, chiropractic appeared to be homogeneous—and hopeless. There was ample reason for regulars to believe that if they'd seen one chiropractor they'd seen them all, and that it was not an edifying sight. To begin with, there was the Discoverer, the self-proclaimed genius who repeatedly issued absurd pronouncements about medical science. All drugs were unmitigated "poison," for example; the army physicians led by Walter Reed, the discoverers of the mosquito as the vector of yellow fever, were "fools"; smallpox vaccination was "the biggest piece of quackery and criminal outrage ever foisted upon any civilized people, . . . the foulest blot on our civilization." (To be fair, Palmer did occasionally demonstrate a flair for intentional comedy. How are surgeons like alley cats, he asked? "Because they mew-til-ate and annoy our patients.")[26]

Other chiropractors seemed no less foolish in their unquestioning faith in the superiority of adjustments. "No method of combating disease has ever deserved to be called scientific until Chiropractic was developed," stated a 1920 advertisement by the Universal Chiropractors Association. "The Chiropractor knows—not guesses—but *knows*—what organs in the body are weak or diseased after he has analyzed the spine," the ad continued, so that "the only reason why a Chiropractor cannot promise a complete cure to every patient in the world—is the possibility that the case has gone so far that Nature herself will not cure it." A chiropractor under oath in a court proceeding in the Midwest answered yes to every question when asked successively if he could cure cancer, tuberculosis, smallpox, diphtheria, scarlet fever, typhoid fever, diabetes, heart disease, insanity, and imbecility by removing subluxations. His only negative response was to the possibility of restoring the drowned to health. The same confidence was voiced by the students from the Chicago chiropractic school who found a way to get into the surgical amphitheater at Cook County General Hospital and badger surgeons with shouts of "Have you tried chiropractic?" B. J. Palmer put chiropractic audacity in a nutshell, boasting to allopaths that "my analysis is better than urinalysis."[27]

Audacity was evidenced in newspaper and magazine advertising as well, a representative specimen of which was the blurb in the *Idaho Falls Times Register* recounting "why his wife left him." It had been because Jack "never had a smile" and "was grouchy with the baby." He "desired to sleep alone" as well, leaving his wife to fear "he had ceased to love her." In truth, Jack did still love her, "but due to nerve pressure in the spinal column, he was not normal sexually." Understandably, his wife eventually left, neither of them realizing that "a happy home could have been made if he had gone to the Busby Chiropractic specialists and had these vertebrae adjusted to normal." One can only hope that Jack's frustrated wife came across the chiropractic advertisement in a Michigan newspaper: "Dear Doctor, Before taking your Chiropractic . . . treatments, I was so nervous that NOBODY could sleep with me. After taking six treatments ANYBODY can sleep with me."[28]

Not infrequently, regular doctors believed, the patient himself went to sleep after a chiropractic appointment—and never woke up. A regular feature of allopathic journals was the notice headlined "Chiropractor Indicted on Charge of Manslaughter," or "Patient Dies in Chiropractor's Office," or "Neck 'Twisted'—Patient Dies," or some such other report of death "due to a dislocation of the cervical vertebrae." Yet much as regular practitioners hated chiropractors and thought them deadly, osteopaths may have disdained them even more. They were certain that the Davenport Discoverer had discovered nothing but merely had imported his ideas and methods from nearby Kirksville; rumors of Palmer having visited the Missouri town, even having shared Still's roof, abounded. Chiropractic, osteopaths scoffed, was at best no more than "the first three weeks of osteopathy," whose "ignorant and unrestrained" practices resulted almost daily in patients' deaths, more rightly recognized as "Chiro Executions." (Not even the Spanish Inquisition, one osteopath suggested, had "a better method of extorting confessions.") "These chiros will kill so many of their patients," it was feared, "that it will cause a revulsion of public feeling against manipulative therapeutics," and osteopathy "will be made to bear the blame of the stupidity and crimes of its counterfeiter." The chiropractic response to this "campaign of venom, viciousness and vulgarity" was to mock osteopaths as paranoid (before long they likely would "be accusing the medical profession with having stolen materia medica and surgery from osteopathy") and as themselves plagiarists: their manipulative methods were nothing but "worked-over massage," with the only shred of originality in Still's work being that "there never has been more junk passed as science."[29]

Legal Battles

Consequently, the first generation of chiropractors had to look over both shoulders, to spot allopaths pursuing them from one direction for practicing medicine without a license, and to look out on the other side for osteopaths chasing them down for practicing osteopathy without a license. They were caught any number of times and regularly convicted of both offenses, becoming martyrs in a grand saga of persecution. "For years," in the telling of this chiropractic epic, MDs

> . . . have ruled the people, as slaves they bowed before them all;
> Their arrogance is great; they forget that pride goeth before a fall;
> These Allopaths would feign believe themselves safe, and as strong as the Czar,
> And that naught could arise to cause them fear, or the ease of their lives to mar.

But at the height of allopathic arrogance there strode forth a hero, a "herculean giant [with] Chiropractic emblazoned on his shield," who so alarmed the "poisoners and butchers" they closed ranks to destroy him. Their weapon was the "Medical Practice Act."

> The devilish doctors now laugh and grin and chuckle in their ghoulish glee:
> "Oh, we are the only, only ones, now, who can touch the sick for a fee.
> We can charge as we wish, and do what we like with poison and knife and saw,
> And should we by chance kill a patient or two, it's in the name of the law;
> The Chiropractors, altho they have brains, we have to acknowledge that fact,
> If they practice, will be heavily fined by our Medical Practice Act."[30]

One of the first to be fined was the therapeutic Hercules himself, arrested in 1905 in Davenport, convicted of violating medical practice laws, and sentenced in 1906 to 105 days in jail when he refused to pay the $350 assessed as penalty: "He will stick with chiropractic to the end," the *Davenport Democrat* reported, and "offer himself as a martyr . . . instead of paying the fine." Palmer had stood trial on the charge once before, incidentally, in his days as a magnetic healer, and had won acquittal then with his defense that his drugless, scalpel-less treatments had nothing to do with medicine and he needed no diploma except the one he already had from "High Heaven." When the gambit failed the second time around, he cheekily proposed that the judge shorten his sentence to spare taxpayers the full cost of his incarceration, and in fact his term was shortened, but by his wife, who paid the fine plus court costs of $39.50 after only twenty-three days of her husband's imprisonment "in Bastile [sic]." The experience had been worth it, the unregenerate Palmer declared, because all the newspaper attention had "stimulated the growth of our business," and consequently "thousands will be benefitted."[31]

Palmer's story was to be repeated thousands of times over the next several decades ("some chiropractors are such confirmed jailbirds that incarceration is no novelty for them whatever"), even though chiropractors devised a range of tactics to throw allopaths off the scent. "In the early days," one chiropractic trailblazer remembered, "it was necessary to protect the 'child' " (Palmer's term of endearment for his science; he called himself "Old Dad Chiro") with innocuous terminology "in order to avoid the chill and ice of the law." DCs did not perform "diagnosis," for instance, they did "analysis"; they did not provide "treatment" but gave an "adjustment"; such non-allopathic euphemisms "were garments to protect the child until legal clothing could be secured." Many chiropractors refrained from hanging diplomas or other DC credentials in their offices. They tried to pass themselves off as masseurs or physical therapists, practitioners less likely to rouse the regulars' wrath, by displaying heat lamps and vibration devices around the office. They practiced behind locked doors or in patients' homes and refused to take on patients who appeared seriously ill and might die and call attention to their treatments.[32]

Above all, they tried to avoid "spotters," people posing as patients while actually cooperating with the authorities. "Before arresting a Chiropractor for practicing medicine or osteopathy," Palmer warned his followers, "it is customary for the prosecuting attorney to hire two sneaks to call upon him for the purpose of getting such information as they desire." As a result, "we . . . are martyrs to chiropractic," a New England practitioner lamented. "It's very hard not knowing whether the next person who comes in your office is OK or not." So hard was the anxiety to take, an Indianapolis chiropractor drew up a document that every patient was required to sign that described all treatments in non-chiropractic terms. Blank forms were made available to the whole profession so they could "be brot [sic] into court to offset any misstatements made by the sneakers."[33]

The sneakers were also thwarted by satisfied patients. It was commonplace in the 1910s and '20s for the clients of arrested chiropractors to show up in court to testify to the benefits they had received from their drugless healer. (In Bucks County, Pennsylvania, in 1928 the two hundred supporters of an arrested chiropractor made such a ruckus at his judicial hearing that proceedings had to be postponed until the afternoon, when state police arrived to impose order.) If despite such efforts the defendant were convicted and jailed, patients sometimes mounted demonstrations of support for the wronged party and even organized parades to celebrate the chiropractor's release when the sentence was up; a 1922 procession in Wichita Falls, Texas, was a "fifteen-block spectacle." The following year, the governor of Ohio intervened to allow a chiropractor who had been jailed for practicing without a license to continue to treat one of his patients, a child who was brought to him in his cell![34]

In most cases, however, spectacles and judicial interventions were unnecessary, as only a small percentage of jury trials went against chiropractors. Jurors generally related to patients who swore that adjustments had helped them and sympathized with arguments that the prohibition of chiropractic was a violation of sacred democratic principles. That explains the reaction of a Massachusetts judge who sentenced a chiropractor to thirty days in jail after a judicial hearing; when the defendant threatened to appeal for a jury trial, the judge suspended his sentence with the explanation that "juries never convict chiropractors." Certainly "almost never" was an accurate enough assessment. One Texas chiropractor, for example, went to trial sixty-six times and lost only once.[35]

When chiropractors did go to jail, they found, as Palmer had in 1906, that it was good for business. Publicly suffering for defending the people's freedom against a monopolistic medical profession was positive press, and chiropractors made the most of it. In the early 1920s there was even a "Go to Jail for Chiropractic" movement, originating in California and spreading across the country, that applied professional pressure for convicted practitioners to follow Old Dad Chiro's example and insist on being incarcerated rather than paying a fine. In at least one instance, a number of chiropractors marched off to jail together singing "Onward Christian Soldiers." Later in that decade an American Bureau of Chiropractic (the ABC) was founded to further educate the public about chiropractic and "to organize laymen to secure and maintain legal recognition" of the system. By 1932 an ABC rally in Madison Square Garden could attract over twelve thousand attendees. Legal counsel, not just laymen, organized for the chiropractic cause, too, with a former lieutenant governor of Wisconsin, Thomas Morris, leading a team that specialized in defending chiropractors throughout the country.[36]

All elements of virtuous chiropractic's courageous struggle against allopathic exploitation of the American people were brought together in particularly engaging form by W. H. Rafferty, DC, in a twenty-one-page novelette composed apparently in the 1920s. Health and Love a la Chiropractic tells the inspiring story of Gracie Woody, beautiful child of a widowed mother, paralyzed by a fall from a playground swing and told by her Wisconsin town's most prominent allopath, "There is absolutely nothing I can do." Sent away from Mercy Hospital in a wheelchair to "her own little home where her Mother toiled over the wash tub," Gracie one day chanced to read a pamphlet that had been pushed under their humble door. It was an announcement of the services provided by a Dr. Justor, the town's newly arrived chiropractor.

(Justor's first name is never disclosed, but it has to have been Ad, perhaps a nickname for Admirable.) With nothing to lose, Gracie's mother took her to see this new type of doctor and was told after an "analysis" that adjustments might help. "Mrs. Woody was too poor to pay," needless to say, "but the Chiropractor waved that objection aside."[37]

The plot darkened that evening when little Gracie was visited by Ella Goodman, the nurse from Mercy Hospital who had vowed to do all she could to make the disabled child's existence tolerable. Being a "refined creature and lovable piece of humanity," Ella held her "rising . . . wrath" within when Gracie told of her visit to Justor, but the very next day she stormed into the chiropractor's office "with fury snapping in her eyes" and venom dripping from her tongue over this charlatan's "presumption to raise such hopes in one so trusting when the best of science knew it to be an utter impossibility." But just as she was poised to strike, "their eyes met. . . . Just for the moment there was that flash from eye to eye that Innate alone knows—the flash of understanding; 'You are the one I am looking for—you are mine.' " The moment passed all too quickly, but so did Nurse Goodman's skepticism as "this young man['s] . . . very sincerity and determination disarmed her." To make the short story even shorter, Goodman ends up getting fired from the hospital when she defends Justor to her allopathic supervisor (he diagnoses her as being "infested with quackitis"), while Gracie responds to the adjustments applied to her third lumbar first by wiggling a toe, then, after several weeks, standing, next walking, and ultimately "she even romped." That, thinks Justor, should "impress a certain little spitfire of a nurse."[38]

The chiropractor's reward for his miracle, of course, is to be arrested, detained on a warrant instigated by Ella Goodman's former supervisor, who was determined that Justor would be made "to suffer for his crime of getting people well without a license." As soon as word of this injustice got out, "quite a few of his patients . . . came forward and offered bond." Justor had no need of their help, however, because he had retained "the wonderful Tom Morris [who] had fought in every court of the land for the rights of the sick." For a man such as Morris the trial was child's play. First he tricked the "State's star witness" into admitting he was one of those spotters or sneaks, a man "hired by the medical interests to get evidence against the Chiropractor." Then he called patient after patient to testify that Justor had cured them without the use of drugs or surgery. In concluding, Morris argued that "the laws that were supposed to protect the people had been misused to deprive them of ways and means to get rid of their ills." It was no surprise, then, that the jury took "just twenty minutes to decide that an adjustment was not a treatment—that Chiropractic was not medicine; that it was personal hatred and not a desire to protect the dear people that was responsible for Justor being hauled before the court." Justor's exoneration was "another victory for humanity, another step toward medical freedom," one more "victory over the Great Medical Trust." (There is an even happier ending in store for Justor, it must be told. Won over by chiropractic, Ella Goodman is in Davenport during Justor's trial, enrolled in the Palmer School. As soon as he is freed, Justor rushes to Iowa to attend the annual reunion and hear B. J. Palmer's lecture on how chiropractic "will liberate mankind from the tyranny of drugs and the knife." Afterward, Justor finally gets Ella alone and confesses he is in torment from a subluxation of the heart. " 'Can you adjust it?' fervently. 'I cannot.' 'Why?' disparagingly. 'I am only a junior,' coquettishly. 'Look at me you Minx. I love you. . . . Say that you love me; that you will be my wife.' 'I do love you and I will be your wife—oh!—you impulsive boy. Let me get my breath.' The End.")[39]

Through popular education projects such as *Health and Love* and the concerted political activities of the American Bureau of Chiropractic, the fledgling profession steadily succeeded in winning licensing protection throughout the country. Kansas fell into line first, in 1913, and over the next decade the total climbed to twenty-two. In some states, chiropractors were able to win recognition as midwives as well as manipulators, following the example of other alternative systems in promoting their approach as surer and safer than allopathic obstetrics, as indeed a method of natural childbirth. D. D. Palmer himself recommended chiropractic adjustments for women brought to bed, though his son stated the point much more forcefully. "Instead of 72 hours of excrutiating pain, tears, lacerations, and often, death," B. J. Palmer declared, chiropractic care "makes childbirth as easy as a nice clean movement of the bowels. . . . Spinal adjustments make it like a pleasant dream." During the 1920s twenty-five more states and the District of Columbia enacted chiropractic licensing laws, so that eventually opponents could despair that "there is a chiropractor at every cross-roads, and in such sinks of imbecility as Los Angeles they are as thick as bootleggers." Not until 1974, however, were chiropractic licensing laws in effect in all fifty states.[40]

Internal Dissension

Like the osteopaths, early twentieth-century chiropractors fought as viciously among themselves as against regulars, fomenting their own version of the "straight" versus "mixer" conflict. Initially, internecine strife centered on adjustment technique, virtually every practitioner finding through trial and error particular ways of manipulating subluxations that worked best for her or him; there were, among other refinements, the Meric, the Torque-Toggle-Recoil, and the H-I-O (Hole-in-One) methods. Some felt their techniques were different enough from those of Palmer as to constitute a distinct system. Such, for example, was neuropathy, the hybrid of chiropractic, osteopathy, and ophthalmology created by A. P. Davis, the second graduate of D. D. Palmer's school. Such also was naprapathy, a splinter group appearing in 1906 that utilized variations on "the traditional Bohemian manipulative arts." There were "impassioned controversies" over these offshoots (Palmer expressed "pity for the ignorance of the author" of neuropathy, whose system was "a mongrel of . . . many breeds"), but these disagreements were as nothing compared to the fireworks set off when some chiropractors decided that all the adjustment techniques in the world couldn't cure everything.[41]

Quite early on, a practitioner named John Howard realized that there were "many conditions to meet [and] pathological tissue changes to overcome which are beyond the reach of spinal technic." To maintain that there were "no limitations" to the power of adjustment, he asserted, "is beyond the scope of truth or reason." By 1915, a textbook of chiropractic could scold the Discoverer for being "overzealous" in promoting adjustment as a panacea. "Naturally," the author continued, "such views could not be subscribed to by anyone with a liberal training in the sciences underlying the art of healing, and especially, one with a knowledge of pathology. . . . Had he possessed such knowledge, he would not have made the claims which he did. . . . Broader views now obtain among the profession as a whole."[42]

"Broader views" meant a broader range of therapies that many chiropractors employed as supplements to vertebral adjustment. A full spectrum of physical methods came into use: massage, vibration, hydrotherapy, electrical stimulation, heat treatments, and so on. Many of these modalities involved the use of mechanical devices and thus struck purist practitioners as perversions of genuine chiropractic; the word meant "done by hand," after all. The use of "mechanical accessories," of "adjuncts," became a hotly controverted issue among chiropractors by the 1910s. "Straights," the disciples of Palmer and simple adjustment, saw "mixers" as dupes of "high-pressure salesmen" of gimcrack machines. Worse, they were traitors, or, in Old Dad Chiro's opinion, "unprincipled shysters," "kleptomaniac scavengers," and "grafters and vampires" who had sold their birthright as "Kiro Kids" to chase after "foul, unclean, filthy, unwholesome" methods; "who would have ever thot [sic] that Chiropractic would have got in such a mixup?" Palmer's feelings were echoed by other defenders of "P., S. & U. chiropractic" (pure, straight, and unadulterated). A "P., S. & U." chiropractor, as described by a 1920 promotion for the Universal Chiropractors' Association (the straights' national organization) "*knows* that the Supreme Architect and builder designed and built the human body and that when the machine does not run properly an adjustment is all that is required." He would never "prostitute his science for money," and in his office would be found no "catch-penny devices . . . no hot lamps to warm the chilly; no violet rays to counteract the blues; no stretching machines to make the short lengthen; no dietetic fads to find the food a weakened stomach will digest; no salts, sulphur or electric baths to forcibly eliminate the poisons; no vibrators to stir the sluggish into life." "To whatever extent one believes in such devices," another straight remonstrated, "he disbelieves in chiropractic."[43]

In reply, mixers ridiculed the narrow-minded backwardness of straights' beliefs. "Is this really the Philosophy of some Chiropractors?"—that "every disease from crabs to leprosy is cured" by adjustment, or that "live gonococci are as innocent as babes in arms, but dead ones, in the shape of a vaccine, kill you quicker than a train. . . . We regret to say, it is." Mixers, those of "broad, liberal and scientific" views, had a "duty to enlighten others" and bring chiropractic into the twentieth century. Adjustment was fine as far as it went, but one could "elevate it" with adjunctive therapies, particularly "the Twentieth Century Appliances" one college of the mixer persuasion boasted; a partial list included "the Solar Therapeutic Lamp and the Electric Light Bath Cabinet, . . . the Arc Lamp, Centrifugal Vibrator, Diet Indicator, Kellogg Douche, Home Douche, Dynometer, Hand Photophore, Kneading Apparatus, Massage Table, Sinusoidal Apparatus, Thermophore and Vibratory Chair." Not least, it would appear, was "the Ampliathrill," whose purpose was to achieve "spinal extension"; it was stated to be "the greatest auxiliary for use in Spinal Treatment of the Twentieth Century," though it is difficult to see how it could surpass the Au-to-chiro-practor, an instrument resembling the medieval rack, by which one could perform spinal adjustments upon oneself. Through Ampliathrills and Au-to-chiro-practors, mixers expanded the meaning of adjustment to embrace the whole patient, not just her backbone. In one proponent's formulation, the full meaning of adjustment was "adjustment of environment, adjustment of the mode of living, and adjustment of contributory causative factors."[44]

Given such house-divided instability, it is something of a wonder that chiropractors were able to obtain licensing laws as quickly as they did, though naturally the range of therapies they were permitted varied from state to state. And, as with osteopathy, the mixer orientation came to dominate. A 1930 survey in which some 1,800 chiropractors participated, found, for example, that 1,124 employed hydrotherapy, 1,173 used light therapy, 1,257 provided electrotherapy, and a full 1,352 trusted in vibration therapy. Alteration of the Discoverer's doctrine extended beyond practice, moreover, to the abandonment of original chiropractic's mystical core. Although "P., S., & U." practitioners maintained their faith in Innate and in their art as a path to spiritual enlightenment ("Chiropractic has investigated and explained that mysterious and elusive thing men call the Soul," one proclaimed, making it "the grandest truth of history"), mixers were inclined to think of Innate Intelligence as electricity or "nerve force." Gradually, use of the term "Innate" disappeared altogether, the soul being pushed aside in favor of the spine as a physical entity that chiropractors had special practical skills at fixing.[45]

B. J. Palmer

One final factor in the dissolution of the original version of chiropractic has to be considered. B. (for Bartlett) J. (for Joshua) Palmer was D. D.'s son by marriage number two, born in 1881 and, by his account, subjected to a wretched childhood. His mother died before he was two, leaving him "at the mercy of three cruel stepmothers, each worse than the one before," and in the hands of a father who alternated neglect with whippings. (He and his sisters "got beatings with strops until we carried welts, for which our father was often arrested and spent nights in jail"; the unfortunate boy thought of himself as "a derelict football being kicked around.") B. J. often was turned out to sleep in the cold, on Mississippi piers or in alleyway crates, and after being permanently expelled from school at age thirteen (for trying to look up female students' skirts), he survived only through income from odd jobs such as scrubbing floors and cleaning spittoons. Not surprisingly, he turned into "a no-account kid-bum . . . one worthless hunk of degenerate boy." From the age of five onward, he claimed improbably, he was a "confirmed and habitual sex-drunkard, dead drunk in the sexual gutter," unaware at such a tender age "that masturbation was the thief of brain food [and] destroyed mental values."[46]

Yet ill used as he was, B. J. followed in Father's footsteps, first working as an assistant in a traveling mesmerism/vaudeville show, then enrolling as a student of chiropractic in D. D.'s school and graduating in 1902. Several months later, when his father suddenly moved to Portland, Oregon, to open another school, Palmer took over the management of the Davenport institution and transformed it into a thriving business. To be sure, the elder Palmer attempted to wrest control of the business back from his son when he returned to Davenport in 1904 from his school-founding ventures in Oregon and Oklahoma. The best he could manage, however, was a partnership with B. J., and even that was lost with his imprisonment in 1906. On being released from jail, the father discovered that through legal maneuvering his son had obtained complete control of the school and would not even allow him to set foot on campus. Insult was then heaped upon injury when that same year B. J. published a textbook—*The Science of Chiropractic*—that D. D. maintained was his own work. "He used to cherish, revere and worship his father's manuscript," the Discoverer related, "so much so, that he rummaged his father's waste basket in order to secure" the material he used for the text; "40 articles, written by my own hand and original with me . . . have been garbled, mutilated and copyrighted by B. J. Palmer." They had been sold, too, marketed as a volume "of unintelligible 'jargonity' . . . not worth the paper they have worse than wasted." It was "an insane effort of a disordered brain" (though only to be expected from a former sex-drunkard), and D. D. found it deeply painful "that my only son would play the Judas, . . . rob me financially and of credit justly due me."[47]

D. D. tried to get back at the ungrateful child, dedicating his own 1910 textbook to B. J. with the tongue-in-cheek hope "that he may honestly and uprightly teach Chiropractic," then returning time and again in the body of the work to excoriate him, charging that "no one Chiropractor has done as much to vitiate, deprave and pervert the principles and philosophy" of chiropractic. The true founder of the healing science was now, however, "advanced in years," as well as "somewhat broken in spirit by acts of traitors," and his days were not to be long. Palmer had left Iowa when turned out by his son, bouncing about from one state to another opening new and short-lived schools. In 1913 he returned to Davenport for the last time, intent on leading a homecoming parade for the now flourishing school he had founded years before. According to one account, B. J. had his father removed from the procession when he refused to ride in an automobile and be sheltered from the sun; according to another, B. J. struck his father with his automobile when he refused to leave. The latter was D. D.'s version, as told in the lawsuit filed when he died three months later in California allegedly from the "reckless, wanton, malicious, intentional, grossly negligent" actions of his son (who, in accord with one of Palmer's last wishes, was barred from attending his father's funeral). Even in death, D. D. was no match for B. J.; the charge was dropped by the grand jury as without merit.[48]

"Like father, like son" nevertheless applied to the pair at least with respect to personality: "The egotism of the man passeth all understanding," one allopath wrote of B. J. ("M.D. Means More Dope—More Death," Palmer shot back.) Indeed, it was that self-esteem, paired with a commercial instinct that would have brought a smile to Barnum, that allowed the younger Palmer to earn the title of the Developer and lead chiropractic to a position of prominence far above what the Discoverer had been able to accomplish. He was an entrepreneurial dynamo, a shrewd eye-on-the-main-chance man whose dictum that the spine supports three things—the head, the ribs, and the chiropractor—was given gilded practical demonstration through every available medium.[49]

At the forefront of Palmer's development projects was the Davenport school he usurped from his father, an institution that when he took it over had only twenty-one students but by 1920 had surpassed two thousand and was not merely the largest of the many schools of chiropractic in America but the largest school of any system of healing in the world. There a faculty of more than twenty experienced DCs (including that "attractive little lady" the director's wife, Mabel, professor of anatomy) put students through a course of study running sixteen months, raised to eighteen in 1921 to qualify graduates to meet the licensing requirements of a greater number of states. Students were drawn to Davenport by advertisements identifying the "Chiropractic Fountain Head" as "the foremost institution of its kind in the world," whose faculty were "the very best brains it is possible to obtain in the Chiropractic world," whose diploma was "the gold standard certificate of efficiency in Chiropractic science," and whose director was a "master-mind." The provision of free adjustments for any student in poor health added to the school's allure, and one can well understand how so many succumbed to the call of "The Trail of the Lonesome Spine." "There's a place on Earth where Truth is taught," a PSC student rhapsodized in 1917;

> Where joy and peace for all is [sic] bought
> There the spirit of brotherly love is caught
> And man to man is the power sought.
> It's a home of love and joy divine,
> At the end of the trail of the Lonesome Spine.[50]

The most attractive facet of the Palmer School of Chiropractic, however, was that it trained its students to be more than chiropractors, to be chiropractic businessmen. "The student is here taught how to act with patients, how to act in and out of the office, how to successfully advertise, etc., and in many other ways is given instruction which is of untold benefit to him in a financial way." Note the ordering of the beneficiaries of PSC training as presented in the school's *Annual Announcement* for 1921: "Our graduates . . . know how best to use [chiropractic] for advantage to themselves and benefit to their patients." ("A year ago one of our students earned $2 a day as a common laborer," one ad for the Palmer School's home study course stated. "Now he has a practice of 30 patients a day who each pay him $5 a week, $150 a week; $7,800 a year!") Even before graduating, in fact, after only eight months of study, "students are granted permission to solicit patients outside of clinic, which cases they may adjust for pay." Successful solicitation was assured by the course titled "Salesmanship," a month of "intensive study" of such disciplines as "Personal Magnetism," "Developing the Will," "Business Relations," "Advertising," "Selling the Patient," and "Keeping Yourself Sold." Completion of the course earned one "a special diploma on 'Personal Efficiency,'" a guarantee of quickly recouping one's tuition payment of $350, "spot cash at hour of enrollment" ("husband and wife . . . $437.50"). Palmer was reported to have explained to a chiropractic convention in Montana that "our school back at Davenport is established on a business and not a professional basis. It is a business where we manufacture chiropractors. . . . We teach them the idea and then we show them how to sell it."[51]

Regular practitioners frowned upon advertising as unethical and unprofessional, so for them the selling of chiropractic was perhaps the most distasteful of all the system's excesses. (It was so excessive that even other alternative practitioners were offended: "The whole world has been flooded with the exaggerated claims of the chiroporactor," a naturopath complained in the 1920s; "no patent nostrum ever received one tenth the amount of advertising as has Chiropractic.") Chiropractors, however, saw self-promotion as essential for financial success and thought of success in the public market as the surest demonstration of truth and merit. Further, as the quickest way to make people aware of the health-giving virtues of chiropractic, advertising was in essence a public service. Churches advertised their services, so "should Chiropractic, which is just as good for the *body* as *religion* is for the *soul*, hesitate to do likewise?" Granted, "the poker joint, the opium den and the red light district do not proclaim themselves to the world," and if allopaths preferred to follow "the same silent tactics," one could hardly blame them. But chiropractors, like Christ, had a moral duty "to go out into the world and proclaim the gospel."[52]

"Early to bed and early to rise—Work like hell and advertise": that was the gospel according to B. J. Palmer, who painted the walls of PSC with that and similar motivational slogans. ("The world is your cow—but you must do the milking.") His teachings had the hoped-for effect. As a pupil from Massachusetts remembered, "B. J. had the students so they could hardly wait until they could get out into practice, to carry chiropractic to the world, and to get sick people well. He filled us with enthusiasm and self-confidence. . . . We were 'miracle'." The inspirational influence of Palmer (who in young adulthood bore an uncanny resemblance to the Jesus of classical depiction) was hardly confined to the classroom, however. B. J. was also the mastermind behind Lyceum, an early form of continuing education program held in Davenport every summer from the early 1910s through the 1950s. A week of lectures, demonstrations, motivational talks, and entertainments culminating in a grand ball, Lyceum was "a gathering of the chiropractic clans." Literally thousands of practitioners (eight thousand in 1921, for example) and their families returned to the Fountainhead at Lyceum time, and it was there, fittingly, that Ella Goodman at last adjusted Justor's heart. (It was also for Lyceum that D. D. Palmer made his fateful 1913 visit to Davenport.) Even if one were unable to make it to Lyceum, all was not lost, for PSC's radio station WOC broadcast the "Wonders of Chiropractic" every day. (One of the five most powerful private radio stations in the world in its time and listened to by more than a million people daily, WOC was the setting in which a young sportscaster named Ronald Reagan began his public career.)[53]

"The only principle added [to chiropractic] by B. J. Palmer," his father wrote, "was that of greed and graft," and eventually B. J.'s greed brought him down. At the 1924 Lyceum, Palmer announced the availability of a new diagnostic device, the neurocalometer, an electrical instrument that supposedly measured (meter) the heat (calo) released by nerves (neuro). According to chiropractic theory, nerves impinged upon by a subluxation became inflamed, which meant that at the level of the spine where the subluxation existed there should be a higher temperature on the impingement side than on the other side of that vertebra. The probe of the neurocalometer was to be slowly moved down the spinal column; when it registered a temperature differential, there must exist a subluxation on the side of higher temperature. By making it possible to detect even the slightest subluxation, the device would revolutionize chiropractic diagnosis and treatment. Such, anyway, was B. J.'s prediction.[54]

Most of his Lyceum audience had a somewhat less sanguine reaction to the neurocalometer. First, Palmer had long been the recognized leader of "S., P. & U." chiropractic. The use of machinery and instruments, however, was one of the trademarks of mixers, what with their vibrators and heat lamps and electrical stimulators. "Your Neurocalometer is an adjunct pure and simple," an outraged DC wrote Palmer. "It is a perversion of all that YOU HAVE advocated heretofore, and through which I was made a 'straight' chiropractor, with thousands of others. It is a slap in your dead father's face." But equally disturbing was Palmer's scheme for introducing the device into practice. It was not to be sold outright but to be leased—from B. J. Palmer—for an advance payment of one thousand dollars followed by monthly installments of ten dollars for a minimum of ten years. The contract stipulated that lessees had to charge patients a minimum of ten dollars per reading, and the machine was not to be offered to members of the recently formed American Chiropractic Association, the national organization for mixers. (This was the scheme of the man who had once defined mixing as a disease whose chief symptom was "an itching in the palm.")[55]

Two thousand chiropractors signed up for neurocalometers within a year, and more than a few others purchased imitations quickly brought to market by opportunists under such trademarks as Neurothermometer, Neuropyrometer, and even Hotbox Indicator. Many more members of the profession, however, reacted vehemently to Palmer's blatant money grab, the most remarkable response coming from B. J.'s own student body, three-fourths of whom withdrew; enrollment at PSC plummeted from more than twenty-three hundred in 1922 to less than five hundred by 1927. Many of those students moved on to a new institution opened in Indianapolis by disaffected faculty from the Palmer School. Attendance at Lyceum also fell off drastically, from the thousands into the hundreds, and although Palmer would continue to make himself prominent among the straights in the profession, his position of dominance had been lost.[56]

Palmer's shameless boosterism tainted chiropractic with a shady mercenary image the profession still struggles to outlive. Yet at the same time, by generating so many new practitioners and attracting so much public attention, his efforts were critical for establishing solid footing for chiropractic within the American medical system. (By 1930, it was estimated, nearly two million Americans a year were receiving adjustments, including a number of athletic celebrities such as Jack Dempsey.) As part of the professional reaction against B. J. Palmer's commercialism, moreover, more serious steps began to be taken in the 1930s to elevate the standards of chiropractic education and practice and lift the profession to a level of respectability during the second half of the century. That development, however, is part of a larger story of alternative medical reformation that must be set aside until another major unorthodox school of healing of the early 1900s—naturopathy—is examined.[57]

9

Therapeutic Universalism: Naturopathy

Toward the end of the 1840s, a young German man who had ruined his health through overstudy for the priesthood came across a volume on hydropathy. Desperate to repair a "withered body" that, according to two regular physicians, was already "on the brink of the grave," Sebastian Kneipp threw himself into the water-cure regimen. Slowly his strength returned, eventually to the point that he could renew his studies and gain ordination. Once a priest, he was assigned to Wörishofen, a remote settlement west of Munich. There parishioners petitioned him to save their sickened frames as he had his own, and water-cure, the "life-boat sent to me by a merciful Providence," worked the same wonders for them. As word spread, Wörishofen began to exert as magnetic a pull on Continental health-seekers as Graefenberg had in an earlier day.[1]

Although inspired by the Priessnitz program of therapy, Kneippism was not simply a restatement of hydropathy. Many of the latter's cold water baths were adopted, to be sure, but Kneipp added hot baths, steam baths, and "gushes" (applications of water to a specific area of the body via a garden watering can; later the garden hose was used). Further, the priest's reading in other natural healing traditions, tested by self-experimentation, had opened his eyes to the therapeutic virtues of plants, and he not only mixed certain botanicals into warm baths but administered herbs orally as well, in the form of teas, extracts, oils, and powders.[2]

Kneipp's understanding of how water healed was essentially the same as Priessnitz's; it dissolved and evacuated "morbid matters," he imagined, and it also served "to strengthen the organism." The second effect was particularly important, to his way of thinking, as modern people were unusually susceptible to sickness due to the softening effects of civilization: "The effemination of

191

the people living now-a-days has reached a high degree." The people needed to undergo "hardening." Their primitive vigor had to be restored through exercise and frequent immersions in cold water; even infants were to be given a quick cold water dip every morning to forestall effeminacy. Most effective of all hardening measures, however, were ninety-minute barefoot walks in snow, when available, or else over wet grass. (Farmers around Wörishofen often complained about their crops being trampled by Kneipp's unshod hordes.)[3]

Kneippism clearly was no walk in the park, yet despite its chilling rigors it attracted thousands of patrons of every social class from peasant to pope (Leo XIII). Kneipp spas sprang up throughout Germany and in neighboring countries, and when the founder published *Meine Wasserkur (My Water-Cure)* in 1882, it was an immediate best-seller that was soon translated into fourteen languages and went through a hundred printings. By the 1890s it could be said without too much exaggeration that "the eyes of the whole civilized world look with admiration on the aged pastor of the humble Bavarian village." Nor did the system's popularity end with Kneipp's death in 1897. His village, today known as Bad Wörishofen, after the style of German spa towns generally, remains one of the most popular *Bads* in Europe, hosting seventy-thousand guests annually. Kneipp herbal bath products still sell well, too.[4]

Origins of Naturopathy

In the early 1890s another German youth found himself on the brink of the grave. In this instance, however, the man—Benedict Lust (1872–1945; Fig. 9.1)—was a recent immigrant to America, having come to New York in 1892 to seek his fortune only to find tuberculosis instead. Given up to die by allopaths ("my death warrant was made out by the doctors in my presence"), he decided to return to his homeland for what days he had left, and there he was attracted to the invalid's haven of Wörishofen. Eight months later he was once again in possession of full health and resolved to use his new strength as an emissary of Kneipp to the New World; indeed, the priest/healer "commissioned" him, Lust said, to "go into the new World and spread the Gospel of the Water Cure."[5]

Lust returned to New York in 1896 and set about fulfilling his commission right away. Part of his responsibility, he believed, was to make the healing system more accessible to Americans. Several Kneipp cures had already been established in the early 1890s, but they were restricted to German immigrant communities and made no appeal to the broader populace; initially, the only public notice taken of American Kneippists was ridicule of their barefoot strolls through Central Park. Thus while Lust began his health publishing ventures

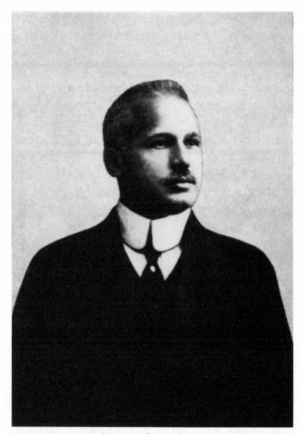

Figure 9-1. Benedict Lust [Benedict Lust, *Universal Naturopathic Encyclopedia Directory and Buyer's Guide Year Book of Drugless Therapy for 1918–19* (Butler, NJ: Lust, 1918), frontispiece]

in the mid-'90s with German-language periodicals, in 1900 he switched to English with his *Kneipp Water Cure Monthly* (though he maintained a small German-language section in each issue). The magazine was different from other Kneipp publications with respect to content as well, for Lust had acquired a faith in several therapies beyond those employed in Wörishofen. Before leaving Germany the second time, he had looked into a number of other components of the rich tradition of "nature cure" that had flourished in that country since early in the century. Various programs of diet, exercise, massage, sunbathing, and other drugless options impressed him as valuable additions to Kneipp's baths and herbs, so the system of care that he publicized in his magazine and provided at the clinic he opened in New York stretched well beyond the boundaries of Kneippism. Even the American-born practices of osteopathy and chiropractic were embraced by Lust (he earned a DO degree in 1898), and it was soon evident that Kneippism was too limited and misleading a designation for his collection of natural remedies. Just how he came up with a new name is not entirely clear (there are several accounts), but by 1901 Lust was calling his approach to healing "naturopathy." (Literally meaning "nature disease," the name was disapproved of by many of Lust's followers, who preferred more accurate designations such as "nature cure," "natural therapeutics," or "physiatrics"; "naturopathy" was the name that stuck, however.) The following year he founded the Naturopathic Society of America (renamed the American Naturopathic Association in 1919), and he served as the organization's only president until his death.[6]

Naturopathic Philosophy

In March 1901 Lust opened the American School of Naturopathy in midtown Manhattan. The first educational institution for the training of practitioners in the new field, it conferred the degree of ND (Naturopathic Doctor) on graduates of its two-term, eighteen-month curriculum. The approach to healing that was taught at the school is presented nicely in a "tree of disease" designed by another leader of naturopathy in the 1910s. There one sees the full range of human infirmities, from colds to cancer, growing out of a trunk impaired by "Accumulation of Morbid Matter in The System" and other disordered states of vitality. The soil from which the trunk of physical impurity rises is one of "Violation of Nature's Laws" of diet, exercise, and other components of hygiene, violations occurring because of humanity's ignorance, indifference, lack of self-control, and self-indulgence. Where regular doctors blamed disease on insults to the body from outside, particularly infection with germs, early naturopaths saw all sickness originating within the body. (Note among the tree's branches that "Germs, Bacteria" are listed as a disease, not a cause.) Rather than the individual being attacked by some alien pathologic agent, each person was responsible for attacking his own body with unnatural habits of life. In brief, all diseases were fundamentally the same, internal poisoning, and thus all therapy had to be directed toward inner cleansing. Nature attempts to eliminate morbid material on her own but sometimes is so overwhelmed by the products of self-indulgence as to require assistance.[7]

Imposing self-control and returning to nature's intended mode of life (hygeiotherapy, in other words) was a necessary first step but was not always sufficient. Then active measures to rid the body of impurities had to be brought into play—but only measures that were friendly to nature by offering support or stimulation. A fundamental principle for naturopathy was that drugs were unfriendly—by definition. Drugs were poison, and to use poison to fight the poison of disease was pitting "Beelzebub against the Devil": "Say Doc," a young boy in a 1913 naturopathic cartoon asks, "does that M.D. you sign after your name stand for much dope?" More than any other system of the early twentieth century, naturopathy utilized and identified with the term "drugless healing": "Drugs have no place in the human body," Lust insisted; "GIVING A SICK MAN THINGS TO MAKE HIM WELL THAT WOULD MAKE A WELL MAN SICK IS STUPID, IGNORANT AND CRIMINAL." ("Criminal" was not just rhetoric for Lust; in one of his more agitated moments he demanded that the drug poisoner should be "where he belongs—in the electric chair or at the end of a rope.") Contempt for drugs did not, however, prevent naturopaths from using healing herbs, remedies that many others thought of as drugs. To their way of thinking, herbs were a gift from heaven (Lust bowed before "Our Lord's Kindness in the Healing Herbs"); they grew from the bosom of nature and were employed in their natural state, not chemically altered or synthesized in the pharmaceutical laboratory by "chuckle-headed scientists [who] believe they are a whale of a lot bigger than Nature herself."[8]

But botanicals had to share space in the naturopathic armamentarium with any number of other restorative agents. An official definition of naturopathy adopted in 1907 included "mechanical, physical, mental and [twenty-seven] spiritual methods, such as mechanical and physical vibration, massage, manipulation, adjustment, electricity, magnetism, earth, water, air, sun and electric light, hot and cold, moist and dry baths, fasting, dieting, physical culture, suggestive therapeutics," and anything else that could be interpreted to strengthen the *vis medicatrix naturae* or remove obstacles to its free functioning; naturopathy, Lust dictated, was a system of "Pathological Monism and Therapeutic Universalism," by which he meant there was only one disease (inhibition of the body's "natural power") but a virtual infinity of healing agents (all of nature's forces).[9]

Healing interventions were not limited to physical modalities, however, for naturopathy was understood to mean not just trusting in nature to heal but striving to return to one's proper place within the natural creation. The "principal object" of naturopathy was "to re-establish the union of man's body, brain, heart and all bodily functions—with nature." True well-being required mental and spiritual health as well, so students also had to master such areas as "Mental and Divine Healing, . . . New Thought, Self-Culture, Mental Regeneration, . . . Pure Love, Soul-Marriage, Pre-Natal Culture, Painless Parturition, . . . Natural Babyhood, Child Culture," and the on-the-face-of-it dubious discipline of "Passionless Fatherhood." For the soul, there were "Physical Immortalism, Spirit-Unfoldment, [and] God-Consciousness."[10]

The same year he established his school, Lust expanded on the philosophy of naturopathic healing in an editorial in *The Naturopath and Herald of
Health*, the recently revised title of his *Kneipp Monthly*. Naturopathy, he explained, aimed for wholeness for its clients. The reason for including such
subjects as self-culture, pure love, and spirit-unfoldment alongside hydropathy
and osteopathy was that the naturopath's goal should be not simply to cure
illness but to promote "ideal living" (or what in recent times has been called
high-level wellness). "Within every human," naturopaths believed, was the
potential for "Massive Muscle, Surging Blood, Tingling Nerve, Zestful Digestion, Superb Sex, Beautiful Body, Sublime Thought, Pulsating Power, . . .
Glorious Freedom, Perpetual Peace, Limitless Unfoldment, and Conscious
Godhood. May These Things Be!" For such things to be, however, people
had to "want to LIVE," Lust exhorted his readers, to live "from your growing
brain to your glowing toes—to conquer Disease and Death—to forget physicians—to roll off the burden of Time—to be free to work out the great,
broad, beautiful destiny that awaits you."[11]

Ideal living was more, of course, than glowing toes and a beautiful
destiny. Ultimately the good life was the moral life. Early naturopathy was
energized by religious undercurrents every bit as powerful as have been seen
with osteopathy and chiropractic, and they frequently surged to the surface.
They were, in fact, much the same currents as those that had flowed through
hygeiotherapy, carrying the conviction that the laws of health were divine
commandments whose honoring earned good favor from the Lord and whose
violation brought punishment: "There is a decalogue and a morality of the
physical," naturopathic educator Henry Lindlahr proclaimed, "as well as of
the spiritual." Lust looked back even beyond the Mosaic commandments, to
the Garden, to frame his physical theology. In Eden, "man did not suffer from
sickness" but lived in perfect health on "what mother Earth produced." Then
came the Fall, an act of disobedience that involved, after all, "a forbidden
meal," an act of unnatural hygiene. Adam and Eve were expelled, and "man
no more remained in direct connection with the earth. . . . In the same measure
as man grew more unnatural and sinful, sickness and all misery arose."[12]

It was not actually a case of unnatural *and* sinful, but unnatural *then*
sinful, for breaking nature's laws of hygiene corroded the spirit as relentlessly
as the body. Early-century naturopaths often sounded like a born-again Trall
in their declarations that not only all bodily infirmity was due to "transgression
of natural law" but "all . . . poverty, misery, worry, vice and crime" as well.
The naturopath, one testified, "believes in his system not only as a science
and an art, but as *a religion that will, if followed, lead humanity to the heaven
of health and happiness*." Thus while MDs might find "the wrenching of a
paltry fee from a trembling patient" enough to satisfy their needs (this is Lust

speaking), NDs could rest content with nothing less than the "loving into wholeness of a triumphant brother." In that context, it was possible for naturopaths to suggest in complete seriousness that one "consider for a moment the greatest Naturopath—Christ." From that perspective, it made sense for Lust to put forward the revolutionary import of his system by observing that approximately every five hundred years a great spiritual upheaval had occurred in Western civilization, beginning with Christ and followed by Muhammad, the Crusades, the Reformation—and now naturopathy. As recently as 1951, a naturopathic text cited "The Holy Bible" as the first item in its bibliography.[13]

Nevertheless, the building of physical vitality was the critical first step toward triumphant life. "With a strong, healthy physique," Lust promised, "man can acquire riches, can conquer the world, can build character, can develop soul-life, in a word, may attain to whatever his heart desires." With health, "his body . . . is in harmony with mind and soul which show him the right way to the wished-for aims." The road to health was paved by the various therapies that reinforced nature's healing power, but fundamental to naturopathic care, as it had been to hygeiotherapy, was education of the public in right ways of living, overthrowing "the unholy trinity of ignorance, self-ishness and self-indulgence." "The naturopathic physician . . . the physician of the future . . . is also a teacher," Lust explained. "He teaches his patients and the public how to live and maintain health"; he teaches "the art of becoming masters of our bodies."[14]

Naturopathic Practice

One could learn the rules of self-mastery from the articles in Lust's monthly journal, which was pitched as much to the laity as to other naturopaths, and could acquire the tools to practice self-improvement at Lust's "health store" in New York, where "a rich and varied stock of health foods" was sold along with health equipment ("vibragenitors, body conformers, respirators, and so forth") and health clothing. The most touted item in the last category was the "health underwear" modeled after vegetable-fiber garments designed by Kneipp as elements of his hardening regime. Lust believed in hardening, too, agreeing that the modes of life fostered by urban, industrial civilization conspired to sap strength and undermine vitality. "Humanity today is an aggregation of bald-heads, glass eyes, false teeth, and wooden heads," he railed, and all because "denatured, devitalized foods, gluttony, sensuality, high heels, corsets, drugs, tobacco, alcohol, over-clothing, over-work, worry, fear, anxiety, etc., is [sic] rapidly sapping the strength of hyper-civilized man." Thus the need for Porous Health Underwear. "Harden your body and learn to enjoy the invigorating winter winds," an advertisement urged; "you will never take cold after you have learned to get along without sticky, stifling, smothering woolens." One could in fact purchase a complete ensemble of health clothing: caps, ventilation shirts, air robes, socks, stockings, sandals, even Porous Suspenders.[15]

Health clothes could be worn anywhere as well as in any season, but they were intended particularly for people residing at what Lust believed was "our best and most important work": Yungborn. What was Yungborn? "Take equal parts of Nirvana, Walhalla, Olympus, Elysium, and Paradise, dissolve in a little morning dew, stir well with a Physical Culture impulse, bake in the quivering rays of the noon-day sun, sprinkle deftly with a few drops of Kneipp's Hydropathic Extract, and add a whiff of Zephyr's summer perfume." That was Yungborn, at least as it appeared to a New York allopath who visited the compound planning to scoff but left with "a new recipe for making the most delicious Sanatorium." The nineteenth century's hygeiotherapy institutes had been sanatoria (from Latin *sanitas*, health), places where patrons learned about and lived by the rules of health. But not even Trall's Hygeian Home put inmates through the hygienic paces expected of those at Yungborn (from *Jungborn*, or fountain of youth, the name of a sanitorium established in Germany's Harz Mountains in 1896 by nature-curist Adolf Just). Just three months after Just opened Jungborn, Lust opened Yungborn, on September 15, 1896, in New Jersey's Ramapo Mountains, near the town of Butler. "The Nature Cure at Butler" was described by a correspondent of *The Naturopath and Herald of Health* as a place of "hope for everyone":

> For Mister Lust can make you well, if you will let him lay
> The plans for what you eat and wear, and his commands obey.
> He's got an Eden out of town, where you will get no meat,
> And walk 'mid trees as Adam did, in birthday suit complete; . . .
> Roast beef, cigars, and lager-beer you'll never want again,
> When you've been healed at Butler, by fruit, fresh air and rain.
> It's very cheap as well as good—this wondrous Nature Cure,
> And if you take it home with you, its blessings will endure;
> For all the ills of all mankind, the cheapest and the best
> Is Mister Lust's great Nature Cure—just put it to the test![16]

But first, Lust's nature cure put its devotees to quite a test. The prescribed day at Yungborn began at five A.M., after eight hours of sleep in either an "air-cottage" or a tent with "sweet mountain air pouring in upon you." Donning a "negligee costume" and sandals, one immediately set out "through a deep forest of majestic pines" on a mile-long hike to the top of Cat's Back Mountain, the high point of Yungborn's sixty-acre preserve. On the way up, a stop for a drink of pure spring water was recommended; on the way down, the stop was at "the men's park" (or at the women's, on the other side of the grounds) to disrobe and "plunge into the running brook and feel the thrill of the delightful reaction that follows." Post-plunge, one dried in the sun, got dressed again, and returned to the central grounds for a half-hour barefoot walk, à la Kneipp, on the dew-covered grass. It was now seven o'clock and time for breakfast, a lacto-ovo-vegetarian repast, as were other meals. (Lust's wife Louisa supervised the kitchen, from which issued "masterpieces of the culinary art" prepared with "the touch of a magician's wand"; her "new and unthought of combinations" that broadened "the gastronomic horizon of the vegetarian" eventually found their way into a *Good Dinner Cook Book.*) After the morning meal, guests walked about at leisure until the eight-thirty bell signaled a half hour of calisthenics and deep breathing. The sexes now sepa-rated again to visit their respective rooms for an hour of Kneipp bath treat-ments, including "the *lightning spray*. Let Felix play that hose on you from head to foot awhile and a 'boiled lobster' has not half as ruddy a glow." Now, with the blood "so wildly dash[ing] through all your arteries and veins," a return visit was made to the men's or women's park to disport in "the garb of Nature," letting the sun and air "do their good offices in our behalf." Mud did good offices, too, sending its "healing magnetism" into those who coated themselves with it and baked it on under the sun. Around eleven A.M. a thorough splashing in the brook washed the mud away, and a game of quoits or ball-throwing filled the hour until dressing for a lunch "so delicious that the only danger is that you will eat too much." The afternoon was essentially a repeat of the morning, though with freedom to swim in a pool, play lawn tennis, and/or exercise on "a running course of a mile through the woods." Dinner was at six, herb tea at eight, and a well-earned lights-out at nine.[17]

That schedule constituted what Lust called the "Regeneration Cure," a regimen that made "vital energy and vital strength return; increased nerve-elasticity and an undreamed-of sensation of powerful health make themselves felt. And," consistent with his holistic philosophy, "with the new creative power there asserts itself a feeling of spiritual . . . rejuvenation and unlimited efficiency." Regeneration, he was certain, could cure any physical ailment or insufficiency, including that of "many a husband who was lacking his best powers [yet] has become a happy father due to our regeneration cure, and many a wife, formerly unhappy, almost despairing, is now a happy mother." All that for only sixteen dollars a week was an offer difficult to resist, at least for the health conscious, and Yungborn was often filled to its capacity of a hundred guests, more than an occasional one from abroad. (A man from Brooklyn who stayed there recalled meeting a count, a Spanish consul, a German artist, a Canadian philosopher, and an ambassador from China whose body was treated everywhere "from cue [queue?] to toe.")[18]

Faith in Nature

Yungborn deserves so much attention because it exemplifies the curious mix
of wisdom and folly that perfused early naturopathy. There is no doubting
that people improved in health during a stay at Yungborn (aside from the risk
of melanoma from all that sunbathing, a danger not understood at the time).
Early to bed, early to rise, eat no meat, and exercise is a prescription for
physical well-being in any location. Nor is there any doubt as to Lust's good
intentions; all that he wrote and all that was written about him attest to his
sincerity in wanting people to achieve the highest vitality and in believing that
his nature cure was the surest path to that end. "Of the men I have met and
the men I would trust," one admirer wrote,

> There are none to excel Dr. Benedict Lust. . . .
> Dr. Benedict Lust is a man thru and thru,
> With conscience and soul for Gentile and Jew.[19]

Yet sincerity and common sense were countered in naturopathy by an
unquestioning faith that every agency of the natural world—be it water, pure
air, or ultraviolet rays—was necessarily productive of benefit because it was
"natural." "Nature is perfect in every way and everywhere," Lust proclaimed
as early as 1900; "the new art of natural healing expects everything from
nature and is convinced that the simple natural remedies employed can only
assist nature to overcome the disease." Such unwavering trust in Mother Nature's kindness resonates throughout naturopathic literature, from a "Naturopath's Creed" that professed belief in nature's "eternal goodness" and "her
perpetual efforts toward ever higher construction" to the quatrains of a naturopathic poet:

> I am getting back to nature, I have strayed from mother earth,
> Have followed many barren paths, since my time of birth,
> I am living close to nature, with the sun, the air, the bath,
> And experience has taught me this, to take 'The Natur-path.'[20]

Naturopaths' reverential absorption in the benevolent mysteries of nature
loosened their minds to jump to intuitive suppositions that had no basis in
objective science—the healthfulness of porous suspenders, for example, and
mud's "healing magnetism." (Children had such fun making mud pies, Lust
explained, because "the child . . . feels within itself the need of the magnetic
surge that sweeps from Nature through man, meets the electric wave that
quivers from Ether through man, and forms the complete circuit comprised
in humanity—from Animal to God.")[21]

Groundless conjecturing was an unfortunate enough weakness. Worse was the willingness to accept into the naturopathic fold any therapeutic modality presented as "natural," no matter how outlandish the method or questionable the motivation of its proponent. One is reluctant to turn to D. D. Palmer for insightful commentary on any aspect of medical care, but he was not far off the bull's eye in his characterization of the naturopathy of his day as "a pick up of anything and everything that their authors find lying around loose." A quick thumbing-through of any volume of *The Naturopath and Herald of Health* (renamed *Herald of Health and Naturopath* in 1916, then *Naturopath* in 1923) will corroborate the chiropractor's appraisal. For a period, for example, the journal had a Phrenological Section. The "science" of reading character by the shape of the skull had been popular among hygeiotherapists in the nineteenth century but had been discredited and largely abandoned by the beginning of the twentieth. Its claim to take in "man's whole organization and mode of life, and how to control and guide it," struck a responsive chord with Lust the holist, however, so phrenology was taken in by naturopathy. There was an Astroscopy Department for a while, too, providing guidance on diagnosis through astrology. To illustrate with one case, the mysterious illness of the son of Tsar Nicholas was correctly determined to be hemophilia—because the boy had been born when the sun was in Leo and the moon in Virgo. An even more popular method of identifying disease was iridiagnosis, or examination of the iris of the eye to discover changes in pigmentation indicative of pathology in some part of the body.[22]

In the realm of therapy and prevention, there was a richness of embarrassments ranging from sand eating, to cure indigestion and constipation, to rectal manipulation, "an absolute cure for chronic headaches and many other diseases supposed to be incurable." One of the most frequently promoted methods was Ehretism, the avoidance of all foods that generated "mucus" inside the body, mucus being a factor in the causation of almost all disease:

> I came home on the 'C-P-R'
> With nothing to eat on the Dining Car
> Except mucus food—and all such junk
> And now my stomach is feeling punk.

An alternative dietary plan was to be discovered in the journal's Apyrotropher Section, where the superiority of "unfired" foods was promoted. Fired, or cooked, food was supposed to ferment in the digestive tract, producing toxins that leached into the blood and played havoc throughout the body. Although apyrotrophers were not necessarily vegetarians (oysters on the half shell and steak tartare were allowable because unfired), their rationale resonated with naturopathic philosophy: "It is a crime against nature to eat foods she provides in any other condition than that in which she provides them." (Lust himself "lived on the unfired diet for six years at one stretch," he claimed.) The raw food philosophy even promoted the spiritual improvement Lust attached to physical health. It was "a new gospel of MORAL DIETETICS":

> The doctor with his knives and drugs,
> The brewer with his steins and jugs
> And all 'ill-fame' will cease to be
> Because of Apyrotrophy.

Even Typhoid Mary could be reformed, one raw foodist proposed, enabled to end her "foul career" if she would just become an apyrotropher.[23]

The advertisements accepted by naturopathic publications demonstrate the same open-mindedness toward all things purporting to be natural. The good (whole wheat bread sticks, strength-building exercise programs) ran side by side with the ridiculous. To select but a few from among the latter group, there was the Parker Vibratory Electric Bath Blanket, which not only warmed the body but "produces vibratory electric effects which are the basis of drugless healing, . . . regulates the action of the heart, [and] equalizes the circulation of the blood"; the Toxo-Absorbent Pack, a container of certain potent minerals that "applied externally searches out the poisons from every organ of the body, draws them to the surface," and neutralizes them, thereby curing pneumonia, tuberculosis, appendicitis, typhoid fever, and cancer; the Golden Sunlight Radiator, which relieved "pains of every description almost instantly" while also making pimples "fade away like flakes of snow under the hot sun"; and the Burdick Infra-Red Generator, a roughly foot-square pack that after being "connected to any light socket" could be applied to any part of the body and there do every bit as much good as the Vi-Rex, an electrical device from the other end of the spectrum whose ultraviolet radiation "penetrates every cell of the entire human system and brings almost instant relief." The grand assortment of literary productions that also found their way into the advertising pages of naturopathic journals stretched from Lust's own works at one end to the booklet "discribing [sic] the inhabitants of the different Planets of this solar system" at the other.[24]

Lust himself was susceptible to blind enthusiasm over unlikely therapies. "I know of nothing that seems to me to hold out such promise of health and long life for the human race," he wrote in the early 1920s, than the "blood washing bath" he had learned about from a young Greek man who had cured his hernia with two long hot showers at the gymnasium. With a bit of experimentation, Christos Parasco had discovered that taking a fine-spray hot shower for eight hours at a time would cure just about anything else, too, and leave one feeling years younger. Lust tested the method on himself at Yungborn and announced that "I am not exaggerating when I say that three of those eight-hour units . . . made me, a man of sixty [fifty-one actually], feel twenty-five years younger." He acknowledged that "it sounds crazy," but in fact "it is as enthralling as an opium dream is said to be. . . . I didn't want to quit when the eight hours were up, but desired to continue until I had experienced a complete return to youth." The results upon his patients were equally extraordinary. A seventy-year-old man who was overweight and suffering with bronchial troubles that had forced him to stop singing took the shower and lost two inches off his waist, and then "with my own ears I heard him render the 'Prologue' from 'Pagliacci' perfectly."[25]

There had to be a reason for the marathon shower's restorative power, and, as with all other drugless therapies, Lust had one. His explanation, further, is additional demonstration of the casual intimacy naturopaths believed they shared with nature. Nature's most profound truths, Lust believed, were revealed rather than discovered, being "vouchsafed" to the receptive mind not through "the cold process of reason but by intuition." Intuition told him that as the tiny droplets of water passed through the air they absorbed molecules of oxygen that had a stimulating effect on the skin when they struck it. This effect was reinforced by the friction created by the water as it pelted the skin unceasingly for eight hours. Surely "electrical reactions of a very mild but very real sort result from that," and electrical stimulation must set the blood into more rapid movement that enabled it to absorb "from the tissues and the joints materials which it ordinarily does not succeed in removing. . . . It is the difference between washing a soiled dish in lukewarm water and directing against it a powerful jet of hot water." (It was in that sense that the shower was a "blood-washing bath.") If the theory were sound, Lust projected, regular prophylactic use of the blood bath could stretch the human lifespan to several centuries, though his vision of erecting "great temples for this new Bath" throughout the country proved, as he feared, "a dream . . . too good to come true."[26]

However much a dreamer Lust was in some respects, he was an insightful realist in others. He was correct in believing that simply giving nature support as it ran its course was the best one could do with many diseases in his day. He was correct in seeing self-abuse as the source of much physical, and emotional, suffering and attacked it with an ardor that MDs would not bring to the task until nearly a century later. Recent medical lamentations over the effects of smoking, sexual promiscuity, and other risky behaviors adopted in the thoughtless chase after pleasure have nothing on Lust's jeremiads: "Walk along Third Avenue or the Bowery . . . some Saturday night," he wrote in 1902, and take note of "the warped features, as they shove in droves for the beer-garden or the theatre or the restaurant. . . . Notice the little squinting selfish eyes, the bestial brow, the coarse animal hair. . . . Observe the dregs of poisoned coffee streaking the muddy complexion, see the cargo of adulterated sweets soured in the acrid expression. . . . Study the huddled posture, the restricted body, the shackling gait, the limp personality. Listen to the fitful, fearful breathing, let the angry throb of passion and hate and greed and malice wrench your whole being . . . in short, live for a single hour in the infinite misery of the average man. Then you will know why naturopathy is." Naturopathy existed particularly for children, whose poor health was so often the result of parental mistreatment or neglect. Today's medical recriminations of parents for letting their children grow soft and fat gobbling Twinkies in front of the television and computer were presaged by Lust, who bemoaned all the forms of overeating and underexercising of his day that "mould most beautifully and harmoniously the helpless babe into a typical American 'kid.' "[27]

Lust was right in reprimanding allopaths for focusing so strongly on disease as to lose sight of the importance of promoting health. (As a colleague put it, regular medicine "has too much school pathology and not enough simple life healthology.") He was right in appreciating the need to "individualize" the treatment of each patient (MDs "lay down before society one coat which must fit Tom, Dick and Harry alike. If it does not fit them, they must go without") and in seeing patient self-responsibility as part of that individualization: there were no nurses on staff at Yungborn because "a nurse adds to your sense of weakness, helplessness and irresponsibility. And the whole idea of the Nature Cure is to make the invalid responsible to himself for every thought, act and emotion of his life."[28]

Growth of Naturopathy

Those were messages that had enough appeal, evidently, to allow naturopathy to expand steadily through the first decades of the century until by 1923 Lust could estimate that there were nine thousand naturopaths, a "vast army of professional men and women" working on all continents to "rejuvenate and regenerate the world." His figures were undoubtedly inflated. An independent survey completed less than a decade later put the number of naturopaths at "possibly 1,500," allowing that if the "allied groups" that advocated drugless healing under other names (physiotherapy, sanipractic) were added on, the total might reach 2,500. Yet whatever their numbers, naturopaths had grown into a force not to be ignored. New schools had appeared, such as the First National University of Naturopathy in Newark and the Lindlahr College of Natural Therapeutics in Chicago, whose ads asserted that "The Demand for Drugless Physicians Greatly Exceeds the Supply" and promised prospective students they could expect to earn from five thousand to ten thousand dollars a year upon graduation. By the end of the 1920s, there were more than a dozen schools of naturopathy in the United States.[29]

A proliferation of naturopathic journals also occurred: *Nature Cure Magazine* ("Devoted to Man-Building on the Physical, Mental and Moral Planes"), *Health Culture, Drugless America, Sanipractic Magazine, The Nautilus, Life and Action, Brain and Brawn*, to cite a few, along with *Nature's Path*, launched by Lust in 1925 to provide more lay-oriented instruction in the rules of health with the hope that naturopaths "can put it on their waiting room tables." But perhaps the most effective periodical for spreading the naturopathic message was *Physical Culture*, the widely circulating publication edited by Bernarr Macfadden. The most colorful health reformer of the first half of the twentieth century, Macfadden concentrated his teaching on the cultivation of physique and strength; the motto of *Physical Culture* magazine was "Weakness is a Crime." Nevertheless, the system of "physcultopathy" espoused by "Body Love Macfadden," the "Bare Torso King," was virtually indistinguishable from naturopathy. He called for sunshine, pure air, and dietary restraint as supplements to exercise and tirelessly attacked the allopathic profession as a "medical octopus" guilty of "unspeakable outrage." Lust himself acknowledged "that Naturopathy and Physcultopathy are the same" and praised Macfadden as "our big brother." Big brother repaid the recognition by publishing articles and advertisements promoting naturopathy in virtually every issue of *Physical Culture*.[30]

The spread of naturopathy was marked by the establishment of more health retreats, too. A Florida Yungborn was opened by Lust in 1913, in the town of Tangerine ("the highest and most healthy spot of the State") so as to allow year-round sunbathing. ("In the sun, life is won" was this Yungborn's motto.) There was a Lindlahr Health Resort in Elmhurst, Illinois, a Biggs Hygienic Sanitarium in Greensboro, North Carolina, and other Yungborn spinoffs too numerous to mention. (In 1923, Lust claimed there were more than 500 such institutions in America founded by graduates of his school alone.) By this point it is unnecessary to point out how all these sanitoria and schools struck regular physicians. Naturopathy, that "medical cess-pool," was nothing more than a "cult [with] no basic idea but to be rather a nature-cure hodgepodge," and, as one of the more succinct appraisals had it, "the absurdity of it all is obvious."[31]

Opposition to Allopathic Medicine

But allopathy was riddled with absurdities, too, naturopaths were convinced, with possibly the silliest being the germ theory, what Lust called "the most gigantic hoax of modern times." Like osteopathy's and chiropractic's, the naturopathic position on bacteria was that they were effect rather than cause, agents that established themselves in the body only after it had already begun to deteriorate "because of our unnatural mode of living." "The healthy body," it was believed, "does not allow undue multiplication of germs. But in the unhealthy body there is so much corruption and waste that the germs start to multiply and flourish." What was the cause of so-called germ diseases, then? One naturopath's interpretation of the great influenza pandemic of 1918–19 will illustrate nicely how drugless healers understood disease and the way it was overcome by their methods. To be sure, other naturopaths would not necessarily have subscribed to every detail of this analysis, but it is representative of the plumb line of naturopathic thought. "We all know that the American nation is a wheat-eating nation," the ND's reasoning began. But restrictions imposed during World War I had forced Americans to substitute barley and corn for much of the wheat they were used to, and their bodies had difficulty digesting and eliminating the waste products of these unaccustomed foods. Even so, "everything went fine until the leaves started to fall from the trees" (the flu did erupt in the autumn of 1918). Falling leaves released "fermentive substances" into the atmosphere, "and as we inhaled these substances . . . the barley and corn-meal products, which loaded our systems, were set into fermentation. . . . Now, everybody knows that barley and corn-meal ferment very readily, and as our systems were not used to handling these 'sticky' substances, their waste products began to clog our cells and tissue-spaces." And that, he submitted, was "the whole 'mystery' of the Spanish influenza." On further consideration, however, more could be seen to the mystery. After all, early in that same autumn there had occurred a few days of unseasonably cold weather that had "scared a number of people into heavier underwear." When warm weather then returned for two full months, many of those who had donned woolen undergarments continued to wear them in anticipation of a return of the cold. "In this manner [they] interfered with the skin elimination" of those sticky cell-clogging wastes of barley and corn. In addition, the "loss of relatives and friends in the great war" had produced much sorrow, which "also undermined the body vitality," while "overwork, which was very common during the war," must have contributed to the lowering of vigor, too. All those disturbing factors taken together had "made the population more susceptible to disease."[32]

In the end, the specifics of the foregoing theory are unimportant. What matters is its exemplification of early naturopathy's approach to the understanding of all disease. Illness was supposed invariably to be the result of interference with the body's ability to purify itself. As this theorist put it, "*elimination* [is] the great principle on which Naturopathy is founded," and "elimination must necessarily be the keynote to the treatment of all diseases."[33]

As long as the *vis medicatrix* worked unimpeded in its efforts to expel meta-bolic refuse generated within the body and morbid matter absorbed from the environment, physiological functioning proceeded smoothly. Whenever any-thing (clogging of tissue spaces, impermeable clothing) interfered with nature's processes of elimination of waste through kidneys, bowels, lungs, and skin, sickness was sure to result. Then, and only then, did germs appear, drawn to the feast of putrid fluids pooling in unpurified tissue. In short, naturopathic etiology was hygeiotherapy's physical Puritanism reborn in the age of bacte-riology. Suppression of elimination, futhermore, resulted every bit as easily from mental and emotional factors as physical ones. In the case of influenza, grief over the loss of loved ones in the trenches of Europe aggravated the disordered digestive process; with other ailments, anxiety or depression or lack of faith might be the inhibiting force. In all conditions, it was the whole person—body, mind, and spirit—that was unstable and negating nature's self-purifying action.

To naturopaths' way of seeing things, one of the worst impurities that could be taken into the body was something that allopaths imposed upon their patients all the time, and it wasn't drugs, poisonous as pharmaceuticals were. It was smallpox vaccine. Vaccination to produce immunity to smallpox had been introduced at the end of the 1700s, in Britain, and had become an ever more common component of public health programs throughout Europe and America over the course of the ensuing century. Experience had demonstrated, however, that, terrible a scourge though smallpox was, many people neglected to have themselves and their children inoculated. Consequently, by the begin-ning of the twentieth century most states had enacted compulsory vaccination laws, requiring young children to be vaccinated before they could enter school. There was considerable resistance to such legislation for political reasons: it was state interference with the right of parents to oversee the health of their children and a violation of the right of citizens to determine how or if they would be medicated; in the opinion of a New York homeopath, vaccination "ranks with human slavery and religious persecution as one of the most fla-grant outrages upon the rights of the human race."[34]

But vaccination was also vigorously attacked on medical grounds as a serious risk to health. From the time of its introduction a century earlier, people had felt uneasy about smallpox vaccine because it was produced from another species, cattle (the term "vaccination" was derived from the Latin word for cow—*vacca*—because the procedure employed vaccinia, or cowpox, virus to generate immunity to the very similar variola, or smallpox, virus). For most, reluctance to undergo vaccination had been largely a matter of distaste for receiving pus from an infected cow's udder. But for those of the Physical Puritan turn of mind, cow pus was more than distasteful; it was dangerous—because it was foreign to the human organism. As early as the 1840s *The Water-Cure Journal* lashed out against "The Sinfulness of Inoculation," condemning vaccination as "a process of poisoning the system" and arguing that "it is incomparably better to live so in accordance with the natural laws, that the poison of smallpox can take no hold of the system."[35]

Anti-vaccine warnings previously issued only sporadically came to be expressed much more frequently and stridently, however, once state governments began to make vaccination compulsory in the late nineteenth century. Indeed, anti-vaccination feeling coalesced as a genuine political movement that strove to have the practice abolished as a threat to public health rather than a boon. In truth, vaccination did pose certain dangers. Vaccines were too often produced under less than scrupulously controlled conditions and became contaminated with other disease pathogens, and vaccinators did not always take adequate precautions to sterilize their instruments; tetanus and streptococcal and staphylococcal infections were in fact not uncommon. More rarely, susceptible individuals suffered severe reactions to the vaccine matter and died. But if vaccination had its risks, anti-vaccinationists were disposed to grandly overstate them: one opponent warned that not only would the "diseases of the cow" be passed on to humans but the bovine's "vices [and] passions" as well.[36]

Predictably, all the alternative medical systems of the turn of the twentieth century joined in the attack on the orthodox profession's backing of vaccination. D. D. Palmer spoke out against "the vaccination wickedness" as early as his pre-chiropractic days as a magnetic healer, while osteopaths of the early 1900s warned that MDs in their zeal to apply vaccine prevention were out to inoculate people with every germ known: "Would you like to have an injection of gonococci tonight?" a prominent DO asked? "Even the pneumococci . . . might be good after every ride in a cold rain!" But none of the period's irregular systems attacked vaccination so vehemently as naturopathy. The idea of adding purulent foreign matter to the body so offended naturopaths' intuitive sense of inner purity as the sine qua non of health as to seem demented. Surely it was "beyond the compass of all sane comprehension how corrupted matter—rotted blood—fostered in purposely infected animals . . . can possibly prevent disease, or restore an afflicted person to a normal state!" Vaccination was "such horrible profanation, such disgusting pollution, such absolute insanity" that one had "to ask in amaze, Can these things be possible in the twentieth century?" To Lust, as late as 1927 compulsory vaccination was "that most heinous of all crimes."[37]

Naturopathic literature over the first three decades of the twentieth century was relentless in its condemnation of vaccination as the destroyer of health. "*Filth-pus vaccination*," according to a California naturopath, was "the most dangerous fraud ever perpetrated under the disguise of science," responsible for "the *worst kind of spreading diseases of all kinds.*" Lust went farther, alleging that "this horrible mass of putrid matter" that constituted vaccine was the cause of "disease, constitutional debility and DEATH. . . . Vaccination sows the seed of Erysipelas, Scrofula, Cancers, Leprosy, Consumption, Eczema and other loathsome diseases," including diseases of the mind. The reason a quarter million veterans of World War I would eventually lose their mental faculties, he submitted, was not because of the horrors the men had endured on the battlefield: "It is not to be thought that the Germans did anything to these brave lads to destroy their minds." Rather the "clue to the situation" was to be found in "the insanity produced by vaccination . . . in those who did not get to the battle front." Combatants and non-combatants alike would lose their minds because the army had forced them to be vaccinated. Not surprisingly, when the Anti-Vaccination League of America was organized in 1910, its constitution was published in its entirety in Lust's periodical *The Naturopath*.[38]

By the early twentieth century a number of other vaccines and anti-toxins had been developed by medical science, and they came in for the same kind and degree of denunciation as smallpox inoculation: "serum therapy," the "criminal experiments" of "crazy serum-quacks," was damned as a physical crime in any form; Lust asserted that every complaint from heart disease and cancer to idiocy and insanity had "enormously increased . . . during the regime of inoculations, serums and vaccines." The reason the human race was "degenerating," he maintained, was because it was being "serumized":

> She was a doctor's child, and he Embraced the opportunity
> From all disease to make her free With absolute immunity. . . .
> "Some various serums of my own I'm rather sure will answer;
> I make them for all troubles known, From freckles up to cancer."
> Alas! alas! for all his pains, The end was scarce desirous:
> She soon had nothing in her veins But various kinds of virus.
> Part horse, part cow, part sheep, part goat, Her laugh was half a whinny.
> "Dear me," said he, "she's half a stoat, And badly mixed with guinea."[39]

The creation of vaccines was branded a crime against the entire animal creation, in fact, for every type of serum therapy had been derived from animal experimentation. Just as vigorous as the anti-vaccination movement at that time was a campaign against the use of animals in medical research. As an organized movement, anti-vivisectionism had its roots in England in the 1870s. It had quickly spread to the United States, however, gathering steam in tandem with the dramatic expansion of medical research in the last quarter of the century and expanding its opposition to all forms of animal experimentation, whether or not actual vivisection (cutting open live animals) was involved; anti-vivisectionism, in fact, was part of a larger movement already employing the phrase "animals' rights" that worked to liberate animals from all forms of mistreatment. To be sure, there was enough work to be done just within the realm of medical experimentation, for while many researchers did administer anesthetics and otherwise protect their animals from excessive suffering, more than a few others were shockingly callous toward their laboratory animals. Anti-vivisectionists nevertheless tended to tar all researchers with the same brush, characterizing the allopathic profession as a band of heartless tormentors bearing "the stamp of atrocity and crime," perpetrators of deeds that were "the fine flower and consummation of barbarity and injustice—the *ne plus ultra* of iniquity in man's dealings with the lower races."[40]

Again, alternative practitioners of every stripe joined in the chorus of condemnation; D. D. Palmer, for example, shamed allopaths for putting animals through "untold hours of agony" under their "cruel, bloodthirsty hands" purely "to satisfy a cruel, depraved appetite." Yet none of the irregular groups matched the volume and intensity of naturopathic attacks on vivisectors. More than any other system, naturopathy respected the kinship of humankind with the animal kingdom: Lust, it will be recalled, praised "the complete circuit comprised in humanity—from Animal to God." Naturopaths' ecological understanding of health—people are whole only when they are integrated into nature's great web of life—made them more susceptible to outrage when so-called healers disrupted that unity and misused other members of the natural community: "Think of the unparalleled atrocities of these medical perverts who are inflicting untold sufferings [on] their innocent, helpless victims, to satisfy their devilish mania for experimenting!" (And worse was sure to come, for it "is a fact" that animal vivisection "is but a stepping-stone to human vivisection.") The whole sorry mess of orthodox medicine was summed up in a naturopathic song about "Regular Allopathic Drug Doctors":

> Sing a song of doctors, A satchel full of dope,
> Four-and-twenty patients, A hundred miles of hope.
> When the satchel opens, the doctors start to guess;
> The patients are about to get some nauseating mess.
> Dosem's in the parlor, Analyzing frogs;
> Cuttem's in the kitchen, Vivisecting dogs;
> Prickem's found another Serum for disease.
> But there's no disagreement When they figure up their fees.[41]

Naturopaths' Fight for Medical Freedom

Offensive as all those components of allopathic *medicine* were, what truly enraged naturopaths was allopathic *politics*, the determination of the majority profession to impose its depraved standards on the public through legislation. Conventional physicians would have described their standards differently, to be sure, but they freely admitted that they were becoming more politically active, working "to stimulate, to restrain, or otherwise to control the law-making power" at every level of government in order to preserve and elevate the health of the public. Leadership in these efforts came from the American Medical Association, in existence since 1847 but not particularly involved politically until the beginning of the twentieth century. One of the AMA's most ambitious projects in the years prior to World War I was the establishment of a national health bureau to implement and coordinate an array of public health programs nationwide (including vaccination and medical inspection of schoolchildren). AMA lobbying resulted finally in Oklahoma's Senator Robert Owen in 1910 introducing a bill to create a cabinet-level department. That first bill did not get past the Committee on Public Health and Quarantine, nor did two subsequent attempts by Owen (in 1911 and 1913) succeed in becoming law. The mere threat of enactment, however, was enough to rally all unorthodox practitioners—homeopaths, eclectics, osteopaths, chiropractors, Christian Scientists, even patent medicine manufacturers—to join arms in resistance to what they saw as the onslaught of allopathic tyranny. Uniting under the banner of a National League for Medical Freedom, they worked tirelessly to stir up the public to fight back against the schemes of MDs to assume complete control of all matters medical and hygienic. ("To defeat paternal, unnecessary, extravagant, un-American medical legislation is the purpose of the National League for Medical Freedom.") No group worked harder or more passionately than the naturopaths.[42]

"Senator Owen of Oklahoma is the tool by which this monster evil [the AMA] hopes to become master of the medical field in the United States," one affronted naturopath charged. "No kingdom or monarchy throughout the world has ever had such a cursed monster to exercise iron sway over the people. It is the infamy of the infamous. It is the horror of this world—the 'Black Hand' of medical robbery and murder." It was, according to this same critic, the desperate ploy of "medical peanut politicians," "intellectual degenerates and moral perverts," "vampires and vandals," a "primping graft-ing affected conglomeration of masculine inanity," "effeminate dudes . . . fops and idiots," and "medical turntits [of] hyena heartlessness." If all that seems a bit hyperbolic, then hyperbole was the norm. Consider the words of other naturopaths on the subject: the Owen bill was "the most pernicious national legislation ever attempted here"; it was a case of "medical men . . . exhausting every resource of cajolery and menace, and ransacking the black books of sophistry" to get their way; it was the "foul conspiracy" of "the stupid allo-pathic trust [that] has hired Senator Owen"; "the national executioner, Senator Owen, is waiting for the signal from Congress to spring the trap that will strangle Liberty!" In the opinion of a speaker at "the monster mass-meeting for medical freedom" held at Carnegie Hall in 1911, "no bolder or more audacious demands for monopolistic privileges were ever put forward" than by these seekers after "pelf and power," these "political doctors" so deranged by "selfishness, greed and arrogance" as to think they can set up "a sanhedrin of medicine, from which there is to be no appeal" and then "cast into utter darkness" anyone "who will not bow down and worship the god of allopathy."[43]

There was no question among naturopaths but that pelf and power, the one of course serving the other, were the true motivations behind organized medicine's desire for a national department of health. It was a well-known fact that the medical profession was overpopulated and that the situation of too many doctors competing for too few patients was generating too little income for many MDs. From the naturopathic viewpoint it was clear that all the protestations of wanting to better protect the public's health were but a "false pretense" to cloak an "overcrowded profession['s] . . . scheme . . . to sus-tain, at the expense of the taxpayers, an army of medical incompetents who cannot without legislation in their favor command enough patronage to keep themselves from starving."[44]

It seemed equally clear to naturopaths that the allopathic plan to get the government to "supply fat jobs for all this army of incompetent political doctors" stemmed as well from fear of the competition of more skilled irreg-ular healers, particularly naturopathic ones. The proposed federal health de-partment was most threatening, therefore, because it portended a prohibition of the practice of drugless healing enacted from the national level. By 1910 and the introduction of Owen's first bill, naturopaths had endured a decade of arrests and prosecutions for practicing medicine without a license. Indeed, the founder of naturopathy was arrested before he had even adopted the name naturopathy. In 1899 Lust was hauled into court after a man to whom he had administered a bath reported him to the authorities. Fortunately the judge who heard the case was taking the Kneipp cure himself at a New Jersey establish-ment on weekends and dismissed the case. But Lust didn't always come out on top the numerous other times he was arrested, and once his fine was as stiff as five hundred dollars.[45]

He and his fellow nature-curers were tormented by the same kind of "spotters" and "sneaks" who turned in so many chiropractors. The New York

County Medical Society, according to Lust, "employed a horde of spies, stool-pigeons, sleuths, spittle lickers and hell servants to embarrass the Nature doctors," and "many a morning" during the first decade of the century "there were over a dozen drugless doctors lined up in the Criminal Court building, and each one found guilty and fined $250." The worst of the hell servants was a Mrs. Frances Benzecry, an acknowledged "investigator" for the county society, a "dirty woman sleuth . . . with an unspeakable name" who ensnared Lust after taking an electric light bath from him; he was fined $250 and had to pay another $250 in legal fees, "enough to make any man boil!" He was but one of many to suffer the wrath of Benzecry. By the time she retired from her twelve-year reign of terror stalking naturopaths, chiropractors, osteopaths, physiotherapists, massage therapists, and Christian Scientists (she was an equal opportunity stool pigeon), she had initiated the arrests of more than eight hundred naturopaths.[46]

Benzecry seems to have held the record for martyring naturopaths, but there were other "dirty stool pigeons," Lust complained, who "harassed and brought hundreds of drugless doctors to court on false evidence." (Some of them, he revealed, were "women of the lowest character. I could not tell you how low these women were—going around in the tenderloin district, to the masseurs, taking treatments, and when they liked one they went out with him at night.") The low women then had the nerve to "go to court, kiss the Bible and testify that she went into the defendant's office, took a bath, and while she took the bath asked the nurse whether baths are good for rheumatism, and as she said 'Yes' she therefore charges the proprietor and the nurse of violating the medical law." It was a point of honor among naturopathic defendants to plead not guilty, but many were convicted nonetheless and given fines and/or jail terms, some being sentenced to as much as a year: "What the drugless doctors suffered in those days only those who were pinched can tell." One woman practitioner "committed suicide . . . in despair, several died with broken hearts in the struggle and many happy homes were ruined." So consumed by hatred were New York allopaths that even "Jesus Christ would be arrested for practicing medicine without a license were He to come to New York State to-day and begin healing the sick and making the blind see."[47]

When in 1921 Lust looked back on those early days of being "shamefully persecuted," he expressed the wish that someday "there will be a time of retribution." He had already gotten a measure of vengeance by being acquitted of a libel charge brought after issuance of certain unflattering remarks about Mrs. Benzecry ("crooked," "a liar," "a disgrace to womanhood," "a woman as mean and dirty as she has never trodden the ground of this free and broad country," and the ominous "her day will soon come"). But the best revenge, as always, was living well, which for the first generation of naturopaths meant securing licensure to practice without having to worry about the Benzecrys of the world.[48]

Naturopaths conducted their offensive against restrictive legislation with the same arguments used by other alternative medical groups, but with the most spirit and thoroughness of any. (One practitioner, San Franciscan A. A. Erz, made the battle for "medical freedom" his area of specialization, laying waste to whole forests of paper in the 1910s with articles such as "Friends of Medical Freedom and Voters, Attention!" and a lengthy (because so repetitious) book telling *The Truth About Official Medicine and Why We Must Have Medical Freedom*. Erz's home state was the first to concede to his arguments, passing a licensing law in 1909; over the next ten years, nine more states would fall into line. Most, however, found naturopathy much more difficult to get a legal handle on than the more sharply defined osteopathy and chiropractic. Even Lust had defined his system as "therapeutic universalism," and the regulation of a profession that potentially employed everything a bountiful nature had to offer seemed a daunting prospect to most legislators. States that did take on the challenge generally did so under the heading of a "drugless healers" act, permitting licensees to do whatever they desired as long as neither drugs nor the knife was involved. The mainstream profession found such allowances ludicrous, of course. When Washington enacted its drugless healers statute in 1919, the editor of *Northwest Medicine* fumed that his state had become the "Mecca of cultism" and that "if there is any fantastic form of practice which has been omitted, this accommodating legislature will doubtless recognize such on request." (The law indeed specified that the Board of Drugless Examiners should consist of eight practitioners: two mechano-therapists, two food scientists, two physcultopaths, and two suggestive therapists.) The majority of state legislatures, however, at first granted naturopaths the right to do little more than massage.[49]

Lust and his compatriots were undeterred, taking the struggle for medical freedom—or at least attempting to—all the way to the White House. In 1920 Lust nominated one W. F. Collins as the Constitutional Liberty League's candidate for the presidency of the United States. That fall, Lust and Collins embarked on "an extensive tour" of the country to stump for the American Drugless Platform. Addressing crowds on the evils of drugs, vaccination, and vivisection, they called on them "to stand up before the world and proclaim ourselves apostles of the new gospel of freedom . . . to stand behind us that our oppressors may know they can no longer dictate our thoughts, our actions and our . . . medical rights." If the people would only unite, they could show the allopaths "what a real fight means." Pride goeth before a fall, but to lose the real fight to Warren Harding must have left a particularly deep bruise on nature-healers' egos.[50]

Relations With Other Alternative Systems

Collins was a chiropractor. That, and his nomination by Lust to head the Drugless Platform, would suggest a rather amiable fellowship among the various systems of drugless healing in the early 1900s. Such was, at least, the ideal for a while. Anyone who saw the folly of drugs, after all, couldn't be all bad, and even though there were many, many alternative medical groups billing themselves as drugless ("fifty-seven varieties" in one naturopath's jocular estimate, including one already calling itself "neo-naturopathy"), there was reason to hope that that common thread could bind all together into a potent force that would at last overthrow the drug-dosing despots of allopathy and usher in a new era: "the age of drugless healing." A National Association of Drugless Practitioners was founded in 1912 (Lust playing an active role), and while the association's object was "to promote interest in the several sciences" of drug-free healing, Lust admitted eight years later that he "cherished a fond dream—the union of all drugless factions [those several sciences] into one great profession." Two years later he described the American Naturopathic Association as a "union for the mutual advancement" of all healers who abjured drug therapies, an organization "under [whose] wings all practitioners, all schools, that use no drugs can find shelter." He backed up his words by running advertisements for other drugless systems in his publications and even by adding an American School of Chiropractic to his American School of Naturopathy. There were a number of schools, in fact, that offered degree programs in both naturopathy and chiropractic, an arrangement that appealed particularly to chiropractic mixers. (A cartoon in *Naturopath* in 1923 shows B. J. Palmer leaping and flailing about in frustration on the steps of the Palmer School of Chiropractic as a herd of cattle each branded "mixers" stampedes toward a naturopathic college glowing in the rays of the rising sun.)[51]

Yet the same year that he summoned all drugless healers to nest under the wings of the American Naturopathic Association, Lust lost his patience with chiropractic. Straight chiropractors, he objected, were not showing the same collegial spirit. They "proclaim from the public platform and through the press that their methods are superior to, and are rapidly supplanting all others." If that were so, he continued snippily, why was it that "leaders in Chiropractic, heads of Chiropractic schools, when sick always go to a Naturopath for treatment[?] Their wives patronize whole chains of nature cure Sanitariums," he claimed, and if they weren't going to be honest enough to openly acknowledge naturopathy's virtue, then "no one cares to join them." (Time did nothing to erode Lust's obduracy toward chiropractic straights. More than a decade later he berated B. J. Palmer as "a showman and exhibitionist of the first water," a man of "colossal gall" who led a "treacherous, slimy crew.")[52]

He didn't much care for mixers anymore, either, having finally come to realize they were "thieves who are taking liberal slices off Naturopathy, without even an 'excuse me,'" without even giving "the Naturopaths credit for the work they have done." Lust felt betrayed. He and naturopathic comrades had for years "neglected their own work" for the sake of promoting "the greater union" of all drugless systems. They had "sacrificed opportunity after opportunity to push their own ideas to the front" so that all would benefit, and this was the thanks they got from those "uncongenial elements." The chiropractors were the most uncongenial of all, he believed, and he (and more than a few fellow naturopaths) minced no words in letting them know how he felt. "Chiropractic is only a passing fad that has grown and thrived like the patent medicine business, on advertising," he sneered. "The so-called Chiropractic philosophy is but a big hoax," as evidenced by chiropractors' propensity for "always producing miracles. They talk about opening the blind eyes, unstopping deaf ears, making the dumb tongue sing and causing the lame man to leap . . . as though it were an hourly occurrence with them." Chiropractors gave no attention to hygiene and natural living, Lust charged, because their true philosophy was " 'Eat, drink and be merry' for tomorrow we have our backs punched. Satisfy all your desires for 'wine, women and hootch,' the punch in the back will atone for all your transgressions." Naturopathy, he finished, "was here many years before Chiropractic was dreamed about and will still be here when Chiropractic ceases even to be read about as an interesting bit of history." Over the course of the 1920s and '30s, naturopathy dropped its association with chiropractic and osteopathy, substituting in their stead procedures known as "naturopathic manipulations."[53]

Lust was ready to wash his hands of the other drugless ingrates, too. "Let the Osteopaths, the Chiropractors, the Mental Therapists and all the rest of the one-track systems go their own separate, independent ways," he urged. "Naturopathy has actually compromised its position by encouraging the growth of these various systems," coming "to be looked upon as a hodgepodge of drugless methods of healing." Naturopathy had to pull itself out of the mire and return to its origins, a concentration on "natural living and healing and less compromise with superficial methods of treatment." After all, "keeping people well is a greater art and a more magnificent work than peddling treatments," though it didn't attract as much business as those therapeutic schemes that promised quick and easy cures. By placing "the blame for disease where it belongs—on the ignorance of the people or their willful disobedience of natural law"—and insisting that "the responsibility for cure [is] on the individual," naturopaths gave themselves a far more difficult task than their drugless rivals, but "the course of duty lies plainly before us. Let us not again be side-tracked from our purpose." In the meantime, "let the factions fight their little fight for supremacy. . . . The time has come when we must attend to our own knitting." Lust would labor to the end of his days to pull naturopaths into a more cohesive entity, yet as will be seen in the chapter to follow, naturopathy became even less unified after its founder passed on.[54]

In the early months of 1943, a fire broke out at the Florida Yungborn. Lust was overcome by smoke; though rescued, he remained unconscious for four days. During that period "I was transformed into a human guinea pig," as MDs "squirted into my blood stream" the recently introduced sulfa drugs to ward off infection. Lust survived but never fully recovered "my customary vigor and pep" and refused to accept that the effects of smoke inhalation on a seventy-two-year-old body could be the cause. It was "those damnable shots—shots that are still in [my bloodstream] and which will never come out during the rest of my life." Indeed, his health declined steadily over the next two years, until he died of cardiac complications in September 1945, a "victim of the sulpha debauchery." Lust fought for naturopathy up to the end, finding the energy less than a week before he died to dictate an address for delivery at the upcoming convention of the American Naturopathic Association. The fight against allopathy he continued even from beyond the grave: the first issue of *Nature's Path* to appear after his death carried his final attack against what he now was calling the "Medical Gestapo." Lust was buried in Butler, New Jersey, close by his first Yungborn.[55]

PART III

The Late Twentieth Century: Holistic Healing

The other day my doctor sat at my bedside—just to talk. He assured me my physical complaints will be eased, and that he will be in regular attendance. We talked frankly of the dying process and the need of living as I am dying— to fully appreciate every moment of life. I liked our conversation—it is hard to come by. Most physicians have lost the pearl that was once an intimate part of medicine—humanism. Machinery, efficiency, precision have driven from the heart warmth, compassion, sympathy, and concern for the individual. Medicine is now an icy science; its charm belongs to another age. The dying man can get little comfort from the mechanical doctor.

Frederick Stenn, MD, 1980

10

From Medical Cultism to Alternative Medicine

The last three chapters have painted a picture of irregular medicine in the early twentieth century very different from the one that future historians will paint of the early twenty-first. Clearly an extraordinary transformation of unorthodox practice and of mainstream medicine's view of unorthodoxy occurred over the course of the 1900s. The change became starkly apparent only during the last decade of the century, but progress toward the new order began in the 1930s and reached a first-stage culmination in the 1970s, the decade during which the term "alternative medicine" began to be used. Quietly but steadily unconventional medicine redefined itself during the middle decades of the twentieth century.

Medical Cultism and Scientific Medicine

The standard definition at the outset of that era, at least in the allopathic lexicon, was "medical cultism." In *The Healing Cults*, a 1932 book published by the Committee on the Costs of Medical Care, mainstream medicine's view of irregulars at that time was expressed as clearly as could be stated. "The founder of each sect launched his theory as an explanation of all disease," author Louis Reed began, "and taught a procedure . . . of treatment which he claimed to be a cure for all disease." Narrow- and simple-minded believers in the all-encompassing truth of their healing revelation, unorthodox practitioners "cling to their particular beliefs with a fervor more characteristic of an evangelistic than a scientific group." Winning converts among the uneducated and uncritical through enthusiastic hellfire-and-brimstone preaching, they exalt themselves as the saviors of the disease-ridden world from the treacherous snares of the allopathic Satan. It was this uncompromising hatred of established medicine, "this close-mindedness, this devotion to" their peculiar "dogmas," that "justifies the title, 'cult' or 'sect,' for all these groups."[1]

"All these groups" included survivors from the first generation of irregular systems; homeopathy, eclecticism, and physio-medicalism still had practitioners in America in the early twentieth century. All three groups were in steep decline, however. The last physio-medical college closed in 1911, the last eclectic school in 1939, and while there were twenty-two homeopathic schools at the beginning of the century, only two were left by 1930 (and none by 1960). When allopathic physicians spoke of medical cults, therefore, what they particularly had in mind was osteopathy, chiropractic, and naturopathy. Whatever the cult, it was particularly offensive to orthodox practitioners who came of age at the turn of the twentieth century. The germ theory had transformed public health and surgery in the 1880s and '90s, and remarkable advances in drug therapy were about to follow. Physicians of the time appreciated that they possessed a scientific sophistication and technical prowess that placed them well above all previous generations of doctors, and they couldn't help feeling the smug superiority that was embodied in the words "scientific medicine." That was their battle cry, a phrase employed over and over in both professional literature and publications directed to the laity to distinguish their generation's "scientific medicine" from the ordinary "medicine" of the past. The allopathic profession assiduously cultivated the image of the new doctor as a highly educated, critical-thinking scientist with lifesaving powers, an enlightened physician who had no truck with the ignorance and superstition of former times. The practitioner of scientific medicine was surely the only kind of doctor any rational person would consult, and thus it was extremely upsetting to those practitioners to see that pre-scientific practices could survive into the new era in the form of irregular systems as benighted as any backwoods religious cult. "Every healing cult," complained the editor of the *Journal of the American Medical Association*, "has interfered with the progress of scientific medicine."[2]

The level of interference was not to be discounted. One expects to hear irregular practitioners claim that their systems were "crowding the 'regular' physician to the wall." But MDs said much the same thing. "The medical profession in this country will be swamped by the cults," worried a speaker for the American Association for Medical Progress (an organization devoted to polishing scientific medicine's public image); "unless stringent legislation [is] enacted" against cultism, a New Jersey practitioner predicted, "dire results to both the public and the medical profession" will follow; the incursions of the cultists, an Illinois medical editor despaired, are so serious that "the medical profession [has] to fight for its very existence."[3] One senses a certain exaggeration in these remarks, normal for spokesmen trying to rally forces to meet a threat. But even allowing for overstatement, the reader is impressed that medical cultism of the early 1900s had enlisted enough converts to make orthodoxy nervous about maintaining its hold on public faith.

How many converts were there? The 1920 census indicated that there were approximately 145,000 allopathic practitioners in the United States and about 20,000 unconventional doctors; an estimate in 1923, however, maintained there were one-fifth as many irregulars as "qualified physicians." With regard to volume of business, one study determined that during the years 1928 through 1931, 5.1 percent of all cases of illness were treated by "non-medical practitioners" (identified as osteopaths, chiropractors, naturopaths, and Christian Scientists). Yet a Philadelphia allopath reported in 1924 that over the past four years he had asked all his patients about their use of medical services of all kinds, and learned that fully a third (34 percent) had within the previous three months "been under the care of agents of one or more of the numerous cults." (For the presumably less educated patients attending a free dispensary in Philadelphia, the figure was only 26 percent.) Philadelphia was a bastion of orthodoxy, furthermore, compared to Chicago, where a survey of nearly seven thousand patients conducted the year before had determined that 86 percent of the public had consulted one cultist healer or another. To be sure, many of those patients had merely "dabbled in" irregular medicine, as the Chicago surveyor put it, and still looked to regular doctors as their main source of care. One should remember, however, that the Eisenberg study cited in the preface, the 1993 article that so shocked the late twentieth-century medical profession with its revelation of the "enormous presence" of alternative medicine in America, found a percentage of patients who experimented with some form of unconventional therapy that was exactly the same as was discovered in the 1924 Philadelphia survey: 34 percent.[4]

Practitioners of "scientific medicine" thought of their rivals as cultists for a number of reasons. Not least was that, as the characterization in *The Healing Cults* had begun, they were intellectually enslaved to the founder of their particular sect. The American Medical Association argued the same point, defining a medical cultist as "one who in his practice follows a tenet or principle based on the authority of its promulgator to the exclusion of demonstration and scientific experience." In truth, there was a cult of personality surrounding the charismatic leaders of each system. Lust was "the father of naturopathy," Still "the old doctor," and the Palmers "the Discoverer" and "the Developer." By virtue of having "dictated [chiropractic's] dogma, trained over half its practitioners, and ruled with benevolent despotism over their kingdom," the Palmers, an MD wrote in the early 1940s, were to chiropractic "what the Mussolinis are to Italy"; they "are without doubt the greatest promoters the healing arts have ever seen."[5]

Unorthodox groups looked like cults also because there was such a multitude of them, like so many splinter denominations each convinced it had been vouchsafed the truth about creation and warring against all dissenting interpretations of scripture. A naturopath in fact described the scene as well as anyone, observing that "chaos prevails" among irregular practitioners. "There is no unification, no standardization, no co-operation. There is no loyalty, even. An osteopath will knife a chiropractor, metaphorically speaking. . . . A dietist will call a mental scientist a fool—and a mental scientist will call a dietist a fleshy materialist. A kneippist [sic] will tell you that fasting is dangerous—and a fast-curist will tell you that Kneipp is out of date." All in all, it was a "choice array of partial lunatics [where] no two agree."[6]

Cultism seemed applicable as well because the one-theory, one-cure systems posited mystical, scientifically unexplainable powers in the human body. Mainstream medicine was already well along the road of reductionism, the conviction that vital phenomena can be reduced entirely to mechanisms derived from the material sciences of chemistry and physics, and was automatically derisive of any theoretical position that smacked of vitalism or forces that transcended the physico-chemical domain. The osteopathic rule of the artery, drawn from Still's faith that Providence had placed all needed remedies within the human bloodstream, and chiropractic's Innate Intelligence, a parcel of divinity that energized and regulated the body, both clashed with the biochemical interpretation of the human frame. Christian Science clashed even more resoundingly, divorcing itself altogether from the scientific worldview by denying that such a thing as the corporeal body even existed; it seemed to be supernaturalism rampant.

The model of irregular vitalism was naturopathy, a system that although it accepted the material body was real, still explained health, disease, and healing in spiritual terms irreconcilable with reductionist science. "Every man has a certain, mysterious power within him," Lust proclaimed, a power that was a "psychic force [that] merely uses the mechanical forces as tools and means to attain its aims." It was only the healer who "understands this power, understands its suggestions," he insisted, who "will bring about a marvelous, successful cure." Words such as "mysterious" and "marvelous" were too close to the language of religion for scientific medicine's comfort. So were statements such as those placing naturopathy's "absolute reliance upon the cosmic forces of man's nature" and describing the "life force" as a cosmic power that was the "primary source of all energy, from which all other kinds and forms of energy are derived," a power "which flows into us from the one great source of all life in this Universe" and "would keep on acting with undiminished force" after death, "through the spiritual-material body." How could serious science be reconciled with a naturopath's statement (one made in a

Nature Cure Cook Book no less) that there was a spiritual-material body that was "an exact duplicate of the physical body ... whose material atoms and molecules are more refined and vibrate at infinitely greater velocities than those of the physical-material body," or the assertion that such a position was "not merely a matter of faith or of speculative reasoning, but a demonstrated fact of Natural Science"?[7]

Naturopaths, in turn, piled scorn on allopathy's "one-sided materialistic system of medicine," a system they took to be at a "most primitive" step of evolution in understanding health and healing. Its materialism "is the kindergarten stage of medicine," one ND scoffed, meaning that conventional medicine, not drugless healing, was "the most unscientific school of medicine in existence." (Other irregulars voiced the same opinion, chiropractors, for example, dismissing regular medicine as backward because it was "atheistic materialism.") That hard-won scientific knowledge could be so breezily tossed aside as kindergarten fluff only strengthened the orthodox medical view of irregular medicine as cultism, as did irregulars' belief that the power of healing was a gift and that when they tended their patients they were, in a sense, possessed by a universal spirit: "The Natural Healer, in whom the true healing faculty is aroused, exercises a control over the vital principle which is not and can not, for obvious reasons, be included in any strictly material system." Thus let the "heartless butchers [win] university honors by demonstration of their great knowledge of anatomical detail"; let those possessed by materialist science "pat themselves upon the chest and cry out: We are great and wise men!" God knew better. "God says to them: "You fools! You fools! You have forsaken me and my work. I will make you vanish from the earth as smoke!"[8] What but fanatical cultism, allopaths asked, could account for such Old Testament vengeance-is-mine inanity?

The scent of cultism hovered as well around unorthodox healers' improbable claims of cure. Lust averred with a straight face that half the seriously ill patients treated by allopaths died, while those who sought out naturopathic help were lost at the rate of only 5 percent (and most of those because of the damages that had already been done by MDs). Chiropractors prided themselves on routinely curing infantile paralysis, a disease that had allopaths stymied. The great influenza pandemic of 1918–19 that killed more than half a million Americans was the occasion for particularly questionable accounts of therapeutic omnipotence. "The mortality rate under routine medical treatment" during the outbreak, a chiropractic publication observed, "was exceedingly high." Chiropractic, however, rang up numbers of cure that "were truly startling in their revelations." Of more than twenty thousand flu patients treated with adjustments, the death rate was a miniscule 0.14 percent, meaning "that Chiropractic is from ten to thirty times as effective in the treatment of influenza as any other method that has been employed." Not so, responded naturopaths, who were capable of a 0.00 percent mortality rate. "Not one of my influenza patrons had the fever over three days," one drugless healer reported; "not one had to remain away from work more than a week, not one had any bad after-effects or any complications. And of course [!], there were no deaths." Although osteopaths crowed that they lost only 2 percent of the more than one hundred thousand influenza cases they treated, next to those other irregular practitioners they looked like bunglers; only allopaths could outbungle them.[9]

Irregular Medical Education

Extravagant statements about curative power ("Naturopaths Now Control Cancer") was evidence to MDs of still another facet of the cultist status of unorthodox medicine—the laughable quality of education that practitioners received yet thought of, as naively as graduates of the most dogmatic and blinkered sectarian school of religion, as a profound gospel. Orthodox medicine was on somewhat shaky ground here, as its own educational system had been nothing to boast of before the twentieth century. Indeed, as late as 1910 only sixteen of the more than one hundred allopathic medical schools required as much as two years of college preparation for admission; about fifty more demanded only a high school diploma or an elastically interpreted "equivalent," and the remaining fifty "ask little or nothing more than the rudiments or the recollection of a common school education." Requirements for graduation were similarly rudimentary at most institutions. Nevertheless, reformers had been pressuring schools to raise their standards ever since the 1840s, and over the last third of the nineteenth century substantial progress had been made. The reform effort came to a head in 1910, with the publication of *Medical Education in the United States and Canada*, a survey of medical schools commissioned by the Carnegie Foundation for the Advancement of Teaching and conducted by respected Kentucky educator Abraham Flexner. The Flexner Report, as the volume quickly became known, was a bombshell that rattled medical and political forces throughout the country with its exposé of the miserable standards obtaining at most orthodox schools. To cite just a few of Flexner's evaluations, a New Orleans institution was "a hopeless affair," and Milwaukee's two schools were "utterly wretched . . . without a redeeming feature"; even so, it was Chicago, with its ridiculous total of fourteen schools, that was "in respect to medical education the plague spot of the country." In the aftermath of the report, which gave unqualified praise only to Johns Hopkins, nearly half the medical schools in the country closed, and requirements at the survivors became much more stringent. By 1930, the majority profession could justifiably take pride in the rigorousness of the four-year programs of training—in scientific medicine—now in place in all American medical schools.[10]

Flexner's survey had not been limited to allopathic institutions. He visited and evaluated schools of homeopathy (fifteen in number), eclectic medicine (eight), physio-medicalism (one), and osteopathy (eight) as well and found none truly adequate and most sorely lacking. In a chapter titled "The Medical Sects," he characterized six of the homeopathic schools as "utterly hopeless" and all the eclectic schools as objects of "utter hopelessness." Osteopathic institutions earned such recognition as "worthless," "absurdly inadequate," and "fatally defective." Chiropractors ("chiropractics," he called them) and drugless healers he deemed not even worthy of consideration. They "are not medical sectarians," he opined, but something even lower; "they are unconscionable quacks, whose printed advertisements are tissues of exaggeration, pretense, and misrepresentation of the most unqualifiedly mercenary character. The public prosecutor and the grand jury are the proper agencies for dealing with them." Medical sectarianism in general simply was not "logically defensible," he concluded, "in this era of scientific medicine."[11]

Meanwhile, schools of chiropractic and naturopathy were proliferating, and though Flexner had not included them in his survey, other representatives of orthodoxy were happy to weigh in with their appraisals. Chiropractic, that "malignant tumor" growing out of osteopathy, was sustained by "trade schools" that catered to "the ignorant and the venal" and quickly sent them forth as graduates knowing "practically nothing of the human body." Mainstream medical literature of the 1910s and '20s in fact ran to overflowing with attacks on the unconscionable sham that was chiropractic education, a collection of alleged educational establishments that were in fact "a disgrace" that could "best serve the public interest by quietly going out of existence." An allopath who made "A Visit to a Chiropractic School" reported that most of the students he met there "had not bridged the stage between the grammar school" and their supposed medical course. An MD discoursing on "Where Chiropractors are Made" discarded the schools as devoted "entirely to financial and not at all to scientific standards" and the students as "intellectual refuse" whose "mental equipment" was in a state of "extreme wretchedness." A New York physician who in the early 1920s actually enrolled in the Palmer School in Davenport to get a look at "Chiropractic From the Inside" found that the only educational requirement enforced was to "insist that you must be able to write. If not, it would lead to all kinds of trouble to cash your check." Finally, a Texas allopath went undercover in the guise of a widow who wrote a school in Oklahoma City lamenting "she" had had only three years of schooling yet wondered "if I can be kirpatic dr. if you can make a kirpatic dr. for how much money I got about 2 thousand dolers." "You have the intelligence . . .

and sufficient education to understand the English language," the head of the school promptly replied, and "you would have no difficulty in getting a knowl-edge of this subject so that you could go out and practice and be efficient. You can enter at any time and in eighteen months, upon making your grades, can be graduated." B. J. Palmer himself confirmed his discipline's dubious educational standards by admitting in courtroom testimony that while anatomy was the basis of chiropractic science, his students' dissection experience was limited to an occasional sheep anatomized in a barn behind the school and the odd cadaver examined at Ed Horrigan's funeral parlor; dissection may have been irrelevant, however, since Palmer also professed to adhere to a system of anatomy that differed from the allopathic standard, *Gray's Anatomy*, "very materially."[12]

Much was made of the lack of formal education of most students admitted to chiropractic schools, which often eschewed entrance requirements on the grounds that innate intelligence and hard work alone could make a skilled practitioner—thus B. J. Palmer, answering a Wisconsin judge's question about the extent of his education:

A. Common sense.
Q. None other?
A. Horse reasoning.
Q. Any other?
A. Good judgment.
Q. Any other?
A. That is enough.

"If you never liked school before," one chiropractic institution's catalog re-assured prospective applicants, "you will enjoy chiropractic from the start, because everything is simplified and made practical from the beginning to the ending." Somewhat like Thomsonianism, chiropractic made its pitch directly to blue-collar workers and farmers, with the result, as the editor of the *Journal of the American Medical Association* pointed out in the 1920s, that it was "black-smiths, barbers, motormen and beauty specialists" who had "turned by the thousand to the chiropractic schools" in search of "an easy road to healing." (Critics of chiropractors' social origins seem to have forgotten that Flexner had complained not that many years before that all too often it was "the crude boy or the jaded clerk who goes into [allopathic] medicine.") The theme was picked up by lay critics of chiropractic, too, Mencken, for example, alleged that "six weeks after [the chiropractic student] leaves his job at the filling-station or abandons the steering wheel of his motor-truck he knows all the anatomy and physiology that he will ever learn in this world. Six weeks more, and he is an adept at all the half-Nelsons and left hooks that constitute the essence of chiropractic therapy," therapy that was nothing more than "an heroic pummeling by a retired piano mover."[13]

Naturopathic schools fared no better in orthodoxy's evaluations, being thrown aside as "small affairs of a fly-by-night character" that were "run by men untrained in and antagonistic to medical science" who taught "fantastic forms of assault . . . devised by the paranoic brains of a hundred cultist prophets." A 1920 advertisement for Lust's American School of Naturopathy typified drugless healers' empty pretensions to learning. "Become a Doctor of Naturopathy," it urged, because that "will qualify you at the same time as Osteopath, Chiropractor, Hydropath, Dietitian, Electropath, Mechanotherapist, Neuropath, Zonetherapist, Mental Scientist, etc." And the American School was the best in its field. Just think of the qualifications of a graduate of a Seattle school who put down responses such as the following on his licensing examination:

Q.   What foods are rich in iron, sulphur, proteids?
A.   Beets, lecttes, spenat, carets is very rich in iron. Eggs is rich in sulphur meats is rich in proteids also brad and of corce meny other foods.
Q.   Why are some of the heartiest eaters thin?
A.   One reason may be that they eats to much more than they can digest and they don't eat the wright combination also eat too fast.

This self-described "Dietitian's" physiology and orthography were worrisome enough, but even more disturbing was the fact that his exam had been passed by the state drugless board with a score of 90 percent! It was thus no great surprise when it came to light in 1924 that the head of Seattle's American University of Sanipractic (as naturopathy was known in the Pacific Northwest) had sold diplomas outright to applicants (on a sliding scale that ran from fifty to six hundred dollars) and had obtained copies of the licensing exam from the drugless healing board for use in a cram course for his "graduates." (There was, need it be said, an additional charge for the cram session.) Court action led to the school being shut down, but there were others, such as the Universal Sanipractic College, to take its place.[14]

The "ignoramuses" and "dumbbells" who matriculated at naturopathic institutions were derided as the same sort of hapless career failures who attended chiropractic schools. Enrollees in a Florida college, for example, included a former hod carrier, a telegraph messenger, a carpenter, a watchmaker, a printer, an ex–window washer, three stenographers, and so on, while the professor of pathology was also an insurance clerk. Even the school's administration was subjected to ad hominen attacks, the dean being mocked as "deaf, nervous and thick-headed." (As one might expect, the dean took exception to such obloquy, and the American Medical Association's *Journal* actually published an apology for the "thick-headed" part of the character sketch.)[15]

Irregular practitioners came across to their critics as cultists in a final sense, that of hypocrites in the mold of Elmer Gantry, whose loud protestations of philanthropy were nothing but a smokescreen to hide their greed. Potential students of sanipractic, to illustrate, were wooed with the assurance that a career in that field would be not only "pleasant" but "lucrative"; armed with a diploma from the American University of Sanipractic, "the confidence and the cash of the community are yours." A prominent naturopath's pitch was that "with a complete Nature Cure knowledge and training, you could start a publishing business, a mail course of instruction, a lecture bureau, a manufacturing company, a chain of restaurants, and a few other kinds of business, all at once"; you could become, in short, "a J. P. Morgan of health promotion." Or a B. J. Palmer, for if chiropractic students were reformed truck drivers and beauty specialists, chiropractic "educators" were bunco artists, allopaths alleged, the halls of their schools being rank with "the stench of commercialism."[16]

Basic Science Laws and Educational Reform

Yet many early-century chiropractors, as has been seen, were genuinely dismayed by the mercenaries among their colleagues, rebelling particularly against Palmer, and a number within the ranks of chiropractic and osteopathy alike had recognized as early as the 1910s that the theories of the founders were simplistic and their therapies less than the panaceas they were touted to be. The reader will recall osteopaths asking whether their discipline was to be developed "as a complete system or science" or "as a creed"(read cult) and chiropractors acknowledging that "many conditions ... are beyond the reach of spinal technic" and some elements of Palmer's theory "beyond the scope of truth or reason." Progressives within naturopathy saw failings in their profession, too, and were perhaps most outspoken of all irregulars over the infiltration of their practice by charlatans looking for easy money. Lust bemoaned the dilution of naturopathy by fakes throughout his long career as drugless healing's pater familias: in the very first volume of *The Naturopath*, in 1902, he complained of the many "pseudo-naturopaths" and "abortioners of naturopathy" and blasted a New York nature cure resort as nothing more than a "hyperbolistic home of heroicism" that brought discredit to the true art; more than four decades later, less than a week before his death, he dictated an address to be read at the American Naturopathic Association convention in which he lamented the number of "woeful misfits" and "outright fakers and cheats masking as Naturopaths." Through the years in between, he was joined by many another naturopath indignant over "the hundreds of so-called drug-less healers who are a disgrace to our calling," all the "money changers [who] clutter up our ranks and despoil our temples," and the fact that "there are as many quack methods prevalent in the Nature Cure as there are in the drug business."[17]

Some irregulars, in other words, were among their own worst critics, and out of that internal discontent grew pressure to raise the quality of education and practice in each system. Professional progress for unconventional systems of practice was not, however, entirely a matter of high-minded self-motivation. A good bit of pressure was brought to bear from the outside by legislation, in particular by the enactment during the middle third of the century of so-called basic science laws. The mainstream profession had found it very difficult to prevent the passage of licensing statutes for irregular systems because of the appeal of "medical freedom" arguments to state legislators. But if opposition to the licensing of any practitioners other than MDs appeared monopolistic and tyrannical, there was a good amount of disinterested reason to be seen in the argument that any person presuming to treat the diseased human body should at least have some knowledge of the basic biological sciences. By the 1920s regular physicians in many states were campaigning for new laws that would require applicants for a license in any field of practice to pass an examination in anatomy, physiology, pathology, and other areas of science fundamental to understanding health and disease before taking the licensing test in their special system of therapy.

To MDs, it was as straightforward a matter as could be. Our "cards are placed upon the table face-up," Oregon's physicians announced, "and the fight is clear-cut as being between scientific and unscientific medicine." Irregular practitioners fought back, not surprisingly, but it was not so easy to paint basic science legislation as an assault on individual freedom as it had been to put restrictions against non-allopathic therapies in that light. Unorthodox healers were not, after all, being barred from practice altogether; they were simply being asked to demonstrate more clearly that they knew what they were doing. "With the education necessary to pass such a board," it was pointed out, "the sincere therapeutic enthusiast, be he osteopath, chiropractor, electrotherapist, faith-healer, or herb-doctor, will probably not do much harm to the individual, or be a source of danger to the public health." The first basic science act was signed into law in 1925, in Wisconsin; within four years, six states and the District of Columbia had followed suit, and ultimately twenty-three states would pass such laws.[18]

At first the laws produced the desired effect. In Washington State, for example, in the two years preceding the 1927 statute there had actually been more chiropractors licensed than MDs (forty-seven allopaths, forty-eight chiropractors, forty-four sanipractors, and thirty-eight osteopaths). In the two years following the act, the numbers were eighty doctors of medicine, six osteopaths, one chiropractor, and no drugless healers. (It should be noted that it was the rule in all states to preclude bias by blinding examiners to the school of practice of individual test takers.) In Nebraska, 122 osteopathic licenses had been granted during the eight-year period immediately before the basic science law, but only twenty-one were issued for the eight years after; for chiropractors, the numbers were 290 before and zero after. For all states with boards in the late 1920s and early '30s, the rates of success on the basic science exam were 90 percent for physicians, 63 percent for osteopaths, and 27 percent for chiropractors. (To B. J. Palmer's way of seeing it, chiropractors' examination difficulties were fully deserved. Their wandering away from simple adjustment into the world of mixing had attracted allopathic attention and "brought the basic science bill upon your heads. . . . The basic science bills are the buckshot which we deserve for trespassing" on others' therapeutic turf, he scolded; "chiropractic is doomed.")[19]

As time passed, however, the medical profession became disgruntled with basic science laws for several reasons, not the least being the problems they posed for allopathic licensing reciprocity between states in which the examinations tested on different subjects. The laws backfired against orthodox medicine in another way, though, by forcing irregulars to sink or swim. They chose to swim, and that meant they had to elevate the level of instruction they provided their students in medical science. Although it was a slow process, osteopaths, chiropractors, and naturopaths did steadily improve their pass rates, and basic science exams became a less effective sieve for separating cultists from scientists. Beginning in 1967, one state after another repealed its basic science law, until the last three disappeared in 1979.[20]

The most rapid progress in educational improvement was achieved by osteopathy, which began its campaign in a serious way in the mid-1930s. Reform was risky, it should be borne in mind, because, unlike mainstream schools, osteopathic institutions received no public funding; they were financed almost entirely (more than 90 percent) by tuition fees, and by raising entrance requirements to the MD standard of two or more years of college, they would sharply decrease the size of their applicant pool. (Until the mid-1930s, osteopathic colleges required only a high school diploma for admission.) But with the basic science exam movement gathering momentum, they had little choice; between 1936 and 1940 all six osteopathic schools adopted a two-years-of-college prerequisite rule. Concomitantly, facilities were expanded, the curriculum lengthened to four years, and more highly qualified instructors in the basic sciences hired. The schools managed to stay afloat financially by intensified fund-raising within the profession and aggressive recruiting of college students, and the evident commitment to improvement paid off in the decade following World War II with the first allocations of funds for osteopathic schools and hospitals from the federal government. Osteopaths' success rate on basic science exams shot up between 1942 and 1953, from 52 percent to 80 percent (physicians' rate was 87 percent in the early 1950s), so forcefully demonstrating the profession's educational advancement as to attract the attention of the American Medical Association.[21]

In 1954 the AMA proposed to conduct inspections of osteopathic colleges comparable to the evaluation visits used for accrediting orthodox schools. One osteopathic institution declined the proposal as condescending, but the rest agreed to the survey, which was carried out early in 1955. The inspection committee, which included three medical school deans, determined that while osteopathic education was still inferior to MD training in several ways, the schools nevertheless were providing a "sound medical education." Students' records had been examined, and it had been found "that all had completed the education requirements for admission to medical school"; even more of a surprise was that "the records indicate that a considerable number could have obtained admission to medical school." Further, the committee observed, since manipulative therapy now played only a subordinate, and declining, role in theoretical and clinical instruction, "the teaching in these colleges does not fall into the 'cultist' category."[22]

Chiropractic underwent a similar evolution, with efforts to upgrade education beginning in the 1910s but making little headway until the mid-1930s and the appearance of the profession's own Flexner, one John Nugent. Nugent had particular reason to shoulder the task of educational reform: in the early 1920s he had been expelled from the Palmer School of Chiropractic for "disrespect and insult to the President." In 1935 the National Chiropractic Association, that "playground for mixers," in B. J. Palmer's eyes, appointed Nugent director of education and charged him with overhauling the profession's training system. For the next quarter century he pressed for entrance requirements of at least a high school education and for standardization of programs at four years of nine months' instruction, with more and better educated faculty and expanded clinical facilities. Nugent pushed for smaller schools to close or merge and for all institutions to be made non-profit. That non-profit part did not set well with many schools' administrators (Nugent became "the most hated name in chiropractic"), but over time he got his way. By 1960 most schools of chiropractic had adopted the Nugent standards, though a 1964 survey by a prominent chiropractic educator determined that most enrollees still had not studied beyond the high school level and teachers were obliged to downgrade their instruction "so that students could pass the courses." Over the ensuing decade, however, several schools put a two-years-of-college entrance requirement in place, and by 1974 educational standards had advanced sufficiently for the U.S. Office of Education to grant approval to an accrediting agency for chiropractic colleges. Henceforth schools accredited by the Council on Chiropractic Education would be eligible for federal funding for their programs, and their degrees would no longer be listed as "spurious" by the Office of Education. Even the Palmer School, advancing under the leadership of B. J. Palmer's son David Daniel, joined the parade of progress.[23]

Naturopaths were initially less successful at raising professional standards, education not having been taken that seriously in the field's first decades. The original naturopathic position was much like Samuel Thomson's and B. J. Palmer's, a faith in the power of common sense and native intelligence alone to guide one to truth. Thus when medical critics in the 1920s ridiculed naturopathic students as uneducated refugees from blue-collar trades, the response was that it was irrelevant that some students had previously been carpenters. So had Jesus, and "when Jesus picked his disciples he didn't hunt for college graduates." "No number of degrees, certificates and diplomas will put intelligence into the brain of an imbecile," another spokesman reminded; "imagine Hippocrates as a college graduate!"[24]

But by 1940 leaders of the American Naturopathic Association had resolved to rid their profession of "driftwood from wrecks of poor schools," and to that end had organized a National Board of Naturopathic Examiners to work for standard requirements of a high school diploma for entrance and a full four years of course work for graduation. As with chiropractic, however, the higher-standards program encountered resistance from the affected schools: "Indeed," one leader of the reform effort lamented as late as 1951, "their direct opposition is surprisingly considerable." That opposition reflected an internal disarray that was for a time, at least, the undoing of naturopathy. To be sure, disarray had been present virtually from the outset, as was shown in the preceding chapter, for "nature cure" was so flexible a concept as to encompass almost anything. As early as the 1920s, many naturopaths were complaining that their system's original purity was being compromised by practitioners who were chasing "after strange gods," after any god, in fact, that called itself drugless. "What have we," one of the field's most prominent practitioners asked, "nature cure or a bag of tricks?" Such a grab-bag approach to therapy, he fretted, was the source of limitless "childish quarrelings and foolish bickerings."[25]

The bickering continued, but by the 1940s it had taken on a more ominous tone. Lust's last years were deeply troubled by all the dissension and dishonesty he saw within the ranks of so-called naturopaths, and he called out repeatedly to the pure at heart among his followers to beware of "the internal enemies" of naturopathy, "the borers from within, the destructionists, would-be dictators, fake legislation promoters, the one-track minds and one-horse theorists, the opportunists, push-bottom machine promoters and snake charmers." These "misdirectors, racketeers and jealous opportunists," he believed, posed "a much more serious threat to our movement" than the external enemies, the allopaths. The threat was not exaggerated. Only six months before his death, Lust confided that "my efforts in establishing a profession for the Nature doctors has been a sad disappointment to me," and after death removed his governing hand factionalism rent naturopathy apart. Within five years two national organizations had been founded to rival the American Naturopathic Association, and before long there would be a total of six. Fragmentation opened the doors even wider to opportunists, of course, and by the 1950s naturopathy's old-time leaders were afraid that the youngest generation of practitioners was being attracted to the field only "as an easy livelihood, as a business; they are speculators rather than servants of God, nature, and man." The trend would not begin to be reversed until the 1970s, and not until 1980, with the founding of the American Association of Naturopathic Physicians, would some measure of cohesion and unity be brought to naturopathy.[26]

Yet despite the chaos, standards at naturopathic schools were steadily raised from the 1940s on, thanks to both professional idealism and the requirements of state licensing laws. A perusal of the statutes of the dozen states in which naturopaths were licensed in the late 1940s reveals that most demanded a high school diploma and a degree from a four-year naturopathic program. (There were nine naturopathic colleges in the United States at that time, another twenty-nine having fallen into the "extinct" category; some chiropractic schools also provided training in naturopathy, but the practice was abandoned during the 1950s.) By the end of the 1950s, several states required two years of college before admission to naturopathic training, although there were then only five naturopathic schools still in operation.[27]

The Emergence of "Osteopathic Medicine"

Meanwhile, another unorthodox system was becoming the first to get at least one foot firmly planted in the medical mainstream, and it is worth considering that development in some detail to appreciate how unconventional medicine's transition from cultism to more respectable status came about. By the middle of the twentieth century, osteopathy had evolved into so close a facsimile of orthodox medicine that practitioners had begun to call it osteopathic medicine. Throughout that period, however, it had met with nothing but resistance from regular medicine. Organized medicine's fight against licensing for osteopaths has been recounted. But opposition took other forms, based on the AMA's Principles of Medical Ethics, which had replaced the association's original code of professional conduct. The old consultation clause was gone, but in its stead was Section 3, which said essentially the same thing. "A physician should practice a method of healing founded on a scientific basis," the section stated, "and he should not voluntarily associate professionally with anyone who violates this principle." As officially designated cultists, osteopaths were in violation of the principle and therefore not to be associated with. On that basis, DOs were denied appointment as medical officers in the two world wars (as homeopaths and eclectics had been denied during the Civil War). In the early 1950s, when the town council of Bay City, Michigan, voted to grant osteopaths practice privileges at the municipal hospital, the seventy MDs on staff at once resigned on ethical grounds and the AMA Council on Medical Education and Hospitals rescinded its approval of the institution. Faced with the loss of the town hospital, Bay City's citizens voted in a referendum to withdraw acceptance of osteopaths. A strikingly similar story played itself out in Wharton County, Texas, in 1956.[28]

But by that year, it will be recalled, an AMA committee had inspected osteopathic colleges and determined that their students were adequately trained and were not being indoctrinated in medical cultism. The AMA as a whole rejected the inspection committee's recommendation that the cultist designation be dropped, but before long regular doctors' actions were speaking louder than their words, and the "cultists" began to be welcomed as colleagues. Rapprochement was nudged along by medical necessity. Osteopaths were much more likely than conventional physicians to go into general practice and to locate in rural areas, meaning that there were many small towns in which the only doctor was a DO. If MDs adhered to the no-consultation rule, patients in such towns could be hurt: "You can't let people suffer," a Kansas physician protested, "because you don't approve of the training of the man who wants to refer them to you." As interactions developed, allopaths discovered that osteopaths "were much better trained than they'd suspected," in one regular's words, and by the late 1950s several state and local medical societies were urging the AMA to abandon the cultist categorization of osteopathy. (In Kansas, relations became "so cordial . . . that the two professions have even joined forces to battle the chiropractors.")[29]

In 1961 the national association yielded, at least with respect to osteopathic physicians who had eschewed the use of manipulation as a major method of treatment. Those who were participating in "the transition of osteopathy into osteopathic medicine" clearly were making "an attempt . . . to give their patients scientific medical care." In those cases—that is, osteopaths who practiced "on the same scientific principles as those adhered to by members of the American Medical Association"—it was now "deemed ethical" to engage in "voluntary professional relationships." Professional interactions were not permissible, the AMA's Judicial Council decided, with DOs who held on to the old faith in manipulating osteopathic lesions: "If he practices osteopathy, he practices a cult system of healing."[30]

That same year the California Medical Association took the leap from "voluntary relationship" to marriage, wooing the California Osteopathic Association into a merger of the two professions that was promoted as a means of hastening the maturation of osteopathic medicine into scientific medicine. By the terms of the agreement, the osteopathic school in Los Angeles was converted into an allopathic institution empowered to grant MD degrees, and to grant them, furthermore, not just to future graduates but to osteopaths already licensed by and practicing in the state. In addition, more than sixty osteopathic hospitals underwent the same conversion. DOs were not *required* to change their title to MD, by any means, but it was an offer difficult to refuse. As MDs they would enjoy more prestige, freely make and receive referrals from their new brethren, be eligible for insurance payments for their patients, and partake of all the other privileges of orthodoxy, not least enhanced income. In July 1961 more than two thousand California DOs—"persuaded that a medical paradise would ensue"—gathered in Los Angeles to be made MDs; they had to pay a sixty-five-dollar processing fee for the transformation.[31]

To the three-hundred-and-some California osteopaths who did not undergo conversion, and to the great majority of DOs in the rest of the country, the processing fee was more accurately thought of as "sixty-five pieces of silver": Judas had been guilty of little worse treachery than those osteopaths who had been taken in by "the California conspiracy" and had, to use the *Old* Testament analogy of another critic, sold "their professional souls for . . . a mess of academic pottage." It is not easy to overstate the anger with which the osteopathic profession reacted to the California debacle. In a reversal of mainstream medicine's consultation clause, those California DOs who had relinquished their degrees were expelled from the American Osteopathic Association; the national osteopathic specialty societies for surgery, anesthesiology, pediatrics, and radiology disowned them as well. Just like the pair who had sampled other forbidden fruit (more Old Testament sermonizing), "those who have partaken of merger 'manna' find themselves cast out." They were mocked for the "inferiority complex" that gave them "the urge to merge," and their new title was laughed off as an "m.d.," the lower-case letters "chosen to accord with the academic stature of the . . . degree." What "m.d." really meant, it was joked, was "merger doctor" and "medical deception"; *m* and *d* were "scarlet letters [that] brand the DO who couldn't make good in osteopathic medicine" and signified membership in a new medical cult that was actually sanctioned by the AMA, "the cult of the new m.d." Like Hester

Prynne, the m.d.'s would "prostitute every dignified and respected standard" in their "headlong pursuit of recognition for recognition's sake," and if other DOs were to follow their adulterous example, the whole profession would shortly be recognized and "accepted and approved into oblivion."[32]

The mergers' medical deception was, like Judas's, an event that had been foretold. No sooner had some osteopaths in the early 1900s fallen for the allure of mixing than purists started warning that such a deviation from Still's narrow path must end badly. "Hodgepodge therapy," one prophet fumed as early as 1910, "is nothing short of osteopathic suicide," and another that same year predicted that if DOs continued to give in to the temptations of surgery and drugs, "twenty years hence, osteopathy will no longer be known by that name. It will be absorbed, suppressed, strangled, and so twisted out of shape by this political-medical trust, that it can no longer be recognized."[33]

Half a century later, osteopaths saw the machinations of a political-medical trust still at work. Ostensibly, the California Medical Association's reasons for promoting amalgamation were to further improve osteopaths' knowledge and skills (by improving their education) and to alleviate public confusion caused by two professions duplicating one another's work: the ideal was "one standard of education, one standard for licensure, and one standard of practice," and there was no doubt much sincerity behind those words. But osteopaths smelled monopolistic greed and attacked the amalgamation plan as "just another of a long series of arrogant actions in an almost fanatical drive to take over the osteopathic profession," an act of "academic piracy" that was "desperate in method and . . . pathetic in intent." By transforming osteopathic schools into allopathic institutions, orthodox medicine could limit osteopaths' numbers and thereby eliminate competition. (In fact, an objective analysis of the California merger effort performed in 1977 by a Yale University professor of economics concluded that indeed "the policies organized medicine employed toward osteopaths [were] consistent with concern over preservation of its monopoly power.") To be sure, the killing-with-kindness strategy was more subtle than the early-century attempts to legislate osteopathy out of existence. Yet while the invitation to merge may have looked "like an olive branch," it was "actually a sprig of poison ivy," one osteopath warned; allopathy may have changed its lyrics, as another metaphor had it, "but the melody remains the same." Osteopaths had to resist the siren song and never forget, the editor of the *Journal of the American Osteopathic Association* enjoined, that "a D.O. degree is a prized possession. A profession has invested its life in it. Let us resolve that we . . . will never sell it for sixty-five pieces of silver."[34]

The situation took on added urgency in 1963 when a more ambitious merger plan was set into motion in Washington State in the form of a "paper school" established by the state medical society in cooperation with dissident osteopaths "solely to confer M.D. degrees on D.O.s who want to merge" (the "school" had no connection with the state medical school at the University of Washington). Because the new institution was willing to confer the MD regardless of an osteopath's state of residence, the scheme threatened to undermine osteopathy nationwide. Washington's supreme court soon intervened and declared the school's program illegal, but even though only fifty-four Washington DOs got transformed into MDs, it was clear to osteopaths that their independence was under siege.[35]

The California conspiracy marked "one of the profession's blackest pages in history." One of the brightest was turned in March 1974, just three months short of the centennial of the day that Still flung "to the breeze the banner of Osteopathy." The occasion was a ruling of the Supreme Court of the State of California on an action initiated in 1968 by eight osteopathic physicians from outside the state. These DOs had discovered on moving to California that they could not be licensed to practice as osteopaths because a statute instituted during the merger period, in 1962, had abolished the osteopathic licensing board (in anticipation of osteopaths henceforth converting to standard medicine). The DOs' argument that the law violated their Fourteenth Amendment rights was acknowledged by the unanimous verdict of the state supreme court that "to try to eliminate the osteopathic profession by the 'California method' is illegal and unconstitutional." The verdict was hailed, incidentally, in terms that could have come as easily from the mouths of Thomson and the other irregular crusaders against licensing laws in the 1830s. The overturned law had been "an affront to the very principles upon which this country was founded . . . a threat to the very foundations of the American way of life." The court's decision was a recognition of the inalienable right of osteopaths to pursue their calling and of the state's citizens to choose the kind of medicine they wanted: "The Supreme Court's ruling in California was a people's victory."[36]

In the meantime, other victories had been registered. The fact that in 1961 the California osteopathic school had overnight and with little change been turned into an accredited MD-granting institution impressed legislators and officials in states other than California, and in Washington, DC, as evidence that there was no longer any basis for thinking of osteopathy as an inferior form of medical practice. One of the most important demonstrations of newfound respect was the opening of state-supported schools of osteopathy, beginning with Michigan State University College of Osteopathic Medicine in 1969. Operating on the same campus as an allopathic medical school, and sharing basic science faculty yet maintaining independence in administration and budget, MSU-COM "gave visible expression . . . that the two medical professions were separate but equal." During the 1970s several more state-funded schools were established; when combined with newly founded private institutions, they gave osteopathy an extraordinary increase from five to fourteen schools in the decade from 1968 to 1978. At the national level, the U.S. Civil Service Commission announced in 1963 a new policy of considering DO and MD degrees as equal, referring specifically to the California merger as justification for the decision.[37]

Three years later, Secretary of Defense Robert McNamara brought an end to one of osteopaths' longest-standing grievances, their exclusion from medical practice in the armed forces. This in fact had been a century-long sore spot for all the irregular systems: in World War I, Lust accused the federal government of "treason" for "keeping drugless physicians out of the country's service." Osteopaths had protested most loudly, however, and after being shut out of two world wars and the Korean conflict, they finally won acknowledgment of their acceptability for military practice just as the American involvement in Vietnam began to escalate. (Denial of the privilege of practicing in the military had actually been a blessing in disguise, as during World War II DOs were granted draft deferrals so they could fill the physician shortage created by so many MDs being taken into the military; the preponderance of osteopaths during the war years made them much more familiar and acceptable to the American public.)[38]

A more telling sign of acceptance had come the year before the opening of military practice, in 1965, when osteopathic medical services were specified for reimbursement under the newly established Medicare system. (Chiropractic and naturopathy also appealed for inclusion in Medicare, incidentally, but were denied.) Osteopathic medicine made still other inroads into the medical establishment in the 1960s and '70s. The American Medical Association extended membership to DOs, and allopathic residency programs began to accept graduates of osteopathic schools. In the process, however, the historic lines between it and allopathic medicine became ever more blurred, until by the end of the 1970s osteopathy had lost its unorthodox identity in many people's minds. It seemed to be only an extension of allopathic medicine. In 1978 one of the first comprehensive reference works on alternative medicine discussed the full range of unconventional approaches to healing, including chiropractic and massage, but not a single mention was made of osteopathic medicine. The same is true of many subsequent works in the genre.[39]

Osteopathic Medicine as Holism

Identity erosion had been warned about since Still's day, but it was the California merger, with its threat of complete absorption into the mainstream, that forced the osteopathic profession to undertake intense self-examination and determine what, if any, reason there was to remain separate from allopathic medicine. The result of that soul-searching was the formulation of a commitment to return to philosophical fundamentals and reinvigorate "the osteopathic concept." Various meanings were to be teased out of the concept, but it was grounded, as it had been for Still, in the power of musculoskeletal manipulation to enhance physical functioning. As osteopathic manipulative technique had evolved over the twentieth century, it had been shorn of the nearly panaceal properties Still had ascribed to it. Indeed, for many practitioners manipulation had by the 1950s been relegated to a minor role, made simply an "unadherent frosting on the cake," the cake of drugs and surgery. Yet in calling for the restoration of manipulative therapy to a central position, osteopathy's mid-century reformers were not merely aiming at making it a more commonly employed method. "It is not just another form of therapy," it was argued; "it is a whole strategy[:] . . . The putting of influences into the whole man through the accessible tissues of the body, influences which deflect his life processes to more favorable paths." Utilized from that perspective, manipulation would not be mere frosting on the cake but would serve as "the 'leaven' throughout the loaf."[40]

The renewed emphasis on manipulation as the invigorating agent in osteopathic practice redoubled the profession's resistance to conventional medicine's overtures. The AMA's 1961 resolution to remove its cultism label from osteopathy, after all, had distinguished between those DOs who had matured into the practice of scientific medicine ("bases his practice on the same scientific principles as those adhered to by members of the American Medical Association") and those who continued to hold on to musculoskeletal manipulative techniques, employing "a cult system of healing." By reviving identification with Still's orientation, osteopaths were consciously flouting the majority profession's judgment of cultism for the traditional version of osteopathy.

Interpretations of the effects of manipulation were, however, far advanced beyond reestablishment of the rule of the artery. Still now came to be thought of not as a practical-minded man who had worked out certain physical procedures for improving body function but as "essentially a medical philosopher"; his use of manipulation, it was maintained, was just one "means of expressing a medical philosophy," a philosophy whose central tenets were "understanding of the unity of the body, the healing power of nature, and the interrelationship between structure and function." Manipulative methods thus had to be analyzed in terms of that philosophical schema, as, for example, techniques that removed "critical impediments to the optimal operation of adaptive, homeostatic, defensive, restorative, and reparative processes."[41]

The language of "adaptive" and "homeostatic" was rich, of course, with implications of dealing with every patient as a whole systemically integrated organism, and that was indeed an outlook that osteopathy had professed from its beginnings. "The osteopathic idea," according to a 1915 statement of principles, is "that the bodily organism represents a wholeness or completeness, biologically," and the "physiological unity of the organism [must] be kept intact." With the professional introspection forced by the 1960s threat of amalgamation, however, the whole person, psyche as well as soma, was brought to the very center of the stage. By then, the field of psychosomatic medicine had grown (since the 1930s) from a recognition that certain physical ailments can be aggravated by emotional stress to an awareness of psychological forces as an element in the multi-factorial etiology of virtually all illness. From the osteopathic viewpoint, the physical processes that could be affected by manipulation had to be subject as well to the influence of a person's psychological state. Thus diagnosis and therapy had "to be precisely 'custom-made' to the patient and his continually changing circumstances." That was "the Hippocratic philosophy of disease" to which osteopaths claimed to give allegiance, as distinct from regular medicine's reliance on "dazzling displays of tactical bravura and technical virtuosity" aimed at obliterating physical disease while remaining heedless of the critical problem of "human need"; any system afflicted with such a "great preoccupation with diseases" while "neglecting the human factors from which they . . . arise, can only be regarded, basically, as a failure." That osteopaths' self-image was not a badly distorted one is suggested by the comments of a Kansas physician who confided in the early 1960s that "now that I'm acquainted with D.O.s, I'm impressed not only with their common sense but with their strong feeling for treating patients, not merely diseases. It's valuable to M.D.s, especially young doctors, to be constantly exposed to this point of view."[42]

Tightly intertwined with that point of view was what osteopaths of the 1960s called "ecological medicine." Allopaths, they maintained, were overly committed to "etiological medicine," meaning that they concentrated on etiology—the external causative agent of infection or other form of illness—and did not give adequate recognition to the internal imbalances that made a patient susceptible to the etiological factor. The osteopathic ecological interpretation of tuberculosis, for example, acknowledged the necessity of the tubercle bacillus as etiology but was less preoccupied with destroying the germ than with establishing a harmonious physiological ecosystem within the patient that was inhospitable to invading bacilli. Restoring and maintaining ecological integrity was the primary purpose of musculoskeletal manipulation.[43]

Close reading of 1960s osteopathic literature uncovers still other differences that DOs believed separated them from MDs. Their ecological orientation made them place more emphasis on patient education and on prevention, for example, and gave them a more positive definition of health as an elevated state of vitality far above mere absence of disease. In sum, the osteopathic profession submitted, their medicine was not only as good as the majority profession's but one that "gives an extra dimension to [the] care of patients." It was the same scientific medicine that MDs practiced but with an added area of scientific theory and therapy that allopathic medicine had not yet recognized. That, osteopaths were saying, was allopathy's loss, and while allopaths could call them what they liked, any objective observer must see that it was time to remove "the cloak of cultism which has hung over its shoulders these many years."[44]

A term other than "cultism" was indeed on the horizon, two terms in fact. During the late 1970s, discussions of unconventional therapies began to refer to them as "alternative medicine," and by the mid-'80s that would be the standard designation. Although "alternative" still indicated these approaches were different from mainstream medicine, and in competition with it, the phrase also connoted a level of acceptability not present in "medical cultism." The suggestion that unconventional systems might legitimately serve as alternatives to orthodox medicine was an acknowledgment of the professional progress that had been achieved by those systems over the past half century.

Recognition of irregular medicine as alternative was due even more, however, to the burst of enthusiasm in the 1970s for an orientation toward health care that utilized a second term. When osteopaths won their 1974 victory in the California courts, they hailed it as a statement by the people of California that "they were looking for physicians . . . who understood and practiced the Still philosophy," who "were trained in the holistic approach to medicine." The "osteopathic concept" and "ecological medicine" were just other ways of identifying a philosophy all alternative systems would soon be espousing as a revolution in healing, the philosophy of holistic medicine.[45]

11

The Holistic Health Explosion: Acupuncture

A crisis of confidence in modern medicine is upon us," Ivan Illich announced near the beginning of his 1975 *Medical Nemesis*. Crisis was in fact the medical leitmotif of the decade. On assuming the presidency in 1969, Richard Nixon had warned Americans that "we face a massive crisis" in medical care, and a national poll conducted a year later found that three-fourths of heads of households agreed with the statement "There is a crisis in health care in the United States." Rising costs and limited accessibility to care were major factors in generating the sense of crisis, but equally important was dissatisfaction with physicians. A wave of books such as *Medical Nemesis*, Thomas McKeown's *The Role of Medicine*, Rick Carlson's *The End of Medicine*, and Marcia Millman's *The Unkindest Cut*, not to mention numerous articles in lay periodicals, repeatedly took the profession to task for a catalogue of sins both committed and omitted. The unifying theme of allopathic medicine's antagonists, voiced so effectively by Illich, was that modern medicine was guilty of a "presumptuous expertise" that required every form of human suffering to be pressed into its narrow biomechanical construct of disease. And just as hubris had been punished by the ancient Greeks through Nemesis, the goddess of retribution, so medicine would get its comeuppance for so arrogantly ignoring the human facets of illness that did not fit easily into the biomedical box.[1] MDs would have to answer, in short, for not treating the whole patient.

The medical world of the 1970s was rocked as well by what Norman Cousins called "the holistic health explosion." To be sure, as a broad concept, holism was anything but new. Many components of the holistic blueprint for reform had long been central precepts for all alternative medical systems. But under the rubric of "holistic medicine," old ideas were reworked into a broad-reaching vision of what medical care ought to be that excited public interest to a degree not previously approached. By 1980 "holistic" had become one of American society's hottest buzzwords, an obligatory descriptor of anything new and good and non-allopathic that was thrown around in conversation and print, one observer quipped, "as enthusiastically as a frisbee in the springtime."[2]

Emergence of Holistic Medicine

"Holism" (from the Greek *holos*, or whole) was coined in 1926 by the South African philosopher Jan Smuts to describe an interpretation of living organisms as systems whose functioning is more complex than the sum of their individual parts: "The synthesis of parts into a whole changes those parts so that they no longer function as they would in isolation." The idea was one that enjoyed considerable favor among biologists of the day reacting against the tendency to reduce animals to simple biochemical machines, and it was contemporaneously embraced by some physicians as a needed reform in the understanding of sick humans. Yet as a term "holism" did not find its way into everyday medical discourse until the 1970s, when it was interjected into discussion primarily by critics of conventional medicine who saw the need for a new model for interpreting disease and healing the sick.[3]

The appearance of the holistic critique signaled the end of a honeymoon between conventional medicine and the American public that had begun with the popularization of "scientific medicine" early in the century, then strongly intensified with the introduction of sulfa drugs in the 1930s and antibiotics in the 1940s. So enamored was society with the "wonder drugs" that by the 1950s it could fairly be stated that "most patients are as completely under the supposedly scientific yoke of modern medicine as any primitive savage is under the superstitious serfdom of the tribal witch doctor." Yet by then it was already becoming evident that wonder drugs were not invariably wonderful, that they could produce side effects of quite serious proportions; the new medicines could not only do more for them, people were coming to see, they could do more to them as well. That was unsettling enough, but a good bit more disturbing was the realization that many physicians were dispensing the potentially hazardous substances indiscriminately, prescribing penicillin as if it were synonymous with panacea. "Antibiotic abandon" was the way an American authority on adverse drug effects described his colleagues' behavior during the 1950s, while the British journal *Lancet* spoofed the profession's heedless enthusiasm by announcing "yet another wonder drug," the compound "3 blindmycin."[4]

The dangers of untoward reactions to drugs would be imprinted upon public awareness even more forcefully by the thalidomide tragedy of the 1960s, after which it became commonplace to attack mainstream medicine as dangerous. Illich's first sentence in *Medical Nemesis*, for example, accused "the medical establishment" of having become "a major threat to health"; shortly after, he referred to doctor-induced illness as an "epidemic." Alternative practitioners of course exploited the new drug anxiety; chiropractors of the 1970s, for example, distributed pamphlets with titles such as *Drug-Caused Diseases* and *Drugs—Dangerous Whether Pushed or Prescribed*. Even the orthodox profession itself admitted that iatrogenic, or physician-induced, illness was a too common result of drug therapy. The title of the chief reference cataloguing the side effects of drugs was the most eloquent acknowledgment of the prevalence of iatrogenic injury: *Diseases of Medical Progress*, Robert Moser called his book. "We have reached a point in medical history when we must reappraise the status of drugs and patients," Moser wrote in the preface of the work's second edition. Nor was it comforting that that 1964 edition ran to 468 pages of text, after the first edition of only five years before had comprised a mere 58 pages; more unsettling, the third edition (1969) would require 821 pages. Well could Moser state in the epilogue of the last edition that " 'diseases of medical progress' will be with us forevermore."[5]

Medicine's critics were bothered not simply by the physical threat posed by new drugs but equally by what antibiotic abandon appeared to say about the physician-patient relationship. Blindmycin (read antibiotics) could be thought of as the successor to calomel: it seemed it was routinely administered for any and all physical complaints, without attention to a patient's individuality, without regard, in a word, for her wholeness. As early as the 1950s complaints were already accumulating that physicians were giving less time to physical examinations and patient histories because the treatment was likely to be the same whatever the diagnosis: this "new generation" of practitioners, an infectious diseases expert objected, was "substituting antibiotics for thinking."[6]

Until the 1970s, however, such misgivings were effectively drowned out by all the huzzahs for scientific medicine. Only then did there at last erupt a full-scale revolt, not just against routine prescribing of drugs and physician indifference toward patients as people but above all against the mindset of biological reductionism that fostered such attitudes. As with any revolt, there was an arch-villain to be overthrown. In this instance it was the renowned French philosopher René Descartes, ingloriously exhumed from the seventeenth century for having drawn a rigid distinction between mind and body that, it was charged, had turned medicine onto a path of denying any influence of the psyche upon the material body. As Carlson, for example, asserted in *The End of Medicine*, allopaths had, thanks to Descartes, "divided the body and mind and chosen the body as [their] focus," and from there "it was only a small step to equate the working of the human organism with the precision of machine function."[7] Machines did not have minds; nor did they have emotions or spiritual qualities. The fundamental meaning of 1970s holism was medicine that repudiated Cartesian dualism to embrace an understanding of human beings as organisms whose mental, emotional, and spiritual powers were fully integrated with, and affected the functioning of, their bodies.

That core meaning was conveyed by the use of the word "wholism," as commonly employed as "holism" in the early 1970s. The alternate spelling soon all but disappeared, however, as the reaction widened to include so many other objections to the conventional orientation beyond neglect of the whole patient. Taken singly, most of these objections were not new; many had been voiced since the 1950s at least. But under the heading of holism they were now combined into a single unified brief against the medical establishment.

First, it was argued, physicians trained as biomedical scientists were unable or unwilling to communicate with patients in terms the lay person could understand and tended to be aloof and superior. (The complaint was an old one; a Chicago woman of the 1920s, for example, related that a physician she had recently seen "was as pompous as a New Zealand devil dancer.") The situation worsened as the century wore on, for the infectious diseases that had previously constituted the most common type of health threat came to be replaced in large measure by chronic ailments such as heart disease, cancer, and diabetes. Infection was an acute problem that usually could be quickly cured with the right antibiotic. Chronic complaints were not only difficult or impossible to cure, but by their protracted and disabling nature they imposed a severe emotional toll on sufferers. Physicians educated according to the model of "scientific medicine," trained for prompt and decisive physical interventions, were ill equipped to provide the sensitive management of personal miseries needed by victims of chronic conditions. One of the memories that haunted an allopathic physician dying of cancer was all the time he had had to spend "upbraiding the medical profession for its callous conduct at the bedside."[8] Chronic ailments such as cancer and AIDS have thus generated patient support for alternative therapies in the same way that acute infections such as cholera and yellow fever did in the nineteenth.

Sensitive personal handling of the sick was further handicapped, it was often charged, by the fragmentation of care resulting from medical specialization, a trend that had accelerated dramatically from the 1930s on. In 1930 more than 80 percent of MDs were general practitioners; by 1960 that had fallen to 45 percent, and the downward trajectory in numbers of generalists was so steep as to augur extinction of the species. Specialist care, by its nature, was episodic, restrained from providing the ongoing personal attention inherent to general practice. As early as the 1940s one encounters frequent statements of exasperation by patients finding themselves batted around between specialists. There was, for example, the schoolteacher who went to a university clinic for evaluation: "The gynecologist blamed dysmenorrhea for her troubles," it was reported, "the endocrinologist blamed a pituitary-ovarian dysfunction, the neurologist blamed severe migraine, the psychiatrist blamed overwork and a poor adjustment to celibacy, the orthopedist blamed a twisted spine, the gastroenterologist blamed 'colitis,' and the surgeon blamed the appendix." By the 1970s explosion of holistic medicine, critics were maintaining that such bewildering runarounds had become the norm.[9]

The fact that decreasing personal attention was being paralleled by increasing costs, and that physicians' income was climbing while organized medicine was steadfastly opposing proposals for national health insurance, further alienated the public from mainstream medicine. The growing expense of medicine figured into public dissatisfaction in still another way, as the 1970s witnessed more and more objections that all that money was not buying all that much health. America, it was pointed out repeatedly, possessed the most technically advanced medical system in the world, yet by measures such as life expectancy and infant mortality the nation finished well down the list of industrialized countries. Even what improvements in health had occurred, critics now argued, were due much more to improved nutrition, environmental hygiene, and limitation of family size than to wonder drugs and miracle surgeries. "When contrasted with all the other factors that demonstrably affect health," Carlson wrote, "medicine plays a minor role, despite being cast for lead"; the contribution of medical care to improved health, in fact, was one of an "insignificance [that] cannot be overemphasized."[10]

Broader social forces pushed the process of alienation forward as well. The "secular humanism" counterculture of the 1960s, with its rebellion against authority, distrust of science and technology, concern for individual rights, and promotion of consumerism, necessarily aroused hostility toward establishment medicine, just as the spirit of Jacksonian democracy had fanned revolt in an earlier age. (The spirit of Jacksonianism has in fact reawakened in the form of attacks on medical licensing as "authoritarian" and "overly restrictive," accompanied by Thomson-like appeals to the "people [to] rely more on their own ability to protect themselves.") At the same time, counterculture rhetoric extolling the virtues of the simple, natural life and toleration of diverse lifestyles and cultures (particularly of the oppressed) burnished the appeal of the medical counterculture.[11]

Holistic Philosophy

All these concerns and values went into the molding of a remarkably broad medical philosophy. Details varied somewhat from one advocate to the next, but one can nevertheless identify certain principles central to essentially all versions of holism. Relating to and treating the whole patient was fundamental, of course, as was the distinction between healing, or making the patient whole, and curing, or eradicating the disease. One could cure without healing, it was emphasized, as well as heal without curing. Just as basic was appreciation that the ultimate power to heal resided in nature. The 1978 *Holistic Health Handbook* was actually dedicated "to the search for the universal healer within us all," while one of the best-selling books in the non-fiction category in the 1970s was Norman Cousins's *Anatomy of an Illness*, in which the editor of *The Saturday Review* told the inspirational story of how he overcame a degenerative illness diagnosed as incurable through the stimulating effects of laughter on his "life-force." (It might be noted that Cousins had been anticipated by a naturopath in the 1910s who had written a book on *The Laugh Cure;* in the 1920s another drugless healer put forward "phobiotherapy," or the "fear-cure." Cousins's illness, incidentally, was later diagnosed by several physicians as probably a rheumatologic problem that generally disappears on its own after a year or two.)[12]

Engaging the healer within implied a deeper involvement of the patient in diagnosis, treatment, and recovery than was usually encouraged or allowed by regular physicians. In his widely read *The Role of Medicine*, McKeown submitted that one of the chief reasons conventional medicine should be thought of as "sinister" was that "it usurps the right of the individual to face, deal with, and bear his own health problems." Biomedicine was inclined to dictate to the patient and impose treatment upon him rather than invite a collaboration. Already in the 1920s a patient had protested that "medicine treats you merely as an objective—a clod of a thing to be worked upon," whereas irregular doctors "make you a factor in your own healing." MDs of the day admitted as much, their attitude toward the patient's ability to comprehend his situation being the one expressed by a representative of the AMA in 1925—in a book written for a popular audience, no less. Imagine the average person "trying to understand how a tubercle bacillus makes a cavity within a human lung!" Morris Fishbein laughed; "to explain these things to him would be as hopeless as explaining the theory of the well-advertised Professor Einstein." Holism was a reaction against the notion that medicine was as far beyond the reach of common intelligence as theoretical physics. Indeed, not only could medicine's intricacies be made comprehensible to the lay person, true healing could not occur, holists insisted, until the patient was recruited as an ally and made to feel responsible for bringing himself back to health by acting on the healer's guidance and encouragement. "The principal contribution" of his physician, Cousins asserted, "was that he encouraged me to believe I was a respected partner with him in the total undertaking."[13]

There were other important elements of 1970s holism, emphases such as prevention of illness through correct living, pursuit of "high-level wellness" instead of mere health, and living in harmony with the cosmos. For the most part, MDs saw all this as generally unscientific and frequently either banal or childish as well. "There is a valuable message in the holistic movement," wrote an editorialist in the *New England Journal of Medicine* in 1979, but "that message [is] distorted by the palpable quackery and silliness of much that calls itself holistic."[14] Nevertheless, by the 1970s there was also a growing conviction within conventional medicine that holism carried a message that was extremely valuable and that it was not being given adequate attention by physicians. This emergence of holistic enthusiasm within mainstream medicine was a potent force in transforming attitudes toward unconventional systems of practice.

Holism Within Orthodox Medicine

To be sure, MDs had occasionally worried that they were losing sight of patients as whole people ever since the advent of "scientific medicine" early in the twentieth century. In 1909, for instance, a Boston medical professor bemoaned the "materialistic viewpoint" of medical students that closed their minds to the human complexity of patients. "The nature of personality is not adequately studied in the medical school," he lamented. "Many phases of the individual are often exhaustively considered, but at present it is no one's business to combine these scattered parts into the wholeness of the individual child or man or woman. And yet," he reminded, "every patient is an individual, a personality, and has a heart and kidneys and nervous system and all the rest only as parts ministering to this personality, the only essential whole." He hopefully predicted that "the tide [of whole patient care] is coming in!" The very next year, however, the Flexner Report was published, and the materialist viewpoint that concentrated on organs over personality was established as the curricular ideal medical schools would aspire to for the next half century. (That orientation, it should be noted, was not entirely in accord with Flexner's prescription, for although he did demand that medical students be given much more rigorous scientific training, he was equally emphatic that the medical graduate should be "first of all an educated man," a broadly learned person possessed of "insight and sympathy" in addition to scientific acumen.) Allopaths had also occasionally recognized that the appeal of alternative medicine derived in great part from its more holistic viewpoint. As an Indiana doctor pointed out in 1923, "irregular healers . . . would not exist if they did not fulfill a kind of need," a need for physicians possessed of talents beyond the "scientific foundation and mental discipline" given them by post-Flexnerian medical training: "The people of this country are demanding of the medical profession something more than shaking up test tubes and looking through microscopes."[15]

Appeals to restore the holistic orientation were infrequent, however, until the 1950s. By then, public restiveness over the personal content of physician-patient interaction had grown to a level that could not be overlooked. In 1954 a New York practitioner could actually ask readers of the state medical journal, "Do Your Patients Really Like You?" and assure them that very often the answer was no. That conclusion had been forced upon him by a survey he had taken in which patients had repeatedly complained that their doctors were attentive only to their anatomy, not to their selves. "A modern patient feels that he has been cheated," the writer observed, "that he has x-ray machines instead of human relationships." This was not to say that sick people wanted to see X-ray machines discarded but only that "on an emotional level" they desired "to come back to the kind of relationship . . . that they used to have with their doctor." As one of the survey respondents said of his physician, "all he did was make me well." That, the author suggested, was "the outcry of a person who feels let down, neglected, and robbed of what he thinks his doctor should have given him—love, interest, and affection." (This being the 1950s, it struck the author that one way of showing affection for patients would be to set out free candy and cigarettes in the waiting room.) Those sentiments would echo through ensuing years; a physician of the mid-1960s, for example, suggested that modern practitioners had become so focused on disease as to create a situation in which "the patient knows how he feels but doesn't know what he's got—while the doctor knows what he's got but doesn't know how he feels." "The milk of human kindness," he worried, "has been curdled by molecular biology."[16]

Molecular biology was the basis of the orthodox medical worldview, an understanding of disease and cure that was commonly characterized as "biomedicine." During the 1960s and '70s biomedicine was constantly glorified as the scientific key to eradicating humankind's physical miseries. Yet at the same time, growing numbers within the profession began to assail the "biomedical model" as an overly narrow, therefore unscientific, way of addressing human ills. Medicine was in "crisis," psychiatrist George Engel argued, because "it assumes disease to be fully accounted for by deviations from the norm of measurable biological (somatic) variables." The biomedical model left no room "for the social, psychological, and behavioral dimensions of illness." Medicine needed a new model, Engel asserted, and largely through his direction an orientation identified as the "biopsychosocial model" of illness emerged by 1980 as the progressive ideal for conventional practitioners.[17]

The biopsychosocial approach advanced along several professional fronts. Vital impetus came, for example, from the development of a new area of specialization in the 1960s, the field of family medicine. While some found the notion of specializing in general practice laughable, most physicians by the 1950s recognized a need for broadly trained practitioners who could treat most complaints themselves, refer patients to the proper expert when specialist attention was needed, and coordinate the activities of all specialists involved in a patient's care. In theory, that was what general practitioners had been doing all along, but the training of generalists had not kept pace with the growing complexity of medical care and the health care system. Not only were old-style general practitioners ill equipped to oversee the handling of patients in this new environment, but their numbers had plummeted in recent times as ever more medical school graduates opted for the greater prestige and pay of specialty practice. Between 1930 and 1960 the number of general practitioners declined from 112,000 to 75,000, and over the next five years the total would fall still farther, to 66,000; by that point only about one-quarter of American physicians were GPs.[18]

The year 1966 was pivotal in the resurgence of generalist physicians, thanks to the publication of the recommendations of two prestigious professional groups. The Millis Commission's volume on *The Graduate Education of Physicians* and the report of an American Medical Association committee on *Education for Family Practice* both demanded the training of more doctors for family practice. Yet in addressing the crisis of too few generalists, protagonists for family medicine concentrated as much on the need for qualitative enhancement as for increases in numbers. The patient must be treated "as a whole," the Millis Commission maintained, and the training of family practitioners should be as much "social and humanistic" as "biological," to enable them to "deal with man as a total, complex, integrated, social being." The AMA committee spoke similarly, asserting that the family physician must be "a personal physician, oriented to the whole patient, who practices both scientific and humanistic medicine."[19]

In the aftermath of these publications, attention to holism only intensified. Thus a 1968 report from the Family Health Foundation of America characterized mainstream medicine as a "modern collection of highly indoctrinated robots, each one of whom knows all there is to know about one part of the body and is highly skilled either in taking it out or restoring it to normal function." But how well, it was asked, did such doctors minister to "the sum total of human suffering"? It appeared that "in the plethora and pride of its scientific accomplishments, American medicine [has] lost sight of its essential objective: to provide continuing comprehensive care to the whole man" and to educate physicians "who know that the whole human being is a more interesting subject than any of the illnesses that afflict him."[20] The commitment to holism deepened yet farther after family medicine gained formal recognition as a distinct field of specialization in 1969.

The same commitment was being advanced with at least equal fervor in the 1970s by the field of psychosomatic medicine. In its fundamentals, the psychosomatic perspective can be traced back to Hippocrates, who understood illness as the product of interaction of mental, emotional, and social forces with a person's material body. Those insights persisted in Western medical thought over centuries, but as laboratory-based biological reductionism rose to dominance in the 1800s, the relation of sickness to psychological state came to be regarded as an unsavory mix of intuition, anecdote, and sentimental speculation. Such ideas were positively tainted, furthermore, by their being preached by Quimby, Eddy, and other questionable proponents of mind cure. Not until the 1920s did psychosomatic medicine experience a revival, being resuscitated by a handful of physicians encouraged by advances in psychiatry and psychotherapy to revolt against their era's excessively mechanistic interpretation of disease.[21]

That initial attempt to construct an empirical foundation for psychosomatics foundered by 1960, however. Its concentration on hard-to-quantify entities such as subconscious emotional conflicts, and its inclination to single out specific conditions (hypertension, ulcerative colitis) as predominantly if not purely psychogenic, subjected the movement to renewed suspicions of scientific softheadedness. Only as attention shifted to more readily studied conscious emotional influences, and psychological state was demoted to the rank of one component among several in the multi-factorial model of disease causation, did psychosomatic medicine begin to gain lasting respect. Just as critical were the introduction of quantitative research methods that produced solid measurements of the physical effects of psychic irritants and the formulation of physiological rationales to explain the psyche's effects. Studies of the impact of emotional stress on physical well-being, especially in the new field of psychoneuroimmunology, were particularly important for finally giving psychosomatic medicine a secure foothold in the 1970s. So was the development— at last—of effective therapeutic procedures such as biofeedback.[22]

By the mid-1970s it was clear that pychosomatic medicine "has staged a spectacular comeback," and it was hoped that its revival signaled "the twilight of the golden age of reductionism." Anti-reductionism was evident in the virtually obligatory inclusion of the language of holism in statements of purpose of the discipline. One goal, to illustrate, was "propagation of a holistic (bio-psycho-social) approach to patient care." (It was generally recognized, incidentally, that in terms of basics this was simply a pouring of old wine into new bottles: "Hippocrates would have been aghast," an MD wrote, "at the notion that the newest of our specialties is psychosomatic medicine.")[23]

Mainstream practitioners' growing sympathy with holism culminated in 1978 in the founding of the American Holistic Medical Association by some 225 physicians. The organization announced itself to be "dedicated to the concept of medicine of the whole person which emphasizes integration of body, mind, and spirit with the environment," and though espousal of such an orientation was no longer news in allopathic circles, organizing a professional society primarily to advance that viewpoint was a novel undertaking. Even more striking, however, was the AHMA's acceptance that "this process of integration may demand combination of both orthodox and non-damaging unorthodox approaches." That hint that the door might be opened to alternative therapies to collaborate in the holistic care of patients was soon made explicit. As early as the third issue of the association's *Journal of Holistic Medicine*, the editor listed ten "interrelated fields of knowledge" that were acceptable as subject matter for articles; these included predictable items (nutrition, exercise, psychotherapy) but also two surprises, acupuncture (which had only occasionally been discussed seriously in mainstream journals before) and homeopathy, that "unclean thing" that allopaths had hitherto regarded as "the death of every upright principle." Further, the editor immediately added that the journal would give "special emphasis" to any of the "less well-known and non-traditional methods of diagnosis and treatment which are safe and effective." For reasons not divulged, homeopathy was dropped from the list of specified fields with the next issue, yet several articles on homeopathy were published by the journal soon after.[24]

Receptivity to alternative approaches was a characteristic as well of the holistic health centers that conventional physicians established in number from the mid-1970s on. In part an outgrowth of the free clinics opened in Haight-Ashbury and elsewhere to serve the disaffected youth of the 1960s, holistic health centers publicly professed to a medical philosophy essentially identical to that of alternative medical systems: addressing the psychological and spiritual needs of patients, catering to the unique needs of each individual, giving preference to therapies that encourage self-healing, promoting wellness through patient education, and the like, including the employment of alternative methods where useful.[25]

There was no shortage of holistic alternative therapies to choose from, for the holistic explosion was not just an explosion of interest in the tenets of holism but an explosion of megaton proportions in the number of therapies set before the public with the label of "holistic medicine" affixed. Reflexology and Rolfing, suggestology and shiatsu, megavitamin therapy and dream work, Native American medicine and Tibetan medicine: all manner of practitioners devoted to freeing the healer within rushed to link arms under the holistic umbrella.

Rediscovery of Acupuncture

Many came from a considerable distance, as the onset of the holistic age coincided with America's discovery that there were still more alternative approaches to healing to be found in the Far East. Both cultural and political change contributed to that realization. The hippie ideology that bloomed in the 1960s fostered an interest in the contemplative, non-violent spiritual traditions of the Orient, while even those most repelled by the hippie lifestyle had their attention turned eastward in the early 1970s by the lifting of the Bamboo Curtain and the reopening of diplomatic relations between the United States and China. In July 1971 journalist James Reston traveled to China to report for the *New York Times* on the renewal of relations between the two countries. While there, he developed acute appendicitis and had to undergo surgery at the Anti-Imperialist Hospital in Beijing (in a ward whose entrance bore Mao's unsettling warning that "there is certainly no escape" for the "running dogs" of capitalism, all of whom "will be buried" in the near future). Conventional anesthesia was employed for the operation. On the second night following, however, Reston was bothered by abdominal discomfort, and an acupuncturist was called to attend him. Within an hour his pain was permanently relieved. A week later, the writer published a front-page account of his experience in the *Times*, along with anecdotal reports of cures of a variety of diseases by Chinese acupuncturists.[26]

Only two months later, four American doctors (one of whom was Paul Dudley White, former physician to President Eisenhower) were invited by the China Medical Association to undertake a medical tour of their country. There the Americans encountered even more surprising applications of acupuncture, most particularly its use as an anesthetic in surgeries ranging from operations on the stomach and lungs to removal of tumors of the ovary and brain. Patients given no anesthesia other than acupuncture were observed to remain conscious and unflinching throughout the procedures, sometimes conversing with the surgeon and even taking food and drink. A man who had a tumor removed from his thyroid was described as draining a glass of milk as soon as the operation ended, then holding up his copy of the little red book and proclaiming, "Long live Chairman Mao and welcome American doctors." He then put on his pajama shirt and walked out of the operating room unassisted. Similar stories were told by British physicians invited to China.[27]

The Chinese surgeons and anesthesiologists who performed these operations had been trained in Western medicine and confessed that they had originally supposed that acupuncture anesthesia must be a "hoax." Experience had convinced them otherwise, however, and they now claimed a 90 percent success rate in cases deemed amenable to acupuncture management. (Many patients were found not suitable and were given chemical anesthetics instead.) American doctors hearing these stories, on the other hand, usually concluded it must surely be a hoax after all. "To any Western-trained physician, the reports seemed incredible," explained Walter Tkach, the personal physician of President Nixon. "Many of us suspected a trick. . . . It simply did not make sense that this illogical 'witch-doctory' " could work. As with homeopathy, acupuncture was initially rejected because it made no theoretical sense. As if it were not implausible enough that sticking needles into the body obliterated pain instead of causing it, the sites at which the needles were inserted "bore no relation to the human nervous system," Tkach objected. "There was no anatomical logic whatever."[28]

Tkach at first agreed with other Western physicians that post-hypnotic suggestion must be the acupuncturists' trick. Then he accompanied Nixon to China in the winter of 1972, charged by colleagues to "take a look at acupuncture to see if I could discern the trick behind the startling reports." Along with an osteopathic physician in the presidential party, Tkach observed several surgeries (on the eye, the ovary, and the thyroid), and "so far as we could tell, there was no trickery." He interviewed patients before and after their surgeries and was convinced that they had not been sedated or hypnotized beforehand. They "obviously [were] suffering no pain or discomfort" during the operations, he concluded, and when the procedures were completed, "the patients got up from the table and walked away with no visible discomfort. To any Western doctor, these things stagger the imagination." His initial skepticism was so thoroughly displaced by the certainty that "the Chinese doctors [were not] trying to put one over on us," in fact, that Tkach expressed willingness to accept acupuncture as anesthesia for any operation on himself. He had "seen the past," he announced, "and it works."[29]

Early History of Acupuncture

That past was a long one. Indeed, one of the justifications for acupuncture frequently offered by proponents was that it had been used in the East for centuries, and it could never have lasted so long unless there was something to it. According to one legend, several thousand years ago a Chinese warrior noticed that pain in one part of his body subsided after he was wounded with an arrow in another part. The hint was pursued by trial-and-error insertion of needles instead of arrows into different locations on the skin, and gradually there evolved a system of not only relieving pain but curing many ailments as well. (The Western term "acupuncture" was derived from the Latin words *acus*, needle, and *punctura*, puncture.) It was eventually decided that needling influenced the flow of qi (pronounced *chee*), the body's vital energy or life force, through a network of channels, the chinglo system, that ran throughout the body. Twelve main meridians, as the chinglo channels came to be called, were traced through the body running from head to fingertips and toes, and each linked to a specific internal organ. Along the meridians, moreover, several hundred points were identified as places where one of the channels was particularly close to the surface of the body and offered a site for efficacious insertion of needles.[30]

Scholars differ on just how far back the practice of acupuncture goes, some proposing so great a distance as seven millennia. The oldest surviving texts discussing the practice, however, date only to the second or first century B.C.E., where acupuncture is set within a cosmology constructed around the Tao, the Way, the power that brought the world forth from chaos and generated the forces of yin and yang. These opposing principles of female and male, negative and positive, dark and light jointly governed the functioning of the material world by maintaining harmony among the five elements of water, fire, wood, metal, and earth. Health depended on a person's living in compliance with the Tao and thus in harmony with all of nature. "Man lives on the breath of Heaven and Earth," according to the *Huang Di Nei Jing* (*The Yellow Emperor's Canon of Internal Medicine*), "and he achieves perfection through the laws of the four seasons."[31]

When one strayed from the Way, there occurred an imbalance between his yin and yang that created a blockage to the flow of qi, causing an excess of the vital energy in some areas and a deficiency in others, thereby bringing on disease. The imbalance could result, furthermore, from emotional distress or moral impropriety as easily as from physical error, so the ancient Chinese philosophy of health was, in a word, holistic. Within that broad philosophy, there were several methods of treatment, including herbal remedies, nutrition, spiritual counseling—and acupuncture. After diagnosing the problem by questioning, visual and aural examination, and, most important, a meticulous reading of the patient's pulse, the acupuncturist determined which points along the meridians needed stimulation and inserted needles—one or several—in accordance. The points generally bore no spatial relation to the site of pain or the affected organ; headache, for example, might be treated with a needle in one of the toes, or a liver ailment with a needle in the knee. Depending on the diagnosis, the needles might be withdrawn immediately after puncturing, left in situ for several minutes, or twirled in place for some time. In addition, the treatment could be supplemented with moxibustion, the burning of small cones of moxa, the powdered leaves of the herb mugwort (*Artemisia vulgaris*). The burning moxa might be placed directly on the skin over an acupuncture point or, more commonly in Chinese practice, used to warm the needle inserted in a point. Alterations and refinements of technique were developed over the centuries, but the basics of practice remained constant. Acupuncture spread outward to Japan and other Asian nations in ancient times.[32]

Acupuncture in the West

When the West discovered acupuncture in the 1970s it was actually a rediscovery, for nineteenth-century European and American physicians had already given a good bit of attention to the practice. Europeans first became aware of the method in the mid-1600s, through the reports of Jesuit missionaries who had spent time in China. Soon after, the first Western physician to investigate acupuncture brought the subject to the attention of the profession. During the 1670s, Willem Ten Rhijne, the doctor at a Dutch trading post in Nagasaki, received instruction in traditional Chinese medicine from local physicians in exchange for teaching them the rudiments of Western medicine. In 1683, after returning to Java to direct a leprosarium, he published a medical treatise that included a section on acupuncture and moxibustion. He there described the methods and explained that practitioners employed them for a wide range of complaints: abdominal pain, headache, arthritis, cataracts, fevers, diarrhea, and gonorrhea, among others.[33]

Several other Western medical writers subsequently discussed acupuncture, and the profession had become generally aware of the practice by the end of the 1700s. Yet the technique seems not to have been given its first clinical application in the West until 1810. (As an English practitioner of the day explained it, "between the frightfulness of running needles into the flesh and the high improbability of any benefit derived from such a practice, a hundred and seventeen years [sic; 127 years] elapsed before any European made trial of it.") In that year, L.V.J. Berlioz, father of the composer, treated a Parisian woman affected by "nervous fever." Subsequently, he claimed success in relieving whooping cough, headaches, muscle aches, and other pains and aroused so much interest that by the mid-1820s French physicians had filed reports of cures of everything from rheumatism and tic douloureux to gout and chronic hiccuping with acupuncture. (Early nineteenth-century European experimenters with acupuncture, incidentally, used ordinary sewing needles, often affixing a ball of wax to the upper end to make them easier to push in and to remove.) In England, clinical experimentation with acupuncture began during the 1820s, with several English practitioners finding it to be of

value in various complaints, rheumatism particularly. But as would happen
with their professional descendants of a century and a half later, doctors were
baffled as to the technique's mechanism of action. There was a certain amount
of speculation about the needles acting as a "lightening rod" to draw off excess
electric fluid in the nerves of the pained part (this was in the wake of Perkins's
tractors), but most physicians agreed with the author of the entry on acupuncture in a British medical encyclopedia that "the modus operandi of acupuncture is unknown." The writer was confident, however, that it did not act
through suggestion or hypnosis, since the needles were as efficacious with
"those who are alarmed" by the prospect of being needled and "those who
laugh at their medical attendant for proposing such a remedy" as with those
"who submit to it with faith."[34]

Although nineteenth-century American physicians gave less notice to
acupuncture than their European counterparts, there was some experimentation
with the technique as early as the 1820s. Most notable was the work done by
Philadelphian Franklin Bache, great-grandson of Benjamin Franklin and a
physician at his state's penitentiary. In 1825 he tested "acupuncturation," as it
was frequently called, on seventeen prisoners whose afflictions ran the gamut
from "chronic pains" and headache to rheumatism and ophthalmia; seven were
"completely cured," he determined, seven more "considerably relieved," and
only three obtained no benefit. The procedure, he concluded, was "a proper
remedy" in any complaint "whose prominent symptom is pain." Several other
American practitioners reported successes with acupuncture treatment over the
next two decades, but the method never caught on with the profession overall.
An authoritative surgical text of 1859 observed that "its advantages have been
much overrated, and the practice . . . has fallen into disrepute."[35]

Acupuncture's disrepute stemmed from several sources. In the days before Listerian antisepsis, puncturing of the skin with needles inevitably produced infections. Administered by people who had only read about it, not
been trained in the technique by Asian adepts, it also often produced pain.
"A great deal of pain" is what one of Bache's subjects experienced; "very
severe pain," a second felt, pain "so severe as to cause the patient to scream
out." Another "was seized with several excruciating paroxysms of pain" so
distressing that he had to be given opium. The odds for experiencing pain
were increased by Bache's practice of leaving needles in the body for several
hours, even up to a full day: "After remaining four hours," he reported in
one case, the three needles in a patient's thigh "became so painful as to require
removal."[36]

European and American practitioners also followed a commonsense rule
of inserting needles at the location of the subject's pain, without regard to the
Chinese system of meridian points that generally called for the needles to be

placed in a part of the body remote from the pain. ("A needle was inserted into the part affected," Bache reported in one case, as if placement were too obvious to require explanation.) An English physician told of an exceedingly corpulent subject whose lumbago he treated by inserting three needles, spaced two inches apart, into his lower back, the locus of the discomfort. Pushing the needles "to the bone," the doctor was surprised to be informed the pain "was instantly transferred to the left gluteus." The needles were at once moved to the buttock, "where the enemy had made a stand," but that only "routed him thence into the biceps"; when the needles were then removed to the upper arm, the enemy fled to the calf, whence he was "ultimately expelled" by the application of a single needle to that muscle. (Other Western practitioners of the time observed that pain sometimes "required . . . chasing from part to part before it vanished.") The patient, Mr. W., expressed "the greatest astonishment" at the "magical effect of the needles," but his assailant was still not done. "Six hours after, the enemy made a faint attack, but was instantly repulsed by one needle, and the patient left in quiet possession of the field."[37]

Commentary on this case by the editor of *The Lancet* reveals the amused condescension the great majority of nineteenth-century physicians exhibited toward acupuncture. The victor in the battle of Mr. W., he joked, should be showered with "all the 'blessings' and thanks which successful generals are wont to receive." Acupuncture was scorned by most, in part because of inconsistent results (Western practice did not adhere, it has been seen, to Chinese guidelines) and in part because of the lack of a satisfactory theoretical explanation; Tao, yin and yang, and the five elements appeared to be metaphysics, not science. Nor did it help acupuncture's cause that one of its most ardent proponents was London surgeon John Elliotson, who also paraded the colors of mesmerism. Even more discredit came from the activities of charlatans who capitalized on popular fascination with the exotic needling technique by offering cures for sexual difficulties that regular medicine was impotent to treat. Erectile dysfunction, premature ejaculation, nocturnal emissions, and other forms of what Victorians categorized as "male weakness" were dealt with by these mountebanks by the insertion of acupuncture needles into the perineum, the anal cleft, and even the prostate.[38]

There was, in fact, a complete system of irregular therapy for all human ills, not just male weakness, that looked so much like acupuncture as to further embarrass the Chinese practice. Baunscheidtism was the discovery of German Carl Baunscheidt, a businessman of no medical ambition whatever until the afternoon in 1848 when several gnats attempted to land on his painful rheumatic hand as he lounged in his rooms. He tried to wave them off, but the insects proved so persistent he "at last yielded to their importunity" and let them alight "to see what they would do. The gnats stung!" Yet no sooner had the pests performed their "obtrusive service" than an "instantaneous change took place in the sick hand": its pain "fled with the flies." If ever there was a gnatural cure, this was it. "The gnat had taught him the great secret," Baunscheidt exclaimed, its bite having "caused an opening in the epidermis just large enough for the fine, volatile, but pathogenetic substances lodged in the skin to exude" and at the same time applying a stimulus to the system "by means of which the diseased organism was enabled to eject the morbid accumulations" (that is, the body was naturally stimulated to heal itself).[39]

Nevertheless, the sick could not be expected to lie about idly waiting for the benevolent insects to seek them out. Nor would it be feasible to catch enough of the fast-flying little creatures, keep them healthy in captivity, and train them to bite invalids' affected areas. For her lesson to be made practicable, nature would have to be imitated, a mechanical gnat would have to be devised. The *Lebenswecker* (life awakener) that Baunscheidt promptly fashioned was in fact a veritable mechanical swarm of gnats. The instrument consisted of a hollow cylinder of ebony or horn, about two inches deep and three across, attached to a hollow wooden handle. In the cylinder's top side rested a steel plate in which there were imbedded some twenty "very keenly-pointed" needles, each two inches long and sharp. A string running from the base of the needles through the handle and out its end allowed the operator to pull the needles down into the cylinder. The retracted, poised needles might then be placed over the affected area of the patient's body. When the string was released, the needles would spring forward, perforate the patient, and open him up for the release of his pathogenetic substances. No gnat could do it better:

> Make not thyself a drug-shop, reader,
> To tap your blood when sick does harm;
> But try the great Resuscitator
> And he will cure you like a charm.[40]

The Resuscitator, the *Lebenswecker*'s English title, did not do the work of cure-all by itself, however. When the gnat bit, Baunscheidt somehow divined, it injected into the body a fluid that "generates . . . a wholesome irritation, which contributes largely to the extraction, and more rapid and efficacious removal of all morbid secretions in the body." That irritating fluid had to be duplicated as well, which it quickly was in the form of "oleum Baunscheidti," an oil "to be applied, with a chicken feather . . . to the parts that have been punctured by the Resuscitator." Unhappily for many patients, the oil did not necessarily catalyze the evacuation of every bit of the morbid secretions with a single puncturing, and those whose symptoms lingered more than a week after the first treatment were urged to return for puncturing every ten days until fully recovered. Rarely, it was promised, did cure require more than six months. According to an advertisement in a Cologne newspaper, Baunscheidt's "universal remedy" was "beyond all price . . . the diamond among the jewels of life; for what Baunscheidtism cannot cure . . . is incurable."[41]

Whether running for six months or six weeks, the Resuscitator was applied each time to the same region of flesh—the lower back of the jaundice victim, the abdomen of the diarrhea sufferer, the loins of the chronic masturbator, between the shoulder blades of the malaria case, behind the ears of the bald man, and so forth. (Application of the resuscitator a dozen or so times over the heart for three successive days could be trusted to determine whether a presumably deceased person truly had passed on and thus to guard against the "unspeakable horror" of loved ones being buried alive. Like more than a few of his contemporaries, Baunscheidt seems to have been agitated by the thought that such a horrifying thing might one day happen to him and couldn't help but worry over "the indescribable torture and agony of one . . . waking to life and consciousness in his firmly-secured coffin, . . . his horrid prison . . . beneath the pressure of more than one thousand pounds of earth"; it was imperative, he insisted, that the officials of every town purchase at least one Resuscitator to prevent premature burial of their citizens.) A provocative illustration of Aphrodite and Adonis, sharing a single fig leaf, was provided to indicate the puncture points associated with each disease; the drawing was not unlike classic Chinese illustrations of acupuncture points.[42]

It was in fact commonly charged that Baunscheidtism was only acupuncture in disguise, but the method's discoverer denied it. Whether an imitation or an original, however, the practice made its way to the United States by the 1860s and, judging by testimonials collected by Baunscheidt, worked the same wonders here as it had in Germany. In the appraisal of an Indiana minister (from East Germantown, so perhaps he was not entirely impartial), "The Resuscitator does more than all the physicians combined." It still does. As recently as the 1970s a modernized, all-metal Resuscitator was being promoted in Germany, under Baunscheidt's name, as *Die Akupunktur des Westens;* "health through skin irritation treatment" was the marketing pitch.[43]

True acupuncture nevertheless continued in use among a few physicians to the end of the nineteenth century. No less renowned an authority than William Osler, first professor of medicine at Johns Hopkins Medical School, professed faith in the technique in his classic text *The Principles and Practice of Medicine* in the 1890s. Acupuncture was the most effective treatment of all for acute lumbago, he recommended ("ordinary bonnet-needles, sterilized, will do"), and was sometimes useful in sciatica. Like his predecessors in the West, however, Osler inserted his three- to four-inch-long needles deeply at the exact site of the pain. This perhaps explains his failure in treating the lumbago of a wealthy Montreal businessman while Osler was still a professor at McGill University. "At each jab the old gentleman . . . ripped out a string of oaths, and in the end got up and hobbled out, no better for his pain." The result was doubly distressing for the professor, for he had hoped a cure might encourage a donation to the university; his lack of success, he sighed, had "meant a million for McGill."[44]

In the meantime, acupuncture had flourished over the centuries in China, only to fall into disuse in the early twentieth century when Western medicine made its way into the country. Although folk healers continued to use the traditional methods of acupuncture and herbs, Chinese health officials vociferously repudiated them as outmoded and unscientific. After the Communist ascent to power in 1949, however, the ancient ways of healing were rehabilitated and restored to a place of honor. There were far too few Western-trained physicians to meet the needs of China's enormous population, and acupuncture and herbs were relatively cheap. In those circumstances, Chairman Mao recognized, in a dictum issued in 1958, that "Chinese medicine is a great treasure house! We must make all efforts to uncover it and raise its standards!" From that date onward, traditional medicine was revived at a professional level and increasingly integrated with the medicine imported from the Western world. By the 1970s most major hospitals were organized into three sections: a department of traditional medicine, one of Western medicine, and one of combined western and traditional medicine, with patients free to choose the department in which they wanted to be treated.[45]

Even the practice of acupuncture evolved as a combination of new and old, for the use of the technique for surgical anesthesia was a development of modern times. In 1957, it has been reported, Mao observed that his country suffered from a shortage of conventional anesthetics and suggested doctors experiment with acupuncture. It made sense, of course, that a procedure that had worked so well for so long as an analgetic might be adapted to serve as an anesthetic. Through clinical experimentation new acupuncture points were found that produced anesthesia when needles were inserted. At first, upwards of eighty needles were required to get the desired depth of pain suppression, but experience demonstrated that effectiveness could be increased by twirling the needles between thumb and index finger, and thus it became possible to operate with far fewer needles; in some cases, one was sufficient. Hand twirling through the duration of an operation was tiring, though, and it soon came to be replaced by the application of low-voltage electricity to the needles. That was the form of acupuncture anesthesia observed by the first visitors from the West in the early 1970s, by which time more than four hundred thousand operations had been performed using acupuncture (though often small doses of analgetics were administered along with the needles). The surgeons themselves, having been trained in Western medicine, were skeptical of the traditional rationale for acupuncture—the freeing up of qi within the chinglo network—but were willing to practice it because it worked.[46]

Conventional Medicine's Reaction to Acupuncture

"Acupuncture: Witchcraft or Wizardry?" was the choice most American and European physicians initially offered to account for how the method "worked." Surely it wasn't science. "Any medical technique based on a Taoist metaphysical principle declares itself immediately outside the province of serious medical science," a Wisconsin practitioner lectured his colleagues. Such "bizarre therapy" should at once "be decisively branded as the cult practice it is," he railed; it should be put into the same category as chiropractic, copper bracelets, and "other enthusiasms of the kooks" and "non-scientific weirdos." If acupuncture were to be admitted into Western medical practice, then doctors might as well "abandon the scientific method. . . . Instead of sending our patients to hospitals," he suggested, "we might send them to Lourdes, . . . or to miracle-working gurus and evangelists. We might have to revert to venesection, the application of leeches or the administration of nice bowls of chicken soup—all of which [also] have respectable records of restoration of health."[47]

Yet if "tales of the supernatural" and "witch doctory" were the reactions of most MDs to the early reports of acupuncture anesthesia, many others acknowledged the phenomenon to be perfectly natural, in the same way mesmerism had been natural. "Of course acupuncture 'anesthesia' works," one doctor explained. It involved a "ceremonial or ritualistic-like approach" that was "a hypnotic procedure per se," one that "mobilizes powerful autosuggestive factors induced by prior indoctrinations. These motivate the patient's beliefs that the acupuncture anesthesia will be successful. . . . The 'needleism' merely acts as a reinforcing stimulus as well as a diversionary maneuver to disguise the presence of a subtle placebo effect. The resultant misdirection of attention further acts to inhibit painful impulses from reaching the cortex." In sum, the combination of "ideological zeal," "evangelical fervor," and "the prior belief shared by therapists and patients" operated together to transform belief in acupuncture "into conviction—Faith." Acupuncture, he decided, was nothing more than "hypnosis in slow motion."[48]

Many another evaluation similarly emphasized "the susceptibility of the patient to suggestion," the "impressive pyschosomatic" nature of "placing a sharp needle in the skin," and the placebo effect: "The fact that acupuncture treatment programs often go on for two weeks or a month and often for such obscure problems as backache, rheumatism, and tired liver makes one highly suspicious that time plus the doctor's attention have a great deal to do with most results." Even "the efficacy of the wisdom of Chairman Mao" was given the credit for acupuncture cures. Nevertheless, there were also many willing to venture that there might be "some margin of truth" to acupuncture's claims. Reputable Western witnesses had sworn there was no hypnotism or other trickery in the operations they had seen in China, and there remained, moreover, the stubborn fact of the technique having been employed for such an extraordinary period of time. "In matters so uncertain," a Western historian of Chinese medicine commented, was it truly rational to breezily suppose "that a treatment that has been engaged in and accepted by so many millions of people for something like twenty centuries has no basis in physiology and pathology?" Was it really more intellectually defensible to assume "that it has been of purely psychological value" (particularly when positive results were reported in the treatment of infants and animals)? As a Wisconsin physician observed in response to the characterization of acupuncture as the work of "kooks" and "unscientific weirdos," "there is nothing less scientific than making up your mind on a subject about which you know next to nothing."[49]

The point was well taken, and many American practitioners quickly moved beyond reflex rejection of acupuncture to a willingness, indeed eagerness, to learn more about it. Whether it was witchcraft or wizardry or whatever else, Western doctors "have been overwhelmed with curiosity about the art of acupuncture," it was soon reported. At the first demonstration of acupuncture technique in San Francisco, in May 1972, the meeting was packed, with "little standing room." The following month, a symposium on acupuncture held at Stanford University drew 1,400 physicians, so many more registrants than expected that the meeting had to be moved to a larger hall. "After nine hours scarcely a physician had left the room, a situation unusual for a June Saturday in California," and by the close of the day "the initial question in our minds"—was acupuncture witchcraft?—"had changed to 'Where can I buy some needles?'" Further kindling interest was the fact that, being so safe, "acupuncture probably will not increase a physician's malpractice rates!"[50]

The Stanford symposium was also described by a medical reporter as having a "somewhat carnival-like" atmosphere, "with hucksters taking orders for acupuncture charts and plastic dolls"; it "was more what one might expect of a congregation assembled to witness Oral Roberts or some faith healer at work." Indeed, opportunists positively leaped onto the acupuncture bandwagon, just as they had pounced upon mesmerism in the mid-1800s and naturopathy in the early 1900s. There was a "proliferative growth" in acupuncture seminars, and correspondence courses in acupuncture soon appeared, along with Caribbean cruises offering physicians "just enough lectures on the needle art to allow the cruisers to write off their trips as a professional, educational expense." Professional watchdogs issued alerts about "fly-by-night 'acupuncturists' " who were "already . . . abroad in the land" and about the "wave of needles loose in the land," and bemoaned the "massive human pincushion promotion" that was certain to follow. The rising wave of needles was disturbing enough to government officials that in the winter of 1973 the Food and Drug Administration began to detain shipments of acupuncture needles at ports of entry on grounds of uncertainty about their safety. Eventually, in March of that year, the FDA issued a ruling that classified the needles as an "experimental device" that could be used only for experimentation and under the supervision of a licensed physician: "FDA is concerned," the agency announced, "that acupuncture does not fall into the category of 'quackupuncture.' " The FDA would not remove the classification of acupuncture as experimental until 1994.[51]

There was particularly deep dismay over the adoption of acupuncture by practitioners of alternative medical systems. An "unfortunate association of the technic with 'irregular' cultists" had developed, it was observed, many of the "graduates" of seminars and correspondence courses being "chiropractors, naturopaths, or others espousing similar philosophies." One chiropractor was reported to have led seminars "in virtually all parts of the United States," to which "chiropractors have flocked," even at "$345 a head." When asked if three days of instruction was sufficient to qualify a person to practice the technique, the chiropractor was supposed to have said, "I can teach you to do it in ten minutes." Such flippancy was no surprise to MDs, of course: "The chiropractic attitude is typical: science be damned." The hazards posed by "acuchiropractors" and their kind was enough to edge one orthodox journal editor into "needling the profession" to establish a firm position on acupuncture "before the technic . . . becomes further entrenched as another tool of health quackery."[52]

The issue of the expansion of health quackery was tied, of course, to questions of licensing. By the laws of most states, procedures in which the skin was penetrated could be performed only by licensed MDs and DOs. Thus not only was it against the law for most alternative practitioners to use acupuncture (many got around this technicality by practicing acupressure instead), but since acupuncturists who had immigrated to this country from China were not licensed as physicians, it was also a violation of the law for the technique to be employed by the only people who were thoroughly trained in it. Such was the interpretation of New York authorities, for example, when the first acupuncture clinic in the United States, on Manhattan's Upper East Side, was opened "to a crowd of eager patients, TV camera crews, and reporters" in the summer of 1972. The Acupuncture Center of New York offered therapy for migraine, arthritis, hypertension, asthma, and a variety of other complaints, the treatments being administered by four "accredited Chinese acupuncturists" (who had theretofore been practicing "underground" in New York's Chinese community), under the supervision of an American MD. It was allowed to operate for exactly one week (and more than three hundred patients) before being closed by the state department of education, the agency charged with overseeing medical licensure. The state's position that "only licensed MD's can apply acupuncture" enraged the center's director, an internist. Practitioners who had undergone six years of training in acupuncture and acquired as much as thirty years of clinical experience, he protested, "are not even granted the courtesy of a temporary license to practice under medical supervision." Yet at the same time, it was accepted as perfectly legal "for any doctor to shove needles into people, regardless of whether he knows where to put them or anything else about acupuncture." Limited sympathy was attracted from colleagues, the bemusement most doctors felt about the exotic therapy being evident in such responses as a medical journal editor's comment that the moxibustion used to supplement acupuncture at the clinic produced "acrid smoke uncannily redolent of marijuana." Moxibustion, he joked, was "cooked-grass-on-skin therapy," and it was a relief to know that "the smell of grass is gone from the [acupuncture center] now."[53]

Professionalization of Acupuncture

Trained acupuncturists, both native Asians and Westerners who had studied the method in the Orient, quickly realized they would have to reenact the struggles of previous generations of alternative practitioners and campaign for licensing statutes of their own. Yet such was the popular fascination with the Orient and its healing arts, and with holistic approaches to treatment, that legislative victories were won in record time. In July 1973, just two years after Reston had reintroduced acupuncture to America, and despite the state medical association's "valiant battle against licensing acupuncturists," the Nevada legislature did just that, granting practice rights to acupuncturists with at least ten years of experience in the craft. That Nevada was the first state to take such a step was only fitting, in the mainstream medical view, for the act was perfectly in keeping with the gambling ethos of Las Vegas and Reno. Acupuncture was just another slot machine, "a Chinese bandit" or, better, a "two-armed bandit," since "it takes two arms to plant the needles dexterously." "The slot machines," it was predicted, "will be moved over to make room for the needle men. Charges will be per needle, and you pay with chips." Further, if Nevada acupuncturists could produce the same miraculous health effects attributed to practitioners in the world's most populous country, there would soon be "800 million Nevadans sprung from acupuncture."[54]

Shortly after, Oregon passed a similar law, and two more western states followed suit the next year. By 1980 eight states had adopted acupuncture licensing laws, and there was spreading acceptance of the sentiments of a Texas judge who in that year spoke against prohibiting the practice of acupuncture to anyone but MDs: Acupuncture "is no more experimental as a mode of medical treatment," he ruled, "than is the Chinese language as a mode of communication. What is experimental is not acupuncture, but Westerners' understanding of it and their ability to utilize it properly." Practitioners who had been thoroughly trained specifically in classical acupuncture were to be preferred, and by the late 1970s the numbers of such people were being augmented by graduates of newly established training programs in the United States. Beginning with institutions opened in Boston and San Francisco in the mid-'70s, schools of acupuncture would grow rapidly in number, reaching fifty by the end of the century. Accredited by a national Council of Colleges of Acupuncture and Oriental Medicine, these schools operated training programs lasting three to four years. Shorter courses of instruction were developed to instruct physicians, osteopaths, and dentists in acupuncture. By 1999 there were an estimated eleven thousand acupuncturists in the United States, three thousand of whom were MDs; well over half the states in the country, as well as the District of Columbia, were by then licensing acupuncturists.[55]

For the great majority of regular physicians, and in all Westernized cultures, not just America, acupuncture and its "Chinese biophilosophic" principles were just a bit difficult to swallow, and skepticism persisted. The "firm scientific stand" taken by the editors of the *South African Medical Journal* was the typical reaction. "Either acupuncture must be subjected to the closest, objective and carefully-controlled study, or we do not want to hear about it again," they wrote. "Mere magnanimous invitations to come and visit exalted centres in China or elsewhere and to witness these wonders, however kind such invitations are, cannot be accepted as adequate. We want this technique investigated under *our* control where *our* doctors can lay down the rules. . . . If such scientific criteria cannot be met, the acupuncturists must go back from whence they came and leave us in peace to practise our outmoded westernized medicine."[56]

In America, reaction to such calls for scientific evaluation was prompt. In July 1972 the National Institutes of Health announced the establishment of funding for research grants for the assessment of acupuncture as anesthesia and for the relief of chronic pain, though experimentation was already underway with a few physicians. Results were mixed. An operation in which acupuncture worked effectively for anesthesia was reported from the United States as early as 1972, and by the end of that year successful surgeries with acupuncture had been announced by at least four hospitals. Over the longer run, however, experimentation with acupuncture as anesthesia was disappointing (one trial, for example, found acupuncture's pain-suppressing effect to be "not the equal of a modest dose of codeine"), and it failed to be adopted as a general practice in American surgery.[57]

Findings were much more promising in the use of acupuncture to treat chronic pain from conditions such as osteoarthritis, tic douloureux, and cancer. (In the last, even patients who had not responded to morphine were reported to benefit.) All along, however, there was an unsettled question that agitated physicians no end. As the director of a Vancouver, British Columbia, acupuncture school explained it, his "worst students" were American doctors trying to learn more about the art. They were "arrogant [and] absolutely hopeless," he complained, because they were no good at "accepting theories that don't fit in with what they were taught."[58]

Whatever evidence of efficacy there might be, Western physicians could never feel entirely comfortable with acupuncture until it had been explained as science instead of philosophy. From the outset of its rediscovery there was much hypothesizing as to how the insertion of needles at certain points might possibly alter human physiology and the experience of pain. Early in 1972 the surgeon who first used acupuncture anesthesia in America stated he would "speculate" that the technique's effect "may be in part due to the physical stimulation on the small nerve endings. Through a certain pathway, the stimuli may jam or sidetrack the higher center to modify or eliminate the pain." Others picked up on the theme, drawing on a theory of pain developed in the mid-1960s, before the great wave of acupuncture awareness, that had posited the existence of a "gate" in the spinal cord that could open or close to allow or block the transmission of pain impulses. In 1972 a "two gate" theory was formulated specifically to account for acupuncture, suggesting a second pain gate seated in the thalamus. Refinements were quick to follow, a sample elaboration being the argument that qi was "in reality . . . a wave of electrical depolarization traveling along a fiber of autonomic nervous system. The meridian, then, is actually an autonomic fiber in which the energy cycle undergoes change via the above polarization process." Yet while a remarkable amount of experimentation and theoretical analysis have been applied to the question over the last quarter century, as of this writing there is no agreement as to the mechanism(s) by which the ancient art of acupuncture works.[59]

12

From Alternative Medicine to Complementary Medicine

"Acupuncture Works," proclaimed the headline of a 1997 article in *Time* magazine. That was the judgment, it was explained, of a panel of international experts appointed by the National Institutes of Health to evaluate the efficacy of acupuncture therapy in a range of complaints. The procedure was "clearly effective," the panel had determined, in relieving postoperative pain and the nausea produced by anesthesia and chemotherapy, and it had been judged "may be effective" in treating the discomforts of migraine, arthritis, and several other common ailments. Best of all, the article suggested, was that acupuncture "has virtually no side effects." Finally, the NIH Consensus Development Panel on Acupuncture had concluded that "further research is likely to uncover additional areas where acupuncture interventions will be useful."[1]

The closing years of the twentieth century bore witness to a striking number of admissions from the medical establishment that alternative therapies of various types—not just acupuncture—"worked" or at least "might be effective." Likewise, there were recurring acknowledgments that alternative treatments might in some instances be preferable to conventional ones because of their lack of side effects. Other medical considerations came into play as well, in such ways as to effect a profound transformation of mainstream medicine's traditional skepticism toward medical alternatives and to give birth to a new willingness to think of long-despised therapies as potential complements to allopathic practice.[2] This process of peacemaking was also furthered by new political and economic pressures. Yet harsh criticism of alternative medicine as unscientific and ineffective continued nonetheless, coupled with opposition to professional cooperation with alternative practitioners. In short, the last decade has constituted a tumultuous era in the history of alternative medicine in America, and one marked by an unprecedented degree of change in relations between medical orthodoxy and therapeutic heresy.

Tumult has resulted in large measure from the holistic health explosion's generation of so many new alternative systems and techniques. There is inadequate space even to begin to take into account all these products of recent history, but consideration of a few of the more prominent examples can provide some appreciation of the rapidly changing face of alternative medicine in the late twentieth century.

The Revival of Homeopathy

One of the new systems only seemed so, being in fact the oldest alternative rival to allopathic medicine. Homeopathy seemed to be a new arrival on the holistic scene because—in America, at least—it had all but disappeared during the middle years of the century. The system of Hahnemann, it will be recalled, had been far the most popular form of irregular practice during the second half of the nineteenth century. From the beginning, however, the seeming absurdity of its principles and practices made regulars confident homeopathy would not survive long. "After living its short day of sunshine," one practitioner predicted as early as the 1840s, "it will follow in the footsteps of . . . all the host of so called rational isms . . . there to rest . . . in a sleep that shall know no awakening."[3]

In truth, the homeopathic profession did fall on lean times by the early 1900s. As the twentieth century opened, there were some ten thousand homeopaths practicing in the United States (nearly 10 percent of the allopathic number) and twenty-two homeopathic medical schools (more than 10 percent of the allopathic total). One of the system's leaders at the time, in boasting of his profession's thirty journals and seventy-nine hospitals, prophesied that "in another generation or two it will constitute one half of the medical world." Yet even then, new recruits were dwindling, not just because regular medicine was more enticing in its glow of youthful germ theory but equally because homeopathy had become off-putting to many, being rocked by internal dissension over issues such as the proper degree of dilution of drugs or whether it was permissible to employ some allopathic drugs in conjunction with Hahnemannian remedies. Professional fragmentation was such that in 1901 the city of Chicago alone was home to four different homeopathic medical societies.[4]

The financial straits experienced by schools as enrollment declined were worsened dramatically by the heightened expectations of state licensing boards following the Flexner Report in 1910. By 1923 only two homeopathic medical colleges remained in existence, graduating fewer than a hundred students a year combined, and though they limped along for some years, neither survived beyond the 1950s. Meanwhile, homeopathic licensing boards had been repealed by state after state, until by the 1950s only Maryland maintained one. The profession's leaders began to prophesy doom: "The precipitous drop in the popularity of homoeopathy," the president of the Connecticut Homeopathic Medical Society sighed in 1948, was "a frightful phenomenon to behold." Ten years later, the president of the American Institute of Homeopathy worried that "homeopathy is a fading institution," and the following year a new president begged the institute's declining membership to awaken to "the gravity of the hour." With the average age of American homeopaths now over sixty, it surely did look as if the profession was facing a sleep that would know no awakening. As recently as 1971, in fact, a monograph on the history of homeopathy concluded that "the future looks grim indeed" and predicted that "unless the trend can be reversed, homeopathy will not survive more than three or four decades."[5]

Three decades later, at the opening of the twenty-first century, homeopathy is a flourishing enterprise. From a low point in the early 1970s, when fewer than one hundred American physicians were still practicing homeopathy, the number rose to one thousand by the mid-1980s. In addition, another thousand practitioners were to be found by then in the ranks of dentists, naturopaths, chiropractors, acupuncturists, veterinarians, and other health professionals. (Veterinary medicine blossomed as an area of homeopathy in the later twentieth century, offering "homeopathic care for the whole animal.") Not only were there many more (and younger) practitioners of the system, but in the early 1980s several states (Connecticut, Arizona, Nevada) reestablished homeopathic licensing boards; in Arizona, for example, the law authorized the licensing of state residents with medical, osteopathic, or dental degrees and a minimum of ninety hours of instruction in classical homeopathy.[6]

Non-prescription homeopathic medicines once again became popular forms of self-dosing, just as homeopathic domestic kits had caught on with nineteenth-century consumers; homeopathic "Home Medicine Kits" were in fact being marketed in the late 1990s, along with veterinary kits and instructional videotapes. Readily available in conventional drugstores, in some instances occupying their own large merchandising section, homeopathic remedies experienced a 1,000 percent growth in sales over the decade of the 1980s and continued to expand at an annual rate of 20 percent or better through the 1990s. Perhaps the surest sign of renewed vitality was intrusion into the homeopathic fold by charlatans seeking to profit off the system's new cachet. In 1979, twenty years after the president of the American Institute of Homeopathy had seen the gravity of the hour demonstrated by falling membership, another president of the institute detected a grave situation in increased numbers of "pseudo-doctors without adequate medical background who have latched onto

Homeopathy." Those "types," he fretted, "do an injustice to a great medicine" and would discredit it in the public eye. Just how severe the injustice could be was demonstrated by the Federal Bureau of Investigation only five years later, when an operation code-named Dip-Scam was made public. No fewer than thirty-eight mail-order "colleges," FBI agents had determined, were issuing phony degrees in homeopathy. Perpetrators of diploma scams go where the money is, and by the 1980s homeopathy was once again a promising business.[7]

Several factors played critical roles in the eleventh-hour rescue of legitimate homeopathy. One was the support offered by another alternative system, naturopathy. During its years in the wilderness, American homeopathy had tried to replenish its ranks by recruiting allopathic physicians (as well as osteopaths and dentists) to post-graduate training programs in homeotherapeutics as a specialty area. Nevertheless, the mailing of thousands of letters explaining homeopathy "in scientific terms of modern medicine" to medical students and physicians, offers of half-price memberships in the American Institute of Homeopathy, and other strategies failed to stanch the bleeding. As interest in holism and natural healing was rekindled in the 1970s and '80s, more conventional practitioners did give consideration to homeopathy, but much more enthusiasm was shown by students of naturopathy. By the 1980s approximately fifty graduates a year from Seattle's John Bastyr College of Naturopathic Medicine, the chief institution for educating naturopaths, made homeopathy a major part of their practice.[8]

Homeopathy's attractiveness to naturopaths stemmed in large part from its profession of natural healing practiced within a holistic framework. These were equally vital considerations in the system's growing acceptance by the public in the 1970s and '80s. Particularly as the eruption of AIDS kindled popular awareness of the importance of immune function, homeopaths' assertions that their drugs were "the primary pharmacological means to stimulate immune and defense responses" brightened the appeal of the system. Just as attractive were assurances that the clinical data "of special interest to the homeopath" were those "spontaneous, characteristic things that each patient longs to tell," subjective matters relating to his whole being that "the busy modern doctor" would pass over as "not sign posts but clutter." Those were the things that to the homeopathic doctor "individualize the case, bringing out the particular patient's reaction to the 'disease' he suffers from." Individualization of both diagnosis and treatment, a process that required giving more time and personal attention to the patient than was commonly extended by allopaths, was homeopathy's strongest selling point. From the allopathic viewpoint, homeopaths maintained, pneumonia is a single disease; but to the follower of Hahnemann there are "as many types of pneumonia as there are people who have it." And each type of pneumonia had its own remedy uniquely effective against the sufferer's total complex of symptoms. As Margery Blackie, homeopathic physician to Queen Elizabeth II, phrased it in the title of her book, *The Challenge of Homeopathy* was *The Patient, Not the Cure.*[9]

Homeopaths sought to counter mainstream medicine's high tech with their own "high touch." That they often succeeded was confirmed by a series of interviews conducted by orthodox physicians in the late 1970s to determine "Why Patients Choose Homeopathy." Most homeopathic patients, it was discovered, suffered from chronic ailments that had not been effectively treated by conventional physicians. "Dissatisfied customers" of regular medicine, they had found satisfaction with homeopathic care in large part because homeopathic practitioners "spend more time with their patients" (typically an hour for the initial visit and twenty minutes for follow-up appointments) and "devote meticulous attention to each symptom, whatever the origin." In contrast to the allopathic effort "to fit symptoms into common diagnostic patterns," homeopaths emphasized "the uniqueness of each person's symptoms"; thus the distinction that Hahnemann had preached so earnestly in the early nineteenth century continued into the late twentieth.[10]

Homeopathy benefited as well from what physicians saw as its most dubious practice, the administration of infinitesimal dilutions as active drugs. Just as the mid-nineteenth-century public was drawn to Hahnemann's spiritual interpretation of drug action, so were enthusiasts of the holistic era attracted by a system of therapy that transcended matter and the laws of physics and chemistry that ruled orthodox reductionism. Late twentieth-century homeopaths no longer claimed to be able to understand how sub-molecular remedies worked: "With homeopathy," a prominent advocate for the practice has admitted, "we have hardly a clue as to how it could work or what the rules it follows might be." As the ease of that confession of cluelessness might suggest, homeopaths are not disturbed by their inability to explain their drugs' action. They remain as resolutely empirical as in the nineteenth century: one "major advantage" of homeopathy over allopathy, it has been stated, is that it "has not got lost in the wilderness of abstract hypothesis. It remains within the realm of the experienceable."[11]

There nevertheless persists a desire to understand how therapeutic experiences so at odds with established scientific rules can occur, and homeopaths have in recent years advanced a number of working hypotheses derived from some of the more arcane reaches of modern physics, chemistry, and immunology. It would require much more room than this book has available, however, to explore such realms as chaos theory and the impression of an "information-carrying pattern" onto water molecules by the serial dilutions of homeopathic drugs. In the end, what matters is whether or not homeopathic drugs do indeed work as anything more than placebos, and the closing years of the twentieth century brought increasing evidence that they well might. In 1991 an analysis of 107 different trials of homeopathic drugs (for an assortment of conditions that included influenza, migraine, hypertension, arthritis, irritable bowel, and duration of labor) determined that in eighty-one of them—more than 75 percent—there was positive evidence of efficacy. Because most of the trials were "of low methodological quality," the authors concluded that evidence was "not sufficient to draw definitive conclusions"; yet they felt they had established that there was "a legitimate case for further evaluation of homoeopathy . . . by means of well performed trials."[12]

Subsequently, several methodologically sound studies again found homeopathic remedies efficacious, and a 1997 meta-analysis of numerous homeopathic trials concluded that results "are not compatible with the hypothesis that the clinical effects of homoeopathy are completely due to placebo." (Meta-analysis is the use of statistical techniques to combine and evaluate data from any number of previous studies on a topic.) Nevertheless, it was added, there was still "insufficient evidence that any single type of homoeopathic treatment is clearly effective in any one clinical condition." Thus while homeopaths at the beginning of the twenty-first century remain unshaken in their confidence that their drugs are effective, they do recognize that more positive trials are needed to convincingly demonstrate that faith to non-believers. Even then, the task will be arduous, for the non-believers' faith is equally strong. A well-designed 1994 study that demonstrated homeopathic medicines to be significantly better than placebo in treating childhood diarrhea (the first homeopathic trial, incidentally, to be published by a peer-reviewed American orthodox journal) was rejected at first, even though two of three reviewers had "very positive" responses to the manuscript; decisive for this initial evaluation was the third reader's reaction, that "I will only accept that homeopathic medicine works if the practitioners of this art can tell me in plausible ways, why they think it works." A physician styling himself "quackbuster" went further, repudiating homeopathy as "complete nonsense—not even worth testing." And just as in the nineteenth century, MDs continue to delight in calculations that demonstrate the absurdity of the notion that a homeopathic preparation could work. A remedy taken to the thirtieth dilution, it has been pointed out, would have only one chance in a hundred billion trillion trillion—"greater than the radius of the universe in centimeters"—of containing a single molecule of the prepared drug.[13]

Therapeutic Touch

One hypothesis advanced for how homeopathy works is that it is due to the influence of some form of "bioelectromagnetic energy" activated by the dilution of a drug below the molecular level. Biological energies of one sort or another in fact came to be espoused as an explanatory mechanism by more than a few therapeutic systems during the holistic era, so many, in fact, that "bioelectromagnetics," or BEM, has won recognition as a distinct category among alternative practices. Within this classification, methods that claim to heal by restoring or stabilizing the bioenergetic field generated by every person have become particularly popular. These "biofield therapies" cover a spectrum running from traditional methods such as Chinese qigong and Japanese reiki to modern discoveries such as polarity therapy.[14]

Perhaps the most commonly employed biofield therapy in the United States today is therapeutic touch, a method initiated in 1972 by Dolores Krieger, a professor of nursing at New York University. Aware of the ancient belief in the healing power of the laying on of hands, and convinced from her nursing experiences that touch had therapeutic benefits, Krieger determined through experiment and clinical trial that she could relieve patients' pain and speed their recovery by passing her hands over them. Eventually, it was realized that the best results were achieved not by actually touching the patient but by keeping the hands two to three inches away from the body's surface and also concentrating on conveying to the patient a sincere intent to heal; without the exercise of intent, the method was unlikely to succeed.[15]

The passing of hands around the body by a practitioner of therapeutic touch looks like nothing so much as one of the techniques commonly used by mesmerists in the nineteenth century. Krieger would not have disputed the connection, as she did recognize that her method was a personalized version of a form of healing that had been employed for centuries in cultures around the world. Nor would she have distanced herself greatly from the sorts of interpretations that mesmerists made of the mechanism of their cures. Although she never spoke of animal magnetism or nervo-vital fluid, she did tie the phenomenon to a similar concept in the ayurvedic medicine of Hindu tradition. (Ayurveda was another of the Asian healing methods that gained a foothold in America in the holistic era.) Prana—the life force, the vital energy—was the entity that she believed she utilized when practicing therapeutic touch.[16]

Prana soon became the "human energy field." In observance of the time-honored alternative practice of formulating a theory after the empirical discovery of a method, Krieger postulated that therapeutic effects obtained without physical contact with the body indicated the existence of an energy field emitted by, and enveloping, the "healee." Illness was the result of "an inbalance in the ill person's energies"; passing the hands around the person served first to sense exactly where the energy field was disturbed, then to "rebalance those energies" so that the body could restore itself to full function. Rebalancing was accomplished partly through channeling of her own energy field to the patient's stricken areas, much as nineteenth-century mesmerists imposed their own magnetic energy upon patients deficient in animal magnetism; Krieger even used Kirlian photography to show that a more intense field of energy surrounded her hands when she was healing than when at rest. And when, like mesmerist predecessors, she was dismissed as having demonstrated nothing more than the power of suggestion, she responded that results were equally good with infants and with patients who were comatose. Suggestion also could not account for broken bones healing in half the usual time. Practitioners of therapeutic touch—or TT—submitted claims of efficacy in the treatment of an extensive range of conditions: pain of all sorts, fever, inflammation, nausea, diarrhea, PMS, thyroid disease, and much more. It was alleged to increase the flow of milk in breast-feeding women, to ease the symptoms of Alzheimer's disease and AIDS, and to comfort the dying. Indeed, Krieger reportedly believed that "there should be no limitation on what healing can be accomplished."[17]

Krieger referred to herself as a "nurse-healer," and it was particularly in the field of nursing that therapeutic touch found practitioners. In 1975 Krieger began teaching nursing students the procedures of therapeutic touch; over the next fifteen years she would train more than seventeen thousand students in the method, while a similar number received instruction from colleague Dora Kunz. Their students, moreover, taught others, so that by the mid-1990s an estimated one hundred thousand American nurses had been instructed in TT, and the technique had become "the fastest-growing alternative nursing practice" in the country. During the 1990s, "energy-field disturbance" came to be accepted as a legitimate diagnosis by the North American Nursing Diagnostic Association.[18]

The nursing profession, in fact, was a hotbed of enthusiasm for holism in general during the last quarter of the twentieth century. That was perhaps only to be expected, as the work of nursing is, by its very nature, involved with patients' anxieties and other emotional states and with support of their natural recuperative powers through the provision of rest, warmth, nourishment, and other physiological needs. The sainted founder of modern nursing herself, Florence Nightingale, wrote in her 1859 definition of the art of nursing that "what nursing has to do is to put the patient in the best condition for nature to act upon him." The point was made most eloquently, however, by American journalist Finley Peter Dunne, commenting in 1901 on the differences between Christian Science and medicine. "If th' Christyan Scientists had some science," his Irish protagonist Mr. Dooley proposed, "an' th' doctors more Christyanity, it wudden't make anny diff'rence which ye call in—if ye had a good nurse."[19]

Visualization

Nurses were also active in promoting the healing technique of visualization, or using the mind's eye to see the source of sickness and to imagine its destruction or elimination. Although the method has come into general use only over the last quarter century, it was prefigured in the Victorian age by practitioners of mind cure. Both Dods and Quimby, for example, claimed to be able to obliterate malignant tumors by effecting a positive mental attitude in their patients: "When the mind is under the influence of confidence, faith, hope, and joy," Dods believed, "organic activity is heightened, and, by keeping the mind upon the tumour while in this happy state, and believing it will disappear, [one] creates a surplus of action at that spot through the voluntary nerves, and this surplus action throws off this surplus protuberance, to return no more."[20]

Visualization returned in the contemporary age with the work of radiation oncologist O. Carl Simonton and his wife Stephanie Matthews-Simonton. While doing his residency in the early 1970s, Dr. Simonton sought to help a man dying of throat cancer by suggesting that three times a day he spend fifteen minutes concentrating on a mental picture of his tumor being attacked by radiation "bullets" and white blood cells; two months later, the cancer had disappeared. Results with other oncology patients who tried visualization were less dramatic but still striking, their survival times being lengthened to more than twice the norm for non-visualizing patients. Heartened by these findings, the Simontons founded a Cancer Counseling and Rehabilitation Center in Fort Worth, Texas, that attracted patients from throughout the country. In 1978 their work was taken more directly to the public via *Getting Well Again*, a book that argued forcefully that negative mental and emotional factors were instrumental in producing cancer and included explicit instructions for generating positive mental imagery to overcome the disease. Visualization's popularity was enhanced still farther by a best-seller of the 1980s, Yale surgeon Bernie Siegel's *Love, Medicine and Miracles*.[21]

Prayer and Healing

In its original form, visualization involved concentrating the power of the mind upon one's own body. During the 1980s, there evolved an expansion of visualization from people treating themselves with encouraging thoughts to their directing their benevolent intentions toward others in need of healing. That kind of activity had been practiced for time out of mind, of course, in the form of prayer; believers in a higher power had always looked above for help for themselves and ailing loved ones, and adherents of Christian Science in particular continue to trust in prayer as the path to true healing and to collect "testimonies" of cure through prayer. In the late twentieth century, however, the efficacy of prayer as a therapeutic agent began to be evaluated for the first time by conventional medical researchers—and with results that indicated that an individual's mind does indeed have the power to help others. In the best-known such study, San Francisco cardiologist Randolph Byrd in 1988 reported a clinical trial in which hospitalized cardiac patients were randomly assigned to two groups, one to be prayed for by various people around the country, the other not to receive any outside prayers. Neither patients nor physicians knew which group was which, nor were those offering the prayers personally acquainted with the patients. The group on whom prayer ("to the Judeo-Christian God") was bestowed suffered significantly fewer complications from their disease and required fewer interventions such as antibiotic therapy and intubation.[22]

Byrd recruited Protestants and Catholics to pray for patients, but other researchers have come up with similar findings with prayer provided by Jews, Buddhists, and other religious groups. (There is, of course, a website to facilitate interdenominational healing; Virtual Jerusalem accepts requests for prayers to be inserted into Jerusalem's Western Wall.) Furthermore, studies have shown prayer to have beneficial effects on animals and plants, even on fungi, bacteria, and red blood cells. These results have been welcomed, naturally, by religious organizations, and over the past decade there has occurred a blossoming of enthusiasm for spirituality as a healing force, bolstered by studies showing a positive correlation between commitment to religious faith and such measures of health as normal blood pressure, freedom from depression, enhanced immune function, and less frequent hospitalization. (To be sure, studies in the just-blossoming field of the "epidemiology of religion" have been criticized for giving inconsistent results, and it has been questioned whether the religious live longer because of their faith or because they adhere to a more wholesome lifestyle.) A conference on "Aging, Health, and Religion" has been sponsored by the National Institutes of Health; more than two dozen American medical schools offer courses on spirituality and health; private national organizations (the John Templeton Foundation, the National Institute for Healthcare Research) have been founded to promote the use of prayer and other spiritual activities in mainstream medical care (the National Institute regards prayer as "the most inexpensive Rx to prevent or mitigate illness" and urges physicians to take a spiritual history as part of each physical exam); and even the *Journal of the American Medical Association* has published articles with titles such as "Getting Religion Seen as Help in Getting Well" and "Should Physicians Prescribe Prayer for Health?" In at least one physician's opinion, "not to use prayer with my patients [is] the equivalent of deliberately withholding a potent drug." "The medicine of the future," another has commented, "is going to be prayer and Prozac."[23]

Yet fortunately for those of us who do not find organized religion appealing, the same benefits of "prayer" have been demonstrated by healers of no particular theological persuasion, fostering the belief that mind can contribute to others' healing without the backing of any deity. Internist Larry Dossey has developed this idea to its fullest, arguing that mind is infinite, rather than localized to an individual's brain; capable of stretching across the expanses of space, and even time, an individual's consciousness can act "non-locally" to spur others toward health or to suppress their disease processes. Dossey sees the discovery of non-local manifestations of consciousness as the advent of a new age of medicine. From Era I, the biomedical phase in which mind was equated with the mechanical functioning of the brain and assigned no role in causation or cure, medicine moved through Era II, the mind-body period of the late twentieth century in which illness came to be understood in psychosomatic terms of mind and emotions affecting the body for ill or good. In Era III, he argues in *Reinventing Medicine* (1999), physicians will act on the knowledge "that consciousness can free itself from the body [and] has the potential to act not just locally on one's own body, but also nonlocally on distant things, events, and people." This "distant intentionality" will consist not just of "intercessory prayer," but also of "transpersonal imagery" and "all forms of distant healing."[24] Era III sounds like an environment in which Phineas Quimby would feel right at home—except that it is not intended to displace the earlier stages of medicine, only transcend them. An accident victim receiving prayer would still be X-rayed and sutured and have her anxieties alleviated; she just would be expected to recover faster than a non-prayed-for casualty.

The "Holistic Hodgepodge"

Dossey states the case for non-local consciousness as an agent of healing most eloquently, but he adds that many physicians are resistant to the idea nonetheless, "usually . . . because they cannot swallow the concept of nonlocal mind." Indeed, it was this concept of consciousness acting over distance that sparked the retort quoted in Chapter 1, "That's the kind of crap I wouldn't believe even if it were true." (Siegel has told of posting a report of Byrd's prayer trial on a bulletin board at Yale Hospital and finding it defaced the next day with the comment "bullshit.") Swallowing concepts not explainable by the biomedical model of disease and therapy has also proven to be too difficult for many contemporary physicians with respect to alternative approaches other than prayer. Thus visualization has been jeered as an attempt to "dream your cancer away," therapeutic touch's manipulation of human energy fields disparaged as "placebo mumbo jumbo," and alternative medicine in general derided as "voodoo science" and "nincompoopery" decked out in "new-age techno-babble."[25]

To be sure, trials of alternative medical claims have more than once made a system look like voodoo. As recently as 1998, for example, the *Journal of the American Medical Association* published a report of an experiment that tested the ability of therapeutic touch practitioners to demonstrably perceive the human energy field they claimed to manipulate. On two different occasions, a total of twenty-one practitioners of TT took turns resting their hands, palms upward, on a table. The table was equipped with a tall screen that fit around the practitioner's forearms, preventing her from seeing her hands on the other side. On that side, the experimenter held her right hand just above one of the practitioner's hands (determination of which hand was decided by a coin flip) and asked the practitioner to announce with which hand she sensed a human energy field. Each practitioner underwent ten such tests. The percentage of correct responses was 47 in the first set of tests and 41 in the second, both lower than the 50 percent one would anticipate as the result merely of chance. "TT claims are groundless," the report concluded, and "further use of TT by health professionals is unjustified." As if that weren't embarrassing enough, it was also revealed that the experiment had been designed and conducted by a nine-year-old girl for use as her fourth-grade science fair project.[26]

Emily's little experiment, as *Time* magazine called it, received network newscast and front-page newspaper coverage throughout the country. But in the eyes of therapeutic touch practitioners, it proved nothing. "It's a cute idea," Krieger responded, "but it's not valid. The way her subjects sat is foreign to TT, and her hands are moving, not stationary. You don't just walk into a room and perform—it's a whole process." Once again, it was the practical process of healing rather than the theoretical rationale behind it that was the make-or-break issue for the alternative side, and on the matter of clinical efficacy, there were several studies to point to as evidence that therapeutic touch worked. Mainstream medicine's reaction to those studies, however, was that they were insufficiently rigorous with respect to design and the use of controls. Comparing therapeutic touch to mesmerism, one physician congratulated TT for finally "catching up with eighteenth-century science."[27]

Unquestionably, much that passed itself off as alternative medicine during the last quarter of the 1900s was no better than eighteenth-century science. The benevolent aura of holism translated into market appeal, and the proponents of any would-be scheme of healing, no matter how far-fetched or hare-brained, were certain to label their practice "holistic." (Such, for example, were the empathologists, practitioners of "Mind/Body Healing" whose empathic relating to clients "facilitates your Personal Truth . . . [and] finds and clears the underlying causes of your life and health issues," including "Toxicity issues," "Allergy correction," "Emotional trauma," "Relationship conflicts," "Money issues," and, in fact, everything else: "There is not an issue that can not be addressed with Empathology.") The "holistic hodgepodge," as one critic described the situation, was bewildering, a promiscuous intermingling of the sound with the spurious, the down-to-earth with the extraterrestrial, in which the spotlight too often shone upon the freaks instead of the conscientious practitioners who had some claim to center stage. And with the development of the Internet, gaining time in the spotlight became easier than ever. "Suddenly it's on the Internet," an MD complained at the outset of the twenty-first century; "articles about some nutrient . . . in some cells in a special cell line in Austria that if the moon is in the right position you get a tumor response in cell culture."[28]

Chiropractic

It nevertheless gradually became apparent to objective observers from the regular profession that some systems theretofore laughed off as freakish had in fact matured and become deserving of respect and even acceptance. Hypnosis, for example, had outlived mesmerism and found a place in psychotherapy by the early twentieth century. Over subsequent decades, it came to be applied effectively to other areas, until by the end of the twentieth century even MDs were using hypnosis to treat a variety of problems, from pain and asthma to warts and skin rashes. (A relic from the days of mesmerism remains nonetheless, as hypnotherapy still attracts charlatans and "stage entertainers," as one physician has recently described them.) A more dramatic transformation occurred with chiropractic, which entered the second half of the twentieth century as despised as ever by the mainstream profession. As recently as 1966 the American Medical Association's House of Delegates decreed that "chiropractic is an unscientific cult whose practitioners lack the necessary training and background to diagnose and treat human disease"; practitioners were further castigated for "their rigid adherence to an irrational, unscientific approach to disease causation." That did not necessarily mean the "cult" was a serious threat, as to some judges it appeared the system was in decline. Chiropractic's imminent demise had in fact been predicted for some time; 1930s MDs, for example, opined that "the hand of death is already visible" and that "chiropractic is doomed . . . a device that in time will pass into limbo with the metallic tractors of Dr. Elisha Perkins." Even into the 1960s there were assurances that "chiropractic is cracking up."[29]

The medical profession's actions spoke much louder than those words prophesying extinction, however, demonstrating an awareness that chiropractic actually was doing quite well and growing more robust all the time. In 1963 the AMA established a Committee on Quackery whose chief assignment was "to contain and eliminate chiropractic." Three years later, the same year as the House of Delegates' condemnation of the system as cultism, the editors of the AMA's journal "sounded an alert for all physicians to be on the lookout for chiropractors who attempt to gain hospital privileges," warning that any hospital that permitted cultists "to use its facilities in any way" would likely lose its accreditation. Three years after that, the association announced it was mailing a hundred copies of a recently published exposé of the dangers of chiropractic (*At Your Own Risk*) to every state medical society, as well as one copy to every county society and to each of the 1,200 largest libraries in the country. Members were regularly reminded that the association's Code of Ethics, revised in 1949, specified that "all voluntarily associated activities with cultists are unethical." And just as the nineteenth-century consultation clause had been directed primarily at homeopaths, so was the modern restriction understood to apply above all to chiropractors.[30]

Conflict with chiropractic came to a head over the issue of coverage by Medicare. The act establishing the Medicare reimbursement system, passed in 1965, covered the services of allopathic and osteopathic physicians only. Chiropractors promptly requested inclusion (as did several other groups of licensed practitioners, such as clinical psychologists and physical therapists— and naturopaths), and in response Congress directed the secretary of Health, Education, and Welfare to determine the merits of the requests. The secretary's recommendation with respect to chiropractic was that it "not be covered in the Medicare program" because its "theory and practice are not based upon the body of basic knowledge related to health, disease, and health care that has been widely accepted by the scientific community." (The chiropractic section of the secretary's report was made available by the AMA free on request.) Chiropractors fought back, using the tactic that had worked so well early in the century in keeping unlicensed practitioners out of jail, that of mobilizing satisfied patients to demand justice. "Manufactured mail campaigns" (the phrase is the AMA's) deluged federal legislators with an estimated twelve million letters and telegrams; "Congressional aides were reportedly astonished over the sacks of prochiropractic mail, which never seemed to diminish"—

and that demanded "health freedom," the right of the public to choose the type of care they received.[31]

"The fallacy of such an argument appears obvious," critics of chiropractic responded; "should we license and give Medicare dollars to alchemists, witches, herbalists, health food therapists, faith healers, etc., on the assumption that the consumer will be wise enough to choose the proper kind of care?" If chiropractors did somehow manage to win coverage, another suggested, they should be dealt with the same as other unquestioned threats to public health: since "chiropractic constitutes a hazard to the public at least as great as smoking cigarettes," practitioners should be required to prominently display in their office a sign stating "Warning: The Department of Health, Education and Welfare Has Determined That the Chiropractic Method (Unscientific Cultism) Is Dangerous to Your Health." Chiropractic nevertheless was granted admission into the Medicare system in 1974, and over the course of the next decade chiropractic services came to be covered by virtually every major health insurance carrier and to be included in all states' workmen's compensation plans; even the Internal Revenue Service began to allow taxpayers to deduct the costs of chiropractic care as a medical expense.[32]

Two years after overcoming allopathic opposition to inclusion under Medicare, chiropractic turned the tables on the AMA, filing suit against the association (along with the American Hospital Association, the American College of Surgeons, and nine other medical organizations, including the American Osteopathic Association) for violation of the Sherman Antitrust Act. The intent of the AMA's Code of Ethics, it was alleged, was primarily economic, an effort to restrain competition. The court battle was a protracted one, dragging on until 1987, but in the end the U.S. District Court for the Northern District of Illinois decided against organized medicine in the case of *Wilk v. AMA*. (C. A. Wilk was one of five Illinois chiropractors who initiated the action.) Although the court allowed that the AMA had fought chiropractic out of "a genuine concern for scientific methods in patient care," it found that the belief that adjustments were unscientific was insufficient to justify "a nationwide conspiracy to eliminate a licensed profession." Further, the court ruled that the association had failed to prove that its repudiation of chiropractic as unscientific was "objectively reasonable." An injunction was issued permanently forbidding the AMA "from restricting, regulating or impeding" any of its members or any hospitals or other medical institutions from associating professionally with chiropractors. The final slap was the requirement that the association publish the injunction order in its journal and send copies—"first class mail, postage prepaid"—to all its members. The AMA appealed the decision but was refused by the U.S. Supreme Court in 1990.[33]

Even before the unfavorable judgment was handed down, however, the AMA had retreated from its exclusionary stand on chiropractic. In 1979 the association adopted a new policy that acknowledged that some chiropractic treatments might indeed be of benefit, despite the unscientific theory behind them, and allowed that not all chiropractors "should be equated with cultists. It is better to call attention to the limitations of chiropractic in the treatment of particular ailments than to label chiropractic an 'unscientific cult.' " The following year, all restrictions on consultation were lifted, members now being left "free to choose whom to serve, with whom they associate, and the environment in which to provide medical services." To be sure, the AMA backed off not so much because of a change of heart on the merits of chiropractic care as out of a desire to avoid costly lawsuits and unfavorable publicity. The effect was nonetheless the same, a new level of legitimacy for practitioners of chiropractic.[34]

Legitimacy was also being won in the arena of education. Chiropractic educational institutions had been derided by allopathic medicine from their very beginnings, and on into the 1960s exposés of lax training standards were a common feature of anti-chiropractic literature. Thus the AMA's Department of Investigation in 1963 revived the phony application ploy of the 1920s, approaching several chiropractic schools with letters of inquiry marked by poor spelling, worse grammar, and sentiments such as the hope of one "applicant" that the institution would equip him to "make a lot of money and still not have to go to school all your life like some doctors." The applications were denied by some schools because the writer admitted to not having completed high school, but other schools admitted him with the promise he would be able to complete his high school equivalency degree the first term. (A high school diploma was the minimum acceptance standard at all chiropractic schools, though by the 1960s many entrants had completed one or more years of college.) In addition to admitting students of questionable qualifications, chiropractic schools in the 1960s suffered from inadequately trained instructors in the basic sciences and limited opportunities for clinical experience. "The substandard and unscientific education of its practitioners" was one of the reasons given for the AMA's 1966 branding of chiropractic as cultism, and part of the justification for initially excluding chiropractic from Medicare was that "the scope and quality of chiropractic education do not prepare the practitioner to make an adequate diagnosis and provide appropriate treatment."[35]

Yet by 1974, it will be recalled from Chapter 9, the U.S. Office of Education would be so impressed by the upgrading of chiropractic schooling as to recognize the Council on Chiropractic Education as an official accrediting agency and to drop the epithet "spurious" as a descriptor of degrees issued by accredited chiropractic schools. Meanwhile, chiropractic training had spread abroad, to Canada in 1945 and England in 1965; in the later 1970s, schools would be opened in Australia and Japan as well. There was escalating activity within the profession, furthermore, devoted to research on the biomechanics and neurophysiology of the spine and the construction of a much more sophisticated scientific rationale for the efficacy of chiropractic treatments. Although one could still find advertisements claiming that vertebral subluxation "is a killer of millions of people yearly," by the 1970s the great majority of chiropractors had abandoned the Palmers' "pinched hose" theory of nerve impingement, along with all the metaphysical trappings of early chiropractic. At the same time, better-controlled clinical trials began to be conducted, and they have yielded considerable support for chiropractic adjustments as the method of choice for relieving low back pain. A final factor in the upgrading of chiropractic's standing was the report of a panel appointed in 1978 by the Governor-General of New Zealand to evaluate chiropractic for coverage of health benefits under the country's Social Security Act. The panel began their deliberations with the impression that chiropractic "was an unscientific cult." On completion of what they believed was "probably the most comprehensive and detailed independent examination of chiropractic ever undertaken in any country," they found themselves "irresistibly and with complete unanimity drawn to the conclusion that modern chiropractic is a soundly-based and valuable branch of health care in a specialized area neglected by the medical profession." (It might be noted parenthetically that the early twentieth-century split between straights and mixers has persisted to the present. Although the large majority of chiropractors today utilize a range of therapies as adjuncts to manipulation—dietary supplements, heat, ultrasound, electrical stimulation, acupuncture, homeopathy—there are enough straights, and even enough "super-straight" members of a third faction, to support national organizations for each group.)[36]

Chiropractic encouraged rapprochement with orthodox medicine also by openly acknowledging unsavory elements in its past. In 1975, for example, the National Institutes of Health recognized the significance of manipulation as treatment by organizing a Workshop on the Research Status of Spinal Manipulative Therapy that included not only physicians and osteopaths but chiropractors, too. (At least one medical representative attended in the "hope this meeting stamps out chiropractic," but the workshop actually led to an ongoing series of interprofessional conferences on spinal therapy.) One chiropractic participant in the workshop opened his address to the mixed audience with an apology for the "mishap" and "overclaim" that had long proliferated in his field and followed with assurances that conscientious chiropractors "are not necessarily proud of those that we are responsible for." He hoped that the workshop's other attendees "will not deny the people of my profession the privilege of progress and ethics." Another chiropractor admitted that for much of his profession's history the three main rules for deciding whether or not to accept a patient as a chiropractic case were: "Does the patient have a spinal column? Does the patient have a nervous system? Is the patient alive?"[37]

By the mid-1970s, however, chiropractors were regularly referring patients to MDs—and 5 percent of physicians occasionally referred patients for chiropractic care. By the end of the 1980s, the percentage of family practice doctors who sometimes sent patients to chiropractors had risen to nearly 60, and two-thirds of doctors surveyed in Washington State responded that they regarded chiropractic as "effective for some patients"; most of the remaining third actually deemed the system "an excellent [!] source of care for some musculoskeletal problems," with only 3 percent still insisting "they are quacks and patients should avoid them." Chiropractors were to be found on staff at a number of hospitals, and at least one chiropractor had gained a faculty position in an orthodox medical school, teaching radiology. In the words of the Washington surveyors, mainstream medicine's attitudes toward chiropractic had largely changed from "hostile" to "hospitable."[38]

Naturopathic Medicine

More recently, a similar transition from adversarial to accepting has occurred with respect to another long-disrespected practice: naturopathy, or, as is now standard, naturopathic medicine. Throughout its first half century, naturopathy's development was retarded by naiveté. Virtually any therapy that could be rationalized somehow as "natural" was avidly embraced by naturopaths, while that same reflex made them steadfastly deny that either truth or benefit was to be found in allopathy. A naturopathic textbook published as recently as 1951 still advised "Walking Barefoot to harden the body and to absorb the life currents from the earth," as well as recommending "Magnetic Breathing, Magnetic Bathing and eating Magnetic Foods." And as to the germ theory— "hysterically SUPPOSED by Medical Science" to explain infection—"what nonsense it all is!"[39]

Professionally, naturopathy was in disarray by the middle of the twentieth century. The spectacular expansion of wonder-drug therapy and biotechnology in conventional practice after World War II did much to draw patients away from the simple methods of natural healers, of course, but naturopaths themselves were deeply implicated in the decline of their movement. There had been factionalism within the ranks from the beginning, but it was kept relatively contained until Lust's death in 1945. Then, much as had occurred with Thomsonianism following its founder's death, naturopathy cracked apart. Contentious personalities vied to assume leadership of the one, true natur-

-educated or churned out by unaccredited diploma mills, these un-Ds, as
s refer to "unlicensable naturopaths," exploit popular enthusiasm for al-
ative medicine and thrive in the "regulatory vacuum" that exists in most
es. These unqualified pretenders act, naturopathy's leaders complain, "to
significant detriment of the public and the profession." Clearing the field
harlatans is at the top of the naturopathic agenda for establishing credibility
maintaining professional standards.[46]

Office of Alternative Medicine

ctitioners of naturopathic medicine point to studies conducted by main-
am researchers and published in allopathic journals as evidence for the
cacy of many of their therapies. Furthermore, some treatments—certain
al remedies in particular—have come to be generally acknowledged by
odoxy as useful (saw palmetto for prostate enlargement, for example, and
John's wort for mild depression).[47] Yet overall, much of what naturopathic
sicians do for their patients has not met the gold standard applied to
odox research, the randomized, controlled, double-blind clinical trial. In-
, by that yardstick, all the major alternative systems of practice come up
rt in demonstrating the effectiveness of their therapies, a fact of which they
frequently reminded.

Alternative practitioners have a threefold response to the criticism that
st of their methods have not been clearly demonstrated to be superior to
acebo response. First, they point out, conventional medicine is guilty of
same shortcoming. Randomized, controlled clinical trials were not adopted
he standard by mainstream medicine until the 1950s. By then there were
y therapies being employed that had not been subjected to controlled trials
that have continued in use, and other treatments and procedures were
pted subsequently without rigorous evaluation. A study by the U.S. Office
echnology Assessment in the late 1970s reported that, in fact, the majority
herapies employed in conventional medicine were unproven: "Only 10 to
percent of all procedures currently used in medical practice have been
wn to be efficacious by controlled trial." A separate study published in
estimated that only 15 percent of all allopathic interventions "are sup-
ted by solid scientific evidence." During the same period, regular physicians
ame increasingly critical of the value of specific practices common among
colleagues (coronary artery bypass surgery, for example). Interestingly,
tors who continued to use therapies not fully validated by clinical trials
so because clinical experience had convinced them that they worked.
re important than scientific studies for me," one MD has recently stated,
what I have seen with my own eyes and . . . what I see with my patients.

opathy, with the result that for a time there were no fewer than six different
national organizations claiming to represent the profession. If that weren't
enough of a deterrent to attracting new practitioners, most of the states that
had previously licensed naturopaths (as many as twenty-five at one point)
withdrew recognition of the apparently foundering system; by 1958 only five
states still licensed naturopaths, though a few others allowed them to practice
under the broad category of drugless healers. Naturopathic schools closed as
well, until by the 1970s only one remained in operation. (Naturopathy's for-
tunes sank so low that in 1955 the chiropractic profession, many of whose
schools had for years also offered naturopathic training and degrees, decided
to abandon its affiliation with naturopathy as part of its campaign to enhance
the chiropractic image.) Part of the reason naturopaths were turned down for
Medicare reimbursement in 1968 was that there were only 553 practitioners in
the country, and their number was "rapidly declining." A survey of the natural
health field in 1971 concluded that naturopaths were "making a last ditch
struggle to survive."[40]

The chief reason for excluding naturopathy from Medicare, however,
was the same as initially given for chiropractic: its "theory and practice are
not based upon the body of basic knowledge related to health, disease, and
health care that has been widely accepted by the scientific community." In
addition (as with chiropractic), naturopathic education was found to be inadequate. Yet both those deficiencies were being addressed by naturopaths by
the 1960s. The issue of the field's lack of a scientific basis, in fact, was at the
heart of the internal dissension that surfaced after Lust's death; disruptive as
were belligerent personalities, principles were more important for fueling naturopaths' intramural battles. On the one side were dyed-in-the-wool believers
in "nature cure" (diet, exercise, water, sun, air) as a revelation straight from
nature, healers disdainful of laboratory science. On the other were the liberal
practitioners belonging to the so-called western group, naturopaths concentrated in the western states who recognized the validity of mainstream medicine's scientific foundation and sought to incorporate biomedical science into
their own system and apply it under the guidelines of naturopathic philosophy.
Critical of the scientific backwardness of old-school practitioners, intent on
using "Scientific Naturopathic Research" to evaluate the common nature-cure
therapies and thereby rid the field of all "fads and fancies," and preferring the
forward-looking designation "naturopathic medicine" to simple "naturopathy,"
they seemed to their critics to be heading down the osteopathic road toward
selling their souls for mainstream acceptance; one of the derisive nicknames
applied to them was the "pseudo-medical group."[41]

A key figure among the pseudo-medicals was John Bastyr. A practitioner
in Seattle since the 1930s, and particularly well known for his advocacy of

natural childbirth, Bastyr recognized the necessity of naturopathy staying abreast of advances in biomedical science and applying those advances "in ways consistent with naturopathic principles" (as agents supporting or stimulating the *vis medicatrix naturae*). In furtherance of his vision of "naturopathy's empirical successes documented and proven by scientific methods," Bastyr opened the National College of Naturopathic Medicine in Seattle in 1956, directing it until its relocation to Portland, Oregon, for financial reasons in 1976. Hardly had the National College moved, however, before three of Bastyr's former students established a new school in Seattle, the John Bastyr College of Naturopathic Medicine, in 1978. (There are three other schools of naturopathy in America at present, as well as institutions in Canada, Australia, Great Britain, and India.)[42]

The short history of John Bastyr College is the most compelling illustration of the triumphant rebirth of naturopathy as naturopathic medicine. Although four new naturopathic schools were opened in the holistic excitement of the late 1970s, Bastyr alone survived. Beginning in space leased from a community college, with only thirty-one students enrolled, the school grew until by the close of the twentieth century enrollment exceeded one thousand, with students from more than three-quarters of the American states and nearly a dozen foreign countries. Now located on its own spacious campus near Seattle, Bastyr University (the name change was made in 1994) provides education in six natural health programs in addition to naturopathic medicine (nutrition, midwifery, and acupuncture and Oriental medicine, among others), though approximately half of all students pursue the ND degree. Applicants to the four-year naturopathic medicine program are expected to have earned a college degree, and the mean grade point average for entering students is above 3.3. Bastyr has been recognized by an independent accrediting agency, the Northwest Association of Schools and Colleges, since 1988.[43]

From the outset, Bastyr's co-founder and first president, Joseph Pizzorno, recognized that "anecdotal and unverified 'cures,' particularly when associated with unusual therapies, do our cause little good." Consequently, instruction at the school "has concentrated more on the scientifically verifiable aspects of natural medicine and less on the relatively anecdotal nature cure aspects." That orientation is evident as well in Pizzorno's co-edited *Textbook of Natural Medicine*, the recent second edition of which comprises two hefty volumes whose chapters contain more than ten thousand citations to articles in conventional biomedical literature; pages are filled with discussions of biochemical and physiological mechanisms, with old-time practices such as astroscopy and iridiagnosis conspicuous only by their absence. The same quantum jump in scientific sophistication is evident in the *Journal of Naturopathic Medicine*, published by the American Association of Naturopathic Physicians. (The AANP

was founded in 1980, at last reunifying naturopathic pra decades of disorganization.) The lead articles in the journa for example, bore the titles "Effects of Colon Irrigation lytes," "Inhibition of Endocrine Function by Botanical rectic and Mood-Altering Effects of Ketosis During Ket articles' arguments were supported, furthermore, with cita journals such as *JAMA* and the *British Medical Journal*, n naturopathic literature. "We must define ourselves as a p is the war cry of the modern ND; "let's not go back to days of naturopathy." There are, of course, throwbacks to days still in practice, men and women who are deeply tre naturopaths find it necessary to cast about for more p diagnosis and treatment." But their numbers are dwindlin reason for them to worry about their future "in a world w is stronger than faith in nature."[44]

Naturopathic medical practice nevertheless is still con therapies backed by faith in nature. Among the most con egories are clinical nutrition, botanicals, homeopathy, a therapy, physical medicine (massage, heat, cold, electrici lifestyle counseling. A primary object of treatment is "de the patient of toxic materials, whether produced internall function or taken in from the environment. Yet detoxifi therapies, is meant to serve the more basic purpose of s *medicatrix*. Naturopathy still means trusting in nature to vention of the American Association of Naturopathic Phy slogan "Naturopathic Medicine—working with nature health") and still means "confidence in the perception of force." Hence today's hydrotherapeutic procedures are ju Lust, or even Trall, would commend: hydrotherapy prov ulation of the vital force. . . . [It is] a method designed to to the digestive and eliminative organs [and] stimulate the

Naturopathic medicine thus retains much of the old based natural medicine," but there are other vestiges of that today's practitioners do not celebrate. Lust, we have s attacking those "imposters and unqualified practitioners w selves to be Naturopathic Physicians," and believed that postors was the primary reason why state licensing law naturopaths. The situation has hardly changed. One of th lems for naturopathic physicians today is the proliferatio turopaths" in states that do not license naturopathic pra pathic medicine was recognized in only eleven states as

And that isn't considered 'scientifically valid.' . . . I'm doing observations, and it's very clear to me that people do get better." Another made the point more directly: "I simply say, 'Goddammit, if this works it works, and that we don't understand it doesn't make any difference.' " A homeopath couldn't have said it better.[48]

Alternative practitioners' second reaction to the paucity of research behind their therapies is that they have been unable to do research at the level demanded for proof. It is not that they have avoided clinical trials for fear that their treatments will be exposed as useless—a common charge leveled by physicians. Rather, they explain, they have been trained as healers, not as scientific investigators. Their schooling does not give them the expertise in research design acquired by mainstream researchers. Nor do they have the time and facilities that people employed specifically to do research have at their disposal. Most of all, alternative medicine has never been taken seriously enough to qualify for the level of funding needed for trials of the size and sophistication required to pass muster before MD inspectors. (There is a problem of economic incentives as well, since many alternative therapies are natural materials or agents that have been used medically for years and thus cannot be patented.)[49]

Finally, alternative doctors maintain that their approaches to healing often are not amenable to the standard research model. Naturopaths, for example, stress that they do not treat patients with a single drug, easily tested against a placebo and easily camouflaged from both doctor and patient to achieve double-blinding. Instead, they use an "approach" that combines several treatments, combined with counseling. A urinary tract infection, for instance, might be treated with a combination of increased consumption of water and fresh fruit juices to increase urine flow and flush bacteria from the urethra; cranberry juice to inhibit the adherence of microorganisms to the bladder and urethral mucosa; citrate salts to alkalinize the urine; vitamins A and C, zinc, echinacea, and elimination of sugar from the diet to stimulate the immune system; and garlic, bearberry, and goldenseal for their specific activity against microbes. The naturopathic approach, furthermore, is carefully tailored to the individual's needs, and individualization of therapy is difficult to reconcile with the standardization demanded by controlled trials. From the perspective of many alternative practitioners, in fact, giving a standard remedy for a standard disease would run so counter to what is regarded as ideal therapy as to make the trial results meaningless. In addition, alternative practitioners commonly use diagnoses that are different from allopathic disease categories; their methods are often difficult to imitate with a placebo; and when special skills are needed for a physical intervention (such as acupuncture or, for that matter, surgery) it is impossible to blind the doctor. In summary, "it is not the fact that a therapy is complementary that poses the problems, but that its nature is such that there is no easy equivalent to the inert tablets routinely used in drug trials." As one commentator summed it up, evaluating therapeutic efficacy for the diverse host of alternative systems is akin to "setting the agenda for a convention of anarchists."[50]

The shortage of hard evidence of efficacy for alternative therapies, combined with burgeoning public interest in alternative medicine, and the hope that low-tech alternative treatments might provide a way to rein in runaway medical costs, led in 1991 to an extraordinary event. The Appropriations Committee of the U.S. Senate, the body responsible for funding that most august of orthodox research establishments, the National Institutes of Health, announced that year that it was "not satisfied that the conventional medical community as symbolized at the NIH has fully explored the potential that exists in unconventional medical practices." The NIH was therefore instructed to appoint a panel to develop a research program to evaluate the effectiveness of "the most promising" alternative therapies and granted an allotment of two million dollars ("a homeopathic level of funding," it was joked) to begin the work. (There was a precedent for this action, it might be noted, as in 1974, the year chiropractic was accepted into the Medicare system, Congress had instructed NIH to allot two million dollars for the investigation of the scientific basis of chiropractic.)[51]

The leaders of NIH were hardly pleased with the grant (the institutes' director resigned), partly because it implied legitimacy for alternative medicine but equally because it was a political decision instead of the result of scientific deliberation. The chair of the Appropriations Committee, Thomas Harkin, an Iowa Democrat who had had two sisters die of breast cancer, was encouraged to press for the action by two constituents with strong ties to unconventional therapies. (Harkin himself soon became an outspoken advocate of bee pollen treatments for allergies.) The new research panel convened in June of the following year under the title of the Office of Alternative Medicine. Some greeted the new office as "the Berlin wall [of medicine] coming down"; others denounced it as only one step removed from an "Office of Astrology."[52]

The OAM's duties with its two million dollars were to develop research methodologies applicable to alternative medicine, help alternative practitioners acquire research skills, promote communication between the alternative practice and biomedical research communities, and fund research studies of alternative treatments. Some grants were to go to small exploratory research projects (thirty thousand dollars each), but the most ambitious program was the establishment of university-affiliated research centers for ongoing studies. In 1994 the first two centers were funded, with $840,000 each distributed over three years. One of the awards was made to the University of Minnesota opathy, with the result that for a time there were no fewer than six different national organizations claiming to represent the profession. If that weren't enough of a deterrent to attracting new practitioners, most of the states that had previously licensed naturopaths (as many as twenty-five at one point) withdrew recognition of the apparently foundering system; by 1958 only five states still licensed naturopaths, though a few others allowed them to practice under the broad category of drugless healers. Naturopathic schools closed as well, until by the 1970s only one remained in operation. (Naturopathy's fortunes sank so low that in 1955 the chiropractic profession, many of whose schools had for years also offered naturopathic training and degrees, decided to abandon its affiliation with naturopathy as part of its campaign to enhance the chiropractic image.) Part of the reason naturopaths were turned down for Medicare reimbursement in 1968 was that there were only 553 practitioners in the country, and their number was "rapidly declining." A survey of the natural health field in 1971 concluded that naturopaths were "making a last ditch struggle to survive."[40]

The chief reason for excluding naturopathy from Medicare, however, was the same as initially given for chiropractic: its "theory and practice are not based upon the body of basic knowledge related to health, disease, and health care that has been widely accepted by the scientific community." In addition (as with chiropractic), naturopathic education was found to be inadequate. Yet both those deficiencies were being addressed by naturopaths by the 1960s. The issue of the field's lack of a scientific basis, in fact, was at the heart of the internal dissension that surfaced after Lust's death; disruptive as were belligerent personalities, principles were more important for fueling naturopaths' intramural battles. On the one side were dyed-in-the-wool believers in "nature cure" (diet, exercise, water, sun, air) as a revelation straight from nature, healers disdainful of laboratory science. On the other were the liberal practitioners belonging to the so-called western group, naturopaths concentrated in the western states who recognized the validity of mainstream medicine's scientific foundation and sought to incorporate biomedical science into their own system and apply it under the guidelines of naturopathic philosophy. Critical of the scientific backwardness of old-school practitioners, intent on using "Scientific Naturopathic Research" to evaluate the common nature-cure therapies and thereby rid the field of all "fads and fancies," and preferring the forward-looking designation "naturopathic medicine" to simple "naturopathy," they seemed to their critics to be heading down the osteopathic road toward selling their souls for mainstream acceptance; one of the derisive nicknames applied to them was the "pseudo-medical group."[41]

A key figure among the pseudo-medicals was John Bastyr. A practitioner in Seattle since the 1930s, and particularly well known for his advocacy of natural childbirth, Bastyr recognized the necessity of naturopathy staying abreast of advances in biomedical science and applying those advances "in ways consistent with naturopathic principles" (as agents supporting or stimulating the *vis medicatrix naturae*). In furtherance of his vision of "naturopathy's empirical successes documented and proven by scientific methods," Bastyr opened the National College of Naturopathic Medicine in Seattle in 1956, directing it until its relocation to Portland, Oregon, for financial reasons in 1976. Hardly had the National College moved, however, before three of Bastyr's former students established a new school in Seattle, the John Bastyr College of Naturopathic Medicine, in 1978. (There are three other schools of naturopathy in America at present, as well as institutions in Canada, Australia, Great Britain, and India.)[42]

The short history of John Bastyr College is the most compelling illustration of the triumphant rebirth of naturopathy as naturopathic medicine. Although four new naturopathic schools were opened in the holistic excitement of the late 1970s, Bastyr alone survived. Beginning in space leased from a community college, with only thirty-one students enrolled, the school grew until by the close of the twentieth century enrollment exceeded one thousand, with students from more than three-quarters of the American states and nearly a dozen foreign countries. Now located on its own spacious campus near Seattle, Bastyr University (the name change was made in 1994) provides education in six natural health programs in addition to naturopathic medicine (nutrition, midwifery, and acupuncture and Oriental medicine, among others), though approximately half of all students pursue the ND degree. Applicants to the four-year naturopathic medicine program are expected to have earned a college degree, and the mean grade point average for entering students is above 3.3. Bastyr has been recognized by an independent accrediting agency, the Northwest Association of Schools and Colleges, since 1988.[43]

From the outset, Bastyr's co-founder and first president, Joseph Pizzorno, recognized that "anecdotal and unverified 'cures,' particularly when associated with unusual therapies, do our cause little good." Consequently, instruction at the school "has concentrated more on the scientifically verifiable aspects of natural medicine and less on the relatively anecdotal nature cure aspects." That orientation is evident as well in Pizzorno's co-edited *Textbook of Natural Medicine*, the recent second edition of which comprises two hefty volumes whose chapters contain more than ten thousand citations to articles in conventional biomedical literature; pages are filled with discussions of biochemical and physiological mechanisms, with old-time practices such as astroscopy and iridiagnosis conspicuous only by their absence. The same quantum jump in scientific sophistication is evident in the *Journal of Naturopathic Medicine*, published by the American Association of Naturopathic Physicians. (The AANP was founded in 1980, at last reunifying naturopathic practitioners after three decades of disorganization.) The lead articles in the journal's first issue (1990), for example, bore the titles "Effects of Colon Irrigation on Serum Electrolytes," "Inhibition of Endocrine Function by Botanical Agents," and "Anorectic and Mood-Altering Effects of Ketosis During Ketogenic Diets." The articles' arguments were supported, furthermore, with citations from orthodox journals such as *JAMA* and the *British Medical Journal*, not just references to naturopathic literature. "We must define ourselves as a practice of medicine" is the war cry of the modern ND; "let's not go back to the nuts-and-berries days of naturopathy." There are, of course, throwbacks to the nuts-and-berries days still in practice, men and women who are deeply troubled that "today's naturopaths find it necessary to cast about for more powerful methods of diagnosis and treatment." But their numbers are dwindling, and there is good reason for them to worry about their future "in a world where faith in science is stronger than faith in nature."[44]

Naturopathic medical practice nevertheless is still comprised of distinctive therapies backed by faith in nature. Among the most common treatment categories are clinical nutrition, botanicals, homeopathy, acupuncture, hydrotherapy, physical medicine (massage, heat, cold, electricity), spirituality, and lifestyle counseling. A primary object of treatment is "detoxification," freeing the patient of toxic materials, whether produced internally by metabolic dysfunction or taken in from the environment. Yet detoxification, like all other therapies, is meant to serve the more basic purpose of strengthening the *vis medicatrix*. Naturopathy still means trusting in nature to cure (the 1989 convention of the American Association of Naturopathic Physicians adopted the slogan "Naturopathic Medicine—working with nature to restore people's health") and still means "confidence in the perception of a vital force or life force." Hence today's hydrotherapeutic procedures are justified in terms that Lust, or even Trall, would commend: hydrotherapy provides "general stimulation of the vital force. . . . [It is] a method designed to stimulate circulation to the digestive and eliminative organs [and] stimulate the nervous system."[45]

Naturopathic medicine thus retains much of the old in its new "science-based natural medicine," but there are other vestiges of naturopathy's past that today's practitioners do not celebrate. Lust, we have seen, spent his career attacking those "imposters and unqualified practitioners who represent themselves to be Naturopathic Physicians," and believed that controlling the impostors was the primary reason why state licensing laws were needed for naturopaths. The situation has hardly changed. One of the most vexing problems for naturopathic physicians today is the proliferation of self-styled "naturopaths" in states that do not license naturopathic practitioners. (Naturopathic medicine was recognized in only eleven states as of 2001.) Whether self-educated or churned out by unaccredited diploma mills, these un-Ds, as NDs refer to "unlicensable naturopaths," exploit popular enthusiasm for alternative medicine and thrive in the "regulatory vacuum" that exists in most states. These unqualified pretenders act, naturopathy's leaders complain, "to the significant detriment of the public and the profession." Clearing the field of charlatans is at the top of the naturopathic agenda for establishing credibility and maintaining professional standards.[46]

The Office of Alternative Medicine

Practitioners of naturopathic medicine point to studies conducted by mainstream researchers and published in allopathic journals as evidence for the efficacy of many of their therapies. Furthermore, some treatments—certain herbal remedies in particular—have come to be generally acknowledged by orthodoxy as useful (saw palmetto for prostate enlargement, for example, and St. John's wort for mild depression).[47] Yet overall, much of what naturopathic physicians do for their patients has not met the gold standard applied to orthodox research, the randomized, controlled, double-blind clinical trial. Indeed, by that yardstick, all the major alternative systems of practice come up short in demonstrating the effectiveness of their therapies, a fact of which they are frequently reminded.

Alternative practitioners have a threefold response to the criticism that most of their methods have not been clearly demonstrated to be superior to a placebo response. First, they point out, conventional medicine is guilty of the same shortcoming. Randomized, controlled clinical trials were not adopted as the standard by mainstream medicine until the 1950s. By then there were many therapies being employed that had not been subjected to controlled trials but that have continued in use, and other treatments and procedures were adopted subsequently without rigorous evaluation. A study by the U.S. Office of Technology Assessment in the late 1970s reported that, in fact, the majority of therapies employed in conventional medicine were unproven: "Only 10 to 20 percent of all procedures currently used in medical practice have been shown to be efficacious by controlled trial." A separate study published in 1991 estimated that only 15 percent of all allopathic interventions "are supported by solid scientific evidence." During the same period, regular physicians became increasingly critical of the value of specific practices common among their colleagues (coronary artery bypass surgery, for example). Interestingly, doctors who continued to use therapies not fully validated by clinical trials did so because clinical experience had convinced them that they worked. "More important than scientific studies for me," one MD has recently stated, is "what I have seen with my own eyes and . . . what I see with my patients.

And that isn't considered 'scientifically valid.' . . . I'm doing observations, and it's very clear to me that people do get better." Another made the point more directly: "I simply say, 'Goddammit, if this works it works, and that we don't understand it doesn't make any difference.' " A homeopath couldn't have said it better.[48]

Alternative practitioners' second reaction to the paucity of research behind their therapies is that they have been unable to do research at the level demanded for proof. It is not that they have avoided clinical trials for fear that their treatments will be exposed as useless—a common charge leveled by physicians. Rather, they explain, they have been trained as healers, not as scientific investigators. Their schooling does not give them the expertise in research design acquired by mainstream researchers. Nor do they have the time and facilities that people employed specifically to do research have at their disposal. Most of all, alternative medicine has never been taken seriously enough to qualify for the level of funding needed for trials of the size and sophistication required to pass muster before MD inspectors. (There is a problem of economic incentives as well, since many alternative therapies are natural materials or agents that have been used medically for years and thus cannot be patented.)[49]

Finally, alternative doctors maintain that their approaches to healing often are not amenable to the standard research model. Naturopaths, for example, stress that they do not treat patients with a single drug, easily tested against a placebo and easily camouflaged from both doctor and patient to achieve double-blinding. Instead, they use an "approach" that combines several treatments, combined with counseling. A urinary tract infection, for instance, might be treated with a combination of increased consumption of water and fresh fruit juices to increase urine flow and flush bacteria from the urethra; cranberry juice to inhibit the adherence of microorganisms to the bladder and urethral mucosa; citrate salts to alkalinize the urine; vitamins A and C, zinc, echinacea, and elimination of sugar from the diet to stimulate the immune system; and garlic, bearberry, and goldenseal for their specific activity against microbes. The naturopathic approach, furthermore, is carefully tailored to the individual's needs, and individualization of therapy is difficult to reconcile with the standardization demanded by controlled trials. From the perspective of many alternative practitioners, in fact, giving a standard remedy for a standard disease would run so counter to what is regarded as ideal therapy as to make the trial results meaningless. In addition, alternative practitioners commonly use diagnoses that are different from allopathic disease categories; their methods are often difficult to imitate with a placebo; and when special skills are needed for a physical intervention (such as acupuncture or, for that matter, surgery) it is impossible to blind the doctor. In summary, "it is not the fact that a therapy is complementary that poses the problems, but that its nature is such that there is no easy equivalent to the inert tablets routinely used in drug trials." As one commentator summed it up, evaluating therapeutic efficacy for the diverse host of alternative systems is akin to "setting the agenda for a convention of anarchists."[50]

The shortage of hard evidence of efficacy for alternative therapies, combined with burgeoning public interest in alternative medicine, and the hope that low-tech alternative treatments might provide a way to rein in runaway medical costs, led in 1991 to an extraordinary event. The Appropriations Committee of the U.S. Senate, the body responsible for funding that most august of orthodox research establishments, the National Institutes of Health, announced that year that it was "not satisfied that the conventional medical community as symbolized at the NIH has fully explored the potential that exists in unconventional medical practices." The NIH was therefore instructed to appoint a panel to develop a research program to evaluate the effectiveness of "the most promising" alternative therapies and granted an allotment of two million dollars ("a homeopathic level of funding," it was joked) to begin the work. (There was a precedent for this action, it might be noted, as in 1974, the year chiropractic was accepted into the Medicare system, Congress had instructed NIH to allot two million dollars for the investigation of the scientific basis of chiropractic.)[51]

The leaders of NIH were hardly pleased with the grant (the institutes' director resigned), partly because it implied legitimacy for alternative medicine but equally because it was a political decision instead of the result of scientific deliberation. The chair of the Appropriations Committee, Thomas Harkin, an Iowa Democrat who had had two sisters die of breast cancer, was encouraged to press for the action by two constituents with strong ties to unconventional therapies. (Harkin himself soon became an outspoken advocate of bee pollen treatments for allergies.) The new research panel convened in June of the following year under the title of the Office of Alternative Medicine. Some greeted the new office as "the Berlin wall [of medicine] coming down"; others denounced it as only one step removed from an "Office of Astrology."[52]

The OAM's duties with its two million dollars were to develop research methodologies applicable to alternative medicine, help alternative practitioners acquire research skills, promote communication between the alternative practice and biomedical research communities, and fund research studies of alternative treatments. Some grants were to go to small exploratory research projects (thirty thousand dollars each), but the most ambitious program was the establishment of university-affiliated research centers for ongoing studies. In 1994 the first two centers were funded, with $840,000 each distributed over three years. One of the awards was made to the University of Minnesota

Medical School, for the evaluation of alternative treatments for substance abuse; the other, for the exploration of alternative therapies for AIDS, was given to Bastyr University. The following year, OAM grants were made to eight more institutions, all mainstream medical schools, including such prestigious representatives of orthodox medicine as Harvard, Columbia, and Stanford. Critics could protest that the government was "buying snake oil with tax dollars" and wasting money studying "superstition masquerading as science," but funding for OAM grew rapidly nonetheless, increasing sevenfold by 1996. For the year 2001, the appropriation was eighty-nine million dollars, still modest by NIH standards but some forty-five times the original budget for the OAM, and hardly homeopathic anymore.[53]

Nor was the office simply alternative anymore. In 1998 Congress upgraded its status from office to center (giving it more autonomy within the NIH infrastructure) and renamed it the National Center for Complementary and Alternative Medicine. Designation as *complementary* by so powerful an institution signaled that indeed "alternative medicine has crossed the barrier reef of cultural resistance and come of age in the United States."[54]

Conclusion:
The Twenty-first Century—
The Age of Curapathy?

The November 11, 1998, issue of the *Journal of the American Medical Association* included two editorials that predicted sharply contrasting futures for alternative medicine in America. "We are in the midst of a fad that will pass," assured the author of the column titled "Leeches, Spiders, and Astrology." "Alternative medicine is here to stay," insisted the director of the Office of Alternative Medicine; the only question in his mind was how "to separate the pearls from the mud."[1]

The course of alternative medicine in the twenty-first century is a matter of strongly differing opinions among physicians. In the public mind, however, there seems to be little doubt about the position of the second editorialist. There clearly is widespread receptivity to the message on the cover of the September 1996 issue of *Life* magazine, where the upper left quadrant of a patient is pictured with a stethoscope held to her chest by one physician's hand and a bouquet of herbs extended toward her by another's. This latest "Healing Revolution," the cover explains, is one in which "M.D.'s are mixing Ancient Medicine and New Science" and using the combination "to treat everything from the common cold to cancer." The story that follows fairly bubbles over with assurances that "signs that allopathic and alternative medicine are happily wedded are everywhere."[2]

Even the happiest unions are still troubled at times by disagreement and bickering, and complaints about this merger have indeed been frequent and pointed on the allopathic side. The proliferation of courses on alternative medicine in medical schools, for example, has left some MDs "appalled" at their profession's buckling before the forces of "political correctness" and elicited calls to stand firm as "the last bastion of science in this sea of pseudoscience that is flooding the airwaves and cyberspace." Political correctness (and political pressure) undoubtedly was a factor in the establishment of the Office of Alternative Medicine, as was the hope that alternative systems' low-tech interventions and emphasis on prevention would result in lower expenditures for health care. But if OAM constituted a shotgun wedding, there were many examples during the 1990s of the two parties joining hands freely. In February 1995 the council for Washington State's King County (which encom-passes Seattle, long a hotbed of alternative medicine) unanimously approved the establishment of a clinic to provide the county's low-income population with naturopathy, chiropractic, massage, acupuncture, and other alternative services, in addition to orthodox therapy. With the collaboration of the Seattle King County Public Health Department, the King County Natural Medicine Clinic opened in 1996, in the town of Kent, self-proclaimed "Wellness Capital of the United States." The first publicly funded, broad-spectrum alternative medical clinic in America, it offered patients care co-managed by MDs and NDs, with all practitioners recording examinations and treatments in the same chart. The contract to manage the clinic was awarded to Bastyr University, even though two large allopathic hospitals also applied for the job.[3]

The state legislature broadened the King County action, passing a law that took effect January 1, 1996, requiring every health insurance plan in Washington to cover claims for services provided by all licensed practitioners, including chiropractors, naturopaths, acupuncturists, and massage therapists. This was the first such law in the United States, but already health maintenance organizations throughout the country were including some alternative procedures (most frequently chiropractic) among their services. By 1999 nearly two-thirds of the nation's HMOs offered coverage of at least one alternative method.[4]

There was much additional evidence of a warming relationship. For instance, allopathic institutions began sponsoring programs that invited alternative practitioners to confer on combining approaches; the Washington State Hospital Association even titled its 1995 colloquium "*Mainstreaming* Alternative Medicine" (emphasis mine). Hospitals across the country began opening "integrative clinics" (twenty-seven by 2001), and since the mid-1990s more than a half dozen new journals have been launched to bring together alternative and allopathic practitioners. In 1993 the dean of the medical school at Columbia University gave his blessing to the founding of a Center for Alternative/Complementary Medicine within the school (funded by a grant from the Rosenthal Foundation). Even the president of the United States got involved in the matchmaking: Bill Clinton appointed a White House Commission on Complementary and Alternative Medicine Policy in March 2000. The commission's charge was to develop "a set of legislative and administrative recommendations to maximize the benefits of complementary and alternative medicine for the general public." "Gone were the acrimonious exchanges of the early years of the NIH Office of Alternative Medicine," observers reported of the commission's meetings; in their stead was "a new feeling of tolerance, compassion, and good humor."[5]

The new tolerance is most evident in the flowering of "complementary" as a designation for certain unconventional methods, a recognition of them as respectable enough to be used in tandem with allopathic therapies, to complete and balance conventional treatments (in Great Britain, "complementary" has been used in place of "alternative" since the 1980s). Even the uninspiring acronym CAM, coined in the mid-'90s to represent "complementary and alternative medicine," reflects growing goodwill; by placing "alternative" within the ambit of complementariness, it subtly transforms the image of alternative from dubious option pursued as a last resort to plausible treatment elected in situations where allopathy is insufficient. Yet another term of recent vintage—"integrative"—goes even farther, proposing that unconventional therapies be fully worked into the orthodox structure. The pioneer of "integrative medicine" is Andrew Weil, a Harvard-trained MD and best-selling writer on optimal health who in 1996 established a Program in Integrative Medicine within the Department of Medicine at a major allopathic medical school, the University of Arizona. Designed to provide two-year fellowships for MDs who have completed residencies in family medicine or internal medicine, the program's goal is "to combine the best ideas and practices of conventional and alternative medicine into cost-effective treatments," without embracing alternative practices "uncritically." Within a year, an author in a prestigious British journal could comment enviously that Weil "has more than 2.5 million hits on his web site each month, rather more than *The Lancet* receives."[6]

Whether through Weil's website or other avenues, orthodox practitioners were demonstrating an extraordinary openness toward alternative therapies by the mid-1990s. Among family practice physicians surveyed in 1995, 80 percent expressed an interest in receiving training in acupuncture, hypnotherapy, and massage therapy; approximately 70 percent voiced the same interest in herbal medicine, chiropractic, and homeopathy. In another survey (1994), nearly one-quarter of family practice physicians reported using some form of alternative therapy in their own practice. And in yet another survey (1998), fully half the faculty of a large state medical school responded they had personally received at least one form of alternative treatment. Clearly there has occurred a remarkable break with the attitudes of the past, when, as William James recalled of his medical student days at Harvard in the 1860s, "we sneered at homeopathy by word of command, and not one of us would have been caught looking into homeopathic literature."[7]

Adherents of unorthodox systems have mellowed in their outlook, too. Through most of the past two centuries, the goal of irregulars was not to integrate with allopaths but to overthrow their misguided system completely and replace it with the one valid method of healing, be it Thomsonianism, homeopathy, or chiropractic. Alternative medical literature bristled with challenges to the medical establishment. "Hydropathy aims not at a reform," one of its champions warned as early as 1846, "but a total annihilation of the present system." Soon after, Trall reiterated the threat, explaining that "hydropathy proposes to demolish the whole vast superstructure of a system built on false principles." Such expectations continued well into the twentieth century. A toast offered to Still at his birthday party in 1911 included the prediction that "when a hundred years shall have rolled away, there will be but one school of practice and that school, Osteopathy. The name that shall be blazoned out of the Skies of Science will not be Hippocrates, the Father of Medicine, but Andrew Taylor Still, the Father of the Healing Art." If there was any integration to be done, irregulars believed, it would be on their terms. "In the future we will have only MDs and NDs," Lust dictated in the 1920s. All "the other pathies pathetically peripatetic, that run their little course," would be taken into naturopathy "if they are biologically correct," or, "if contrary to nature, superstitious, dangerous, criminal in their practices and results, they are sure to belong to regular medicine—regular licensed quackery."[8]

Yet throughout the decades of confrontation, conciliatory voices were occasionally to be heard. Regulars "see much to condemn in our opponents," a physician stated at the turn of the twentieth century, "but gentlemen, withal, let us be modest in our claims, for we ourselves are not yet scientifically perfect, our enemies find much in us for criticism, and there is not a specialist or a surgeon or a consultant of any kind anywhere who has not discovered by actual experience that ignorance of this or that well-known medical truth is not confined entirely to irregulars." The mollifying gestures of regular doctors, moreover, were not restricted to admissions of imperfection in their own practice; sometimes they even entertained the idea that some alternative therapies might actually work. "We avow ourselves of such a catholic spirit," a mid-nineteenth-century physician wrote, "as to be ready to grasp any proffered good in the way of HEALING, whosoever may be the offerers, and wheresoever they may have found it." After all, he reminded fellow MDs, "it is not the demerits of the donor or the birthplace of the gift, that, in such a case, we are bound to look to—but simply whether it is qualified to aid us in our glorious and divine mission of soothing the pains of our fellowmen. . . . A saint," he added to drive the point home, "may sing the devil's tunes without contamination."⁹

Nevertheless, as has been shown, for most mainstream physicians the idea that any of the irregular devils' tunes were worth singing was blasphemous, and the uselessness of alternative therapies seemed so obvious that MDs could think of no way to account for their popularity except the ignorance and stupidity of much of the public. Whether in the 1830s (the patrons of homeopathy "swallow with as great gusto at this day as great absurdities as in the reign of magic and witchcraft") or the 1910s ("no doctrines are too ridiculous, no practices too pernicious, to be greedily accepted by the undiscriminating public"), human credulity has been the reflex explanation of the ability of alternative systems to attract clients. The argument has been rounded out by emphasis on the heightened intellectual vulnerability of people who are ill and anxious, particularly those who have already undergone orthodox treatment and failed to get better. Quite recently, the head of the National Council Against Health Fraud, organized in 1984 to combat quackery and unproven therapies, has attributed the enthusiasm for alternative medicine to the fact that "people are desperate and easy to deceive."¹⁰

No doubt many people are easily deceived, yet orthodox physicians have also believed that people can be shown the light and led out of their delusions. Campaigns to educate the public about the unscientific nature of alternative therapies have been a constant feature of the allopathic effort to contain irregular medicine, and every decade has seen confident predictions of the dissolution of alternative systems as the people are made more knowledgeable. One of the first critics of homeopathy in America included in his 1835 *Remarks on the Abracadabra of the Nineteenth Century* a statement of confidence that "not one American will henceforth be duped by homoeopathia, after becoming more intimately acquainted with . . . the superstitious features of its practice." Time and again, MDs have shrugged off alternative medical systems as—in the words of a mid-nineteenth-century physician—"airy gull-traps [that] will pass away and be numbered with the things that were."¹¹

Physicians have expected education to serve as a vaccine to immunize people against making bad medical decisions. Yet in practice it has acted as an allergen. As people have become more conversant with medical science, they have grown more sensitive to alternative medicine's critique of orthodoxy. A number of studies have shown that the clients of alternative practitioners today are of above average education and economic status, anything but the ignoramuses of conventional opinion. (One survey has determined that one-half of people with graduate degrees have employed some form of alternative therapy.)[12] At least some of the airy gull-traps, it seems, are here to stay.

Nevertheless, the clients of alternative practitioners rarely abandon orthodox medical care. Rather, they use it in combination with CAM therapies, in effect creating their own integrative system. They are in fact encouraged to integrate by alternative doctors, who, having outgrown the notion that allopathic medicine could be demolished or annihilated, now readily praise MDs for their skills in handling surgical conditions, trauma, and acute infections. As a practitioner of naturopathic medicine has put it, "if I get into a serious accident, take me directly to the hospital emergency department. Do *not* take me to a naturopathic physician." But, she continues, "once they stop the hemorrhaging, I want the hospital to call my naturopathic doctor, because then I want to integrate. I want the best of both medicines."[13]

Integrative medicine strives to combine the best of both worlds, but it has mountainous obstacles yet to overcome. There are complicated practical questions to resolve with respect to such matters as licensure, reimbursement, referrals, organization of clinics and other sites for delivery of care, legal liability, and education. (There are presently more than 650 schools in the United States offering education and training in one or another CAM therapy; standardizing and accrediting programs will not be easy.) Also at issue is the question of degree of professional autonomy of alternative practitioners. Hard as they have fought to reach this point, unconventional doctors understandably are nervous about the next step, over the threshold of the allopathic stronghold. They worry that, given historic disregard for their talents, they will be pressed into servitude, expected to follow MDs' orders as if they were nurses or physical therapists. Proud of their professional patrimony and jealous of their independence, they aspire to the respectability and freedom of practitioners such as dentists and psychologists, clinicians who cooperate with physicians but are not under their control. Such an arrangement will no doubt be easier to achieve for chiropractors and others who deal with specific diseases or areas of the body than for naturopaths and homeopaths, whose scope of practice duplicates that of the conventional family doctor. All have to be concerned, furthermore, about becoming buried in the paperwork that clogs the mainstream system of reimbursement and decreases the time practitioners can spend with patients; devotion of adequate time to the sick is a cornerstone both of alternative philosophy and of alternative medicine's popular appeal.[14]

Fundamental to gaining equality, of course, is presentation of a convincing demonstration of the efficacy of their therapies. Alternative medicine's task, if it is to move into the realm of integrative medicine, is to meet the requirement set by Flexner at the beginning of the twentieth century. "Scientific medicine," he wrote, "brushes aside all historic dogma. . . . Whatsoever makes good is accepted, becomes in so far part, and organic part, of the permanent structure." As the *Journal of the American Medical Association* has recently editorialized: "There is no alternative medicine. There is only scientifically proven . . . medicine supported by solid data or unproven medicine, for which scientific evidence is lacking." Alternative practitioners today are grappling with the challenge of designing clinical studies that meet the standards of scientific proof while remaining true to the principles of a medical philosophy that evaluates illness and healing on the basis of individual patients instead of the large populations demanded by randomized trials.[15]

Also vital for alternative practitioners' becoming part of the permanent structure of medicine is continued elevation of their educational standards along the lines of the allopathic model in mastery of the basic biological sciences as well as the science of diagnosis. One of the chief objections to alternative healers historically has been that their training exposes them to too few patients and too narrow a range of disease conditions to equip them to diagnose patients adequately. Inability to detect cancer, and consequent failure to refer the patient to the proper specialist, could be as deadly as the administration of toxic drugs. Allaying suspicion about their diagnostic skills, as well as their overall scientific education, is the last measure needed for alternative medicine to put behind an unsavory past that, after all, has been a major barrier to being accepted as complementary instead of rejected as cultist. "Even today," a chiropractor lamented as recently as 1983, his profession had "not entirely pulled away from the heavy hand of the past, for it claws and tears, like an eerie specter from a graveyard of history, reluctant even now to release victims from its grasp." Chiropractors and other alternative practitioners have made remarkable advances in training and practice over the last half century, yet, they feel, their progress is generally overlooked by the orthodox profession, which continues to judge them by outdated perceptions. They are being blamed for the sins of their fathers, unconventional healers protest, and the injustice is compounded by the fact that allopaths' fathers were guilty of the same sins. Not all that long ago MDs were bleeding and purging patients, and most of their educational institutions were laughable still in the early twentieth century. In truth, any skeleton in alternative medicine's closet can also be found in the allopathic closet. Alternative doctors thus see themselves as simply repeating a course of evolution that all professions must pass through, one not significantly different from the evolution undergone by regular medicine. (In the words of one of the founders of Bastyr University, "naturopathic medicine has followed the developmental stages that health care professions typically undergo while becoming accountable to the public.")[16]

As alternative medicine becomes more scientific, its champions argue, mainstream medicine has to become more philosophical and give more serious attention to the holistic interpretation of health and healing if genuine integration is to be accomplished. From the alternative perspective, the philosophy behind the practice remains of critical importance. Naturopathic medicine illustrates this point well. Toward the end of his career, John Bastyr passed the torch to the next generation of naturopaths with the injunction to "keep on with the scientific research, but don't forget the philosophy." In obedience, the American Association of Naturopathic Physicians in 1989 formally recognized that naturopathic medicine is ultimately defined "not by the therapies it uses but by the philosophical principles that guide the practitioner." The six principles adopted by the association as the bedrock of naturopathic practice included respect for the healing power of nature, avoidance of harm to the patient, concentration on the underlying cause of illness rather than treatment of its symptoms, regard for the patient as a whole person, emphasis on prevention, and promotion of wellness. Soon afterward, a seventh principle was added, that the healer must be a "teacher," the meaning of the Latin *doctor*. (To be sure, sensitivity to these principles has increased among MDs over the past decade, fostered by the ever-tightening constraints of managed care and the frustrations of working within a system that rewards practitioners for performing procedures but not for listening and empathizing.)[17]

Naturopathy's philosophical principles are standard holistic philosophy, of course, but are also only a restatement, somewhat fleshed out, of the Hippocratic ethos embraced by all unconventional systems of healing over the past two centuries. Avoiding injury to the sick, for example, was a fundamental rule of practice for Hippocrates ("make a habit of two things," the great physician taught, "to help, or at least to do no harm") and was the motivation for nineteenth-century irregulars' condemnations of calomel. Naturopathic teaching today pays homage to the principle by arguing that therapies should be judged not just by their positive effects but by their negative ones as well and demanding that the patient's quality of life be factored into the evaluation of efficacy. The point has been acutely sharpened most recently by the 1998 publication in the *Journal of the American Medical Association* of a study estimating that as many as a hundred thousand patients die in hospitals each year from adverse drug reactions; that would make death by conventional therapy the fourth leading cause of mortality in the United States. The study has been criticized for placing the number of fatalities too high, but it is generally agreed that there is still an unconscionable number of victims of untoward drug reactions and that "there must be more attention given to the risk side of the equation."[18]

The Hippocratic tradition also placed heavy emphasis on the significance of the individual's level of vitality for his susceptibility to illness. Poorly nourished and inadequately rested people fell sick more easily and, because of a weakened *vis medicatrix*, recovered with more difficulty. It is this lowered state of physiology that naturopathic medicine today addresses with its dictum to find the cause of disease. For the naturopathic physician, the final cause of illness is not some external agent that attacks and invades the body but rather the source of internal malaise that makes the body vulnerable to the attack. Naturopaths identify with nineteenth-century physiologist Claude Bernard, whose response to Pasteur's germ theory was that "the microbe is nothing, the terrain is all." The condition of the terrain, the individual's body, has been the focus of naturopathy from the beginning. Belief that the terrain was all inspired extreme denials of the importance of microbes on into the middle of the twentieth century ("NO ONE WHO IS CLEAN AND HEALTHY IN-SIDE CAN BE AFFECTED BY GERMS OR BECOME THE VICTIM OF GERM INFECTION"), and even though naturopathic physicians at present take a more balanced view of infection, physiological integrity—an intact terrain—remains in their view the best insurance against disease. "Naturo-pathic medicine," a practitioner has recently stated, can be defined as "total respect for what is already there." But Thomson might have defined his system the same way, as might have Trall, Still, or Palmer. Respect for what is already there in the body in a state of health has been the central principle of alter-native healing philosophy all along and was summed up nicely by physio-medical practitioners when they organized the Reformed Medical Association of the United States in 1852: "Resolved, That the fundamental principles of true medical science are not pathological but physiological."[19]

The principle is central to Asian healing traditions as well. "The medical naturalism of Eastern medical thought," one scholar explains, was "a formu-lation in which disease was a function of internal factors, of the malfunctioning of the self, and in which one's own bodily and vital energies were implicated in both the genesis and the treatment of disease." As Asian medical thought has made its way into American culture in recent decades, there has developed an appreciation that the Hippocratic heresy is in truth global, not just a cre-ation of Western history. There has emerged in just the last few years the concept of a "world medicine" that strives to embody the healing wisdom and techniques of all civilizations from antiquity onward and to overcome the spiritual poverty of the biomedical model of disease. World medicine is made compelling also by the planet's growing population and shrinking resources. "Sustainability," the economic imperative of the new millenium, applies to medicine as much as any other endeavor. Continued reliance on expensive technological solutions to poor health, we are warned, "will result in health care costs consuming national finances and stifling national economic growth" in developing and industrialized countries alike.[20]

That said, the proponents of world medicine do not recommend the abandonment of biomedicine's achievements. Technological solutions are seen as having a role but as replaceable in many instances by simpler interventions and in need of being humanized with holistic philosophy. Bastyr University presents itself as the ideal: "a unique institution, where the knowledge of modern science and the wisdom of ancient healing methods are equally valued." What world medicine requires, in essence, is that ancient healing methods, and ancient healing philosophy, be recognized as amenable to modern science, and that will require a more liberal interpretation of science. "What is unscientific about trying to consider the whole person and his or her environment?" a physician has recently asked colleagues critical of alternative medicine as unscientific. Science, he chided, "is a painstaking search for truth, whether truth about haptoglobin or human relationships." By the end of the twentieth century, the protagonists of holistic healing were turning the tables on "scientific medicine," charging that in fact *it* was the endeavor lacking in science. "I have always felt that the only trouble with scientific medicine is that it is not scientific enough," René Dubos wrote two decades ago. "Modern medicine will become really scientific only when physicians and their patients have learned to manage the forces of the body and the mind that operate in *vis medicatrix naturae*."[21]

The holistic medicine movement has been laboring for thirty years to establish such an interpretation of medical science, and the effort is at last bearing fruit. For the time, at least, mainstream and marginal medicine have reached a condition of entente, sometimes cordial, more often wary, but withal holding some promise that their two-hundred-years' war might be about to end—and might conclude not in a sterile truce but with an actual alliance. "We find ourselves," the editor of *The Integrator* has recently written, "in an era beyond the polarization of alternative medicine and conventional medicine," with "an opportunity to become a seamless part of an integrated system that might rightfully be called, simply, *health care*."[22]

This is a turn of events that could not have been easily imagined through most of the past two centuries, yet CAM was not entirely beyond conceiving. Walter Johnson, erstwhile allopath turned homeopath, petitioned all sides as early as the 1850s to "join hands and endeavour each of us to improve, as far as in us lies, the department of practice which each specially cultivates; and instead of degrading ourselves by contemptible bickering, devote our whole energies to the relief of suffering humanity." He hoped "earnestly," he avowed, "for the dawn of that day, when the ephemeral systems which we now practice, shall be absorbed by a new revelation, and cease from affording a pretence for sectarian dissension." About the same time, John Bovee Dods also imagined a time when there might be a single scheme of natural healing, when "Allopathy, Thompsonianism [sic], Homeopathy, Hydropathy, Electropathy [will not] be made to exist as so many separate medical schools; but the excellences of them all, so far as they are applicable to the relief of human sufferings [will] be combined into one grand system TO CURE, and be called CURAPATHY."[23]

The difficulty of achieving that utopian vision was not to be underestimated, however, for the road from cultism to curapathy has been exceedingly long and rocky. And if indeed medical sectarianism should at last give way to ecumenism, it would be so unanticipated a resolution to the historic conflict between orthodoxy and heresy as to amaze all but the very latest generation of combatants. Early in the twentieth century, a naturopath playfully indulged in a fantasy in which he proposed "that the American Medical Association and the American Naturopathic Association each appoint a representative or committee whose sole duty will be to ascertain the points of greater wisdom and excellence *in the other association*. The A.M.A. could say to the A.N.A.— 'We are doubtless making serious mistakes, which your superior knowledge would enable us to correct. Please inform and reform us.' Then the A.N.A. would reply to the A.M.A.—'Not so, brothers. We, verily, are the bunglers— will you not graciously condescend to show *us* the better way?' Each would thus become a regular Alphonse of courtesy to the other's Gaston of humility." At that point, the good doctor came to his senses, realizing how absurd a vision he had conjured. "I have to stop here," he sighed; "such a spectacle takes my breath entirely away, and I must needs recover from the shock."[24]

Abbreviations

The following abbreviations are used for medical and historical journals cited in the notes.

ACM	Academic Medicine
ACT	Alternative and Complementary Therapies
AIM	Archives of Internal Medicine
AJCM	American Journal of Chinese Medicine
AJMS	American Journal of the Medical Sciences
AJP	American Journal of Psychiatry
AJPH	American Journal of Public Health
AM	American Medicine
AMCT	Antibiotic Medicine and Clinical Therapy
AS	American Surgeon
AT	Alternative Therapies
ATHM	Alternative Therapies in Health and Medicine
BHM	Bulletin of the History of Medicine
BMJ	British Medical Journal
BMSJ	Boston Medical and Surgical Journal
BNYAM	Bulletin of the New York Academy of Medicine
CAH	Canadian Hospital
CH	Chiropractic History
CJP	Canadian Journal of Psychiatry
CM	California Medicine
CMP	Culture, Medicine and Psychiatry
CWM	California and Western Medicine
DA	Drugless America

DMJ	Delaware Medical Journal
DNS	Diseases of the Nervous System
DS	Dental Survey
FM	Forum on Medicine
HCQ	History of Childhood Quarterly
HHN	Herald of Health and Naturopath
HM	Health Messenger
HP	Health Psychology
IJCEH	International Journal of Clinical and Experimental Hypnosis
IJHS	International Journal of Health Services
IM	Integrative Medicine
IMJ	Illinois Medical Journal
JA	Journal of Anesthesiology
JABFP	Journal of the American Board of Family Practice
JACM	Journal of Alternative and Complementary Medicine
JAIH	Journal of the American Institute of Homeopathy
JAMA	Journal of the American Medical Association
JAMWA	Journal of the American Medical Women's Association
JAN	Journal of Advanced Nursing
JAOA	Journal of the American Osteopathic Association
JCP	Journal of Clinical Psychiatry
JFP	Journal of Family Practice
JHBS	Journal of the History of the Behavioral Sciences
JHM	Journal of Holistic Medicine
JHMAS	Journal of the History of Medicine and Allied Sciences
JHSB	Journal of Health and Social Behavior
JISMA	Journal of the Indiana State Medical Association
JMP	Journal of Medicine and Philosophy
JMSNJ	Journal of the Medical Society of New Jersey
JNM	Journal of Naturopathic Medicine
JO	Journal of Osteopathy
JRCGP	Journal of the Royal College of General Practitioners
KWCM	The Kneipp Water Cure Monthly
MA	Medical Anthropology
MCP	Mayo Clinic Proceedings
ME	Medical Economics
MH	Medical History
MMFQ	Milbank Memorial Fund Quarterly
MR	Medical Record
MS	Medical Sentinel
MWN	Medical World News

NAMSJ	North American Medical and Surgical Journal
NEJM	New England Journal of Medicine
NHH	The Naturopath and Herald of Health
NJH	New Jersey History
NM	Northwest Medicine
NP	Nature's Path
NR	Nursing Research
NT	Nursing Times
NYJM	New York Journal of Medicine
NYSJM	New York State Journal of Medicine
PAH	Perspectives in American History
PAM	Psychology and Medicine
PBM	Perspectives in Biology and Medicine
PH	Pharmacy in History
PHR	Public Health Reports
PM	Pennsylvania Medicine
PR	Psychoanalytic Review
PRSM	Proceedings of the Royal Society of Medicine
SAMJ	South African Medical Journal
SGO	Surgery, Gynecology, and Obstetrics
SMJ	Southern Medical Journal
SMSJ	Southern Medical and Surgical Journal
SSM	Social Science and Medicine
TC	Technology and Culture
VH	Vermont History
VMHB	Virginia Magazine of History and Biography
WCJ	Water-Cure Journal
WCJHR	Water-Cure Journal and Herald of Reforms
WJM	Western Journal of Medicine
WIMJ	Wisconsin Medical Journal
WMJ	World Medical Journal
YJBM	Yale Journal of Biology and Medicine

Notes

PREFACE

1. *New Yorker* (September 26, 1994), 85.

2. David Eisenberg, Ronald Kessler, Cindy Foster, Frances Norlock, David Calkins, and Thomas Delbanco, Unconventional medicine in the United States. *NEJM* (1993) 328: 246–52, p. 251; David Eisenberg, Roger Davis, Susan Ettner, Scott Appel, Sonja Wilkey, Maria Van Rompay, and Ronald Kessler, Trends in alternative medicine use in the United States, 1990–1997. *JAMA* (1998) 280:1569–75, p. 1575.

3. Spalding Gray, *Gray's Anatomy* (New York: Vintage, 1994), 39.

4. James Harvey Young, The development of the Office of Alternative Medicine in the National Institutes of Health, 1991–1996. *BHM* (1998) 72:279–98; Eisenberg, Unconventional (n. 2), 249, 252; Miriam Wetzel, David Eisenberg, and Ted Kaptchuk, Courses involving complementary and alternative medicine at U.S. medical schools. *JAMA* (1998) 280:784–7.

5. Phil Fontanarosa and George Lundberg, Complementary, alternative, unconventional, and integrative medicine: Call for papers for the annual coordinated theme issues of the AMA journals. *JAMA* (1997) 278:2111–2; *JAMA* (1998) 280:1553–1631.

6. Joseph Pizzorno and Pamela Snider, Naturopathic medicine. In: Marc Micozzi, editor, *Fundamentals of Complementary and Alternative Medicine* (New York: Churchill Livingstone, 2001), 159–92, p. 173; Walter Strode, An emerging medicine: Creating the new paradigm. In: Herbert Otto and James Knight, editors, *Dimensions in Wholistic Healing: New Frontiers in the Treatment of the Whole Person* (Chicago: Nelson-Hall, 1979), 65–76.

7. Dan King, *Quackery Unmasked; or, A Consideration of the Most Prominent Empirical Schemes of the Present Time* (New York: Wood, 1858), 332–3; C.R.B. Joyce, Placebo and complementary medicine. *Lancet* (1994) 344:1279–81, p. 1279.

8. Englishman quoted by Robert Fuller, *Mesmerism and the American Cure of Souls* (Philadelphia: University of Pennsylvania Press, 1982), 27; Jacob Bigelow, On the medical profession and quackery. In: Bigelow, *Nature in Disease* (New York: Wood, 1855), 113–33,

p. 129; John Forbes, A review of hydropathy. In: Roland Houghton, editor, *Bulwer and Forbes on the Water-Treatment* (New York: Fowlers and Wells, 1851), 51–119, p. 119.

9. Joseph Jacobs quoted by Baynan McDowell, The National Institutes of Health Office of Alternative Medicine. *ACT* (1994–5) 1:17–25, p. 22; Walter Johnson, *Homoeopathy: Popular Exposition and Defence* (London: Simpkin, Marshall, 1852), iii.

CHAPTER 1

The section-opening poem is from The death-knell of calomel. *Physio-Medical Recorder* (1864) 28:89–90 (quoted by John Haller Jr., *Kindly Medicine: Physio-Medicalism in America, 1836–1911* (Kent, OH: Kent State University Press, 1997), 70–1.

1. *Thomsonian Botanic Watchman* (1834) 1:8.

2. Benjamin Colby, *A Guide to Health* (Nashua, NH: Gill, 1844), v.

3. J. W. Heustis, Remarks on the endemic diseases of Alabama. *AJMS* (1828) 2:26–42, pp. 41–2; Thomas Mitchell, Calomel considered as a poison. *New Orleans Medical and Surgical Journal* (1844–5) 1:28–35, pp. 31–2; John Warren, *A View of the Mercurial Practice in Febrile Diseases* (Boston: Wait, 1813), 2, 7, 13, 32; Benjamin Rush, *An Account of the Bilious Remitting Yellow Fever* (Philadelphia: Dobson, 1794), 251. Also see John Haller Jr., Samson of the materia medica: Medical theory and the use and abuse of calomel in nineteenth-century America. *PH* (1971) 13:27–34, 67–76; and Guenter Risse, Calomel and the American medical sects during the nineteenth century. *MCP* (1973) 48:57–64.

4. Oliver Wendell Holmes, Currents and counter-currents in medical science. In: Holmes, *Medical Essays, 1842–1882* (Boston: Houghton Mifflin, 1899), 173–208, 204; Calomel in the army. *Chicago Medical Journal* (1863) 6:310–20, p. 316.

5. George Monroe quoted by William Rothstein, *American Physicians in the Nineteenth Century: From Sects to Science* (Baltimore: Johns Hopkins University Press, 1972), 49. For more on early nineteenth-century therapy, see Charles Rosenberg, The therapeutic revolution: Medicine, meaning, and social change in nineteenth-century America. *PBM* (1977) 20:485–506.

6. J. Marion Sims, *The Story of My Life* (New York: Appleton, 1884), 150.

7. Elisha Bartlett, *An Essay on the Philosophy of Medical Science* (Philadelphia: Lea and Febinger, 1844), 290; student notebooks quoted by John Warner, *The Therapeutic Perspective: Medical Practice, Knowledge, and Identity in America, 1820–1885* (Cambridge, MA: Harvard University Press, 1986), 18.

8. Bartlett (n. 7), 290; Worthington Hooker, *Physician and Patient* (New York: Baker and Scribner, 1849), 37; Jacob Bigelow, On self-limited diseases. In: Bigelow, *Nature in Disease* (New York: Wood, 1855), 13–63. For a thorough discussion of the role of nature in healing as seen by a mid-nineteenth-century physician, see John Forbes, *Of Nature and Art in the Cure of Disease* (New York: Wood, 1858).

9. Holmes (n. 4), p. 183; John Harley Warner, "The nature-trusting heresy": American physicians and the concept of the healing power of nature in the 1850s and 1860s. *PAH* (1977–8) 11:291–324, pp. 320–1; Warner (n. 7); Worthington Hooker, *Rational Therapeutics; or, The Comparative Value of Different Curative Means, and the Principles of Their Application* (Boston: Wilson, 1857).

10. Physician quoted by John Harley Warner, Medical sectarianism, therapeutic conflict, and the shaping of orthodox professional identity in antebellum American medicine. In: W. F. Bynum and Roy Porter, *Medical Fringe and Medical Orthodoxy, 1750–1850* (London: Croom Helm, 1987), 234–60, p. 246. Warner's article explores in depth the allopathic profession's identification with heroic therapy as the basis of its orthodoxy.

11. Walter Johnson, *Homoeopathy: Popular Exposition and Defence* (London: Simpkin, Marshall, 1852), 39; Colby (n. 2), 30.

12. Louisa Burns, The old doctor's new book. *JAOA* (1910–11) 10:91–3, p. 93; Benedict Lust, The principles and program of the nature cure system. In: Lust, editor, *Universal Naturopathic Encyclopedia Directory and Buyers' Guide Year Book of Drugless Therapy for 1918–19* (Butler, NJ: Lust, 1918), 13–25, p. 13. For examples of irregulars' ceding of trauma care to surgeons, see Simon Abbott, *The Southern Botanic Physician* (Charleston: Author, 1844), v; and Horton Howard, *Howard's Domestic Medicine* (Philadelphia: Duane Rulison, 1866), 30–2.

13. A. A. Erz, *The Medical Question: The Truth About Official Medicine and Why We Must Have Medical Freedom* (Butler, NJ: Erz, 1914), xxv.

14. Physio-medical quoted by John Haller Jr., *Kindly Medicine: Physio-Medicalism in America, 1836–1911* (Kent, OH: Kent State University Press, 1997), 108.

15. Haller (n. 14), 92.

16. Anonymous, Preface. In: Samuel Thomson, *A Narrative of the Life and Medical Discoveries of Samuel Thomson* (Boston: Author, 1822), 6; Alex Berman, The Thomsonian movement and its relation to American pharmacy and medicine. *BHM* (1951) 25:405–28, 519–38, p. 426.

17. Benedict Lust, *The Fountain of Youth* (New York: Macfadden, 1923), 99. For detailed analysis of one system's "alternative science," see Steven Martin, "The only truly scientific method of healing": Chiropractic and American science, 1895–1990. *Isis* (1994) 85:207–27.

18. Colby (n. 2), 37. For an illustration of the differing uses of "empiricism," see Roland Houghton, Observations on hygiene and the water treatment. In: Houghton, editor, *Bulwer and Forbes on the Water-Treatment* (New York: Fowlers and Wells, 1851), 203–58, p. 239.

19. Alphonse Teste, *A Practical Manual of Animal Magnetism* (Philadelphia: Brown, Bicking and Guilbert, 1844), 25; Nicholas Greene, This is no humbug—or is it? *JA* (1972) 36:101–2, p. 101; Carla Selby and Bela Scheiber, Science or pseudo-science? Pentagon grant funds alternative health study. *Skeptical Inquirer* (July-August 1996) 20:15–7, p. 17.

20. David Reese, *Humbugs of New York* (New York: Taylor, 1838), 15. Conventional medicine's refusal of therapies that can't be readily explained has been satirized as "the tomato effect": James Goodwin and Jean Goodwin, The tomato effect: Rejection of highly efficacious therapies. *JAMA* (1984) 251:2387–90.

21. Mr. Wansbrough, Acupuncturation. *Lancet* (1826) 10:846–8, p. 848; Samuel Rosen quoted by Jacques Quen, Acupuncture and western medicine. *BHM* (1975) 49:196–205, p. 202; Horatio Dresser, editor, *The Quimby Manuscripts* (New Hyde Park, NY: University Books, 1961), 91.

22. Nathan Bedortha, *Practical Medication; or, The Invalid's Guide* (Albany, NY:

Munsell and Rowland, 1860), 68; Henry Lindlahr, *Nature Cure*, 12th edition (Chicago: Nature Cure Publishing, 1919), 10.

23. G. G. Sigmond, Address delivered before the Medico-Botanical Society of London. *Lancet* (no. 1, 1837–8): 769–76, p. 774; Durham Dunlop, *The Philosophy of the Bath*, 4th edition (London: Kent, 1880), 447.

24. Wendell Holmes, *Elsie Venner: A Romance of Destiny* (Boston: Houghton Mifflin, 1861), 211. For a concise discussion of the objectification of disease, see Stanley Reiser, The era of the patient. *JAMA* (1993) 269:1012–7.

25. Daniel Cherkin and Frederick MacCornack, Patient evaluations of low back pain care from family physicians and chiropractors. *WJM* (1989) 150:351–5, p. 354; Robert Kane, Donna Olson, Craig Leymaster, F. Ross Woolley, and F. David Fisher, Manipulating the patient: A comparison of the effectiveness of physician and chiropractor care. *Lancet* (no. 1, 1974): 1333–6, p. 1336; Anne Hawkins, Restoring the patient's voice: The case of Gilda Radner. *YJBM* (1992) 65:173–81, pp. 174, 175.

26. Rascality of a mesmerist. *Lancet* (no. 2, 1850): 181; Thomas Graham, *The Cold-Water System*, 2d edition (London: Simpkin, Marshall, 1843), vii; Abraham Jacobi quoted by James Burrow, *Organized Medicine in the Progressive Era: The Move Toward Monopoly* (Baltimore: Johns Hopkins University Press, 1977), 68; Edward Ochsner in discussion of Buda Keller, The laity's idea of the physician. *IMJ* (1923) 44:13–20, p. 19.

27. Johnson (n. 11), iii–iv; Caleb Ticknor, *A Popular Treatise on Medical Philosophy; or, An Exposition of Quackery and Imposture in Medicine* (New York: Gould and Newman, 1838), 17. For another example of the allopathic reply to the Galileo argument, see Dan King, *Quackery Unmasked; or, A Consideration of the Most Prominent Empirical Schemes of the Present Time* (New York: Wood, 1858), 54–5.

28. Harris Coulter, *Divided Legacy: A History of the Schism in Medical Thought* vol. 3, *ce and Ethics in American Medicine*, 1800–1914 (Washington, DC: McGrath, 1973), 157–8; Martin Kaufman, *Homeopathy in America. The Rise and Fall of a Medical Heresy* (Baltimore: Johns Hopkins University Press, 1971); the painting is by Henry Monnier.

29. Jerome McAndrews, Foreword. In: Walter Wardwell, *Chiropractic: History and Evolution of a New Profession* (St. Louis: Mosby Year Book, 1992), v.

30. Julius Dintenfass, *Chiropractic: A Modern Way to Health*, 2d edition (New York: Pyramid, 1970), 152; E. R. Booth, *History of Osteopathy and Twentieth-Century Medical Practice*, 2d edition (Cincinnati: Jennings and Graham, 1905), 212; Haller (n. 14), 150.

31. William Osler, Medicine in the nineteenth century. In: Osler, *Aequanimitas With Other Addresses to Medical Students, Nurses and Practitioners of Medicine* (Philadelphia: Blakiston, 1927), 227–77, p. 272. For a discussion of the placebo effect, see Howard Brody, The lie that heals: The ethics of giving placebos. *Annals of Internal Medicine* (1982) 97:112–8.

32. Robert Burton, *The Anatomy of Melancholy* (New York: Empire State, 1924), 168; K. B. Thomas, General practice consultations: Is there a point in being positive? *BMJ. Clinical Research Edition* (1987) 294:1200–2; Cherkin and MacCornack (n. 25), 354. Also see Marjorie White and James Skipper, The chiropractic physician: A study of career contingencies. *JHSB* (1971) 12:300–6.

33. James Harvey Young, *The Toadstool Millionaires* (Princeton, NJ: Princeton Uni-

versity Press, 1961), 16–30; Jacques Quen, Elisha Perkins, physician, nostrum-vendor, or charlatan? *BHM* (1963) 37:159–66.

34. Young (n. 33), 27, 30; Oliver Wendell Holmes, Homoeopathy and its kindred delusions. In: Holmes, *Medical Essays, 1842–1882* (Boston: Houghton, Mifflin, 1899), 1–102, p. 15.

35. Young (n. 33), 27–9.

36. Christopher Caustic [Thomas Fessenden], *Terrible Tractoration!! A Poetical Petition Against Galvanising Trumpery, and the Perkinistic Institution*, 2d edition (London: Hurst and Ginger, 1803), 101–2; Jacques Quen, Case studies in nineteenth-century scientific rejection: Mesmerism, Perkinism, and acupuncture. *JHBS* (1975) 11:149–56.

37. Steve Austin quoted by Jared Zeff, The cornerstones of naturopathic medicine. *JNM* (1998) 8:62–5, p. 63; Paul Wendel, *Standardized Naturopathy* (Brooklyn, NY: Wendel, 1951), 27. Irregulars' "scientific empiricism" is discussed by Charles Vincent and Adrian Furnham, *Complementary Medicine: A Research Perspective* (New York: Wiley, 1997), 2–3.

38. Matthew Ramsey, Alternative medicine in modern France. *MH* (1999) 43:286–322, p. 289. The argument that the effort to suppress medical cults is a political act aimed at increasing majority practitioners' professional unity, social status, and cultural authority is made most fully by Susan Smith-Cunnien, *A Profession of One's Own: Organized Medicine's Opposition to Chiropractic* (Lanham, MD: University Press of America, 1998).

39. Richard Cabot, One hundred Christian Science cures. *McClure's Magazine* (1908) 31:472–6, p. 475; *Lancet* editorial quoted by James Harris, History and development of manipulation and mobilization. In: John Basmajian, editor, *Manipulation, Traction and Massage*, 3d ed. (Baltimore: Williams and Wilkins, 1985), 3–21, p. 6; John Coulehan, Adjustment, the hands and healing. *CMP* (1985) 9:353–82, p. 360; Dan Cherkin, Frederick MacCornack, and Alfred Berg, Family physicians' views of chiropractors: Hostile or hospitable? *AJPH* (1989) 79:636–7, p. 637.

40. John Nichols, Medical sectarianism. *JAMA* (1913) 60:331–7, p. 335.

CHAPTER 2

1. Samuel Thomson, *New Guide to Health; or, Botanic Family Physician* (Boston: Author, 1835), 7; Thomson, *A Narrative of the Life and Medical Discoveries of Samuel Thomson* (Boston: Author, 1822), 16.

2. Roberts Bartholow, *A Practical Treatise on Materia Medica and Therapeutics*, 3d edition (New York: Appleton, 1880), 433; Thomson, *Narrative* (n. 1), 16.

3. Thomson, *Narrative* (n. 1), 20–22.

4. Thomson, *Narrative* (n. 1), 24.

5. Thomson, *Narrative* (n. 1), 25.

6. Thomson, *Narrative* (n. 1), 27.

7. Thomson, *New Guide* (n. 1), 7–9.

8. Thomson, *Narrative* (n. 1), 9, 45; Benjamin Colby, *A Guide to Health* (Nashua, NH: Gill, 1844), 56.

9. Thomson, *New Guide* (n. 1), 152; Reuben Chambers, *The Thomsonian Practice of Medicine* (Bethania, PA: Author, 1842), 87; Thomson, *Narrative* (n. 1), 93.

10. Thomson, *New Guide* (n. 1), 38, 48, 54; Chambers (n. 9), 239–40.

11. Thomson, *New Guide* (n. 1), 59, 62–3.

12. Thomson, *New Guide* (n. 1), 65, 84–5.

13. Thomson, *New Guide* (n. 1), 21; James Breeden, Thomsonianism in Virginia. *VMHB* (1974) 82:150–80, p. 172; Chambers (n. 9), 86.

14. Frank Halstead, A first-hand account of a treatment by Thomsonian medicine in the 1830s. *BHM* (1941) 10:680–7, pp. 681–2; Breeden (n. 13), 158.

15. Halstead (n. 14), 682–3.

16. Alex Berman, The Thomsonian movement and its relation to American pharmacy and medicine. *BHM* (1951) 25:405–28, 519–38, pp. 405–9; G. C. Howard, On calomel and gangrenopsis. *BMSJ* (1835) 12:411–3, p. 412; Chambers (n. 9), 129.

17. Caleb Ticknor, *A Popular Treatise on Medical Philosophy; or, An Exposition of Quackery and Imposture in Medicine* (New York: Gould and Newman, 1838), 209–10.

18. Preface. *Thomsonian Recorder* (1833) 2:v (also quoted by Ronald Numbers, Do-it-yourself the sectarian way. In: Guenter Risse, Ronald Numbers, and Judith Leavitt, editors, *Medicine Without Doctors* (New York: Science History, 1977), 49–72, p. 55.

19. Worthington Hooker, *Physician and Patient* (New York: Baker and Scribner, 1849), 115; Ticknor (n. 17), 211.

20. John Thomson quoted by Robley Dunglison, *On Certain Medical Delusions* (Philadelphia: Merrihew and Thompson, 1842), 29.

21. Arthur Schlesinger, *The Age of Jackson* (Boston: Little, Brown, 1945).

22. Quoted by Joseph Kett, *The Formation of the American Medical Profession: The Role of Institutions, 1780–1860* (New Haven, CT: Yale University Press, 1968), 14; Richard Shryock, *Medicine and Society in America, 1660–1860* (Ithaca, NY: Cornell University Press, 1960), 33. For a more thorough discussion of the evolution of medical licensing legislation in the United States, see Richard Shryock, *Medical Licensing in America, 1650–1965* (Baltimore: Johns Hopkins University Press, 1967).

23. H. Shepheard Moat, *Practical Proofs of the Soundness of the Hygeian System of Physiology*, 3d edition (New York: Author, 1832), 31; Alexander Wilder, *History of Medicine* (New Sharon, ME: New England Eclectic Publishing, 1901), 508–9, 511; James Harvey Young, *The Toadstool Millionaires: A Social History of Patent Medicines in America Before Federal Regulation* (Princeton, NJ: Princeton University Press, 1961), 55; Martin Kaufman, *Homeopathy in America: The Rise and Fall of a Medical Heresy* (Baltimore: Johns Hopkins University Press, 1971), 23; Lemuel Shattuck, *Report of the Sanitary Commission of Massachusetts, 1850* (Cambridge, MA: Harvard University Press, 1948), 58; Gonzalvo Smythe, *Medical Heresies: Historically Considered* (Philadelphia: Presley Blakiston, 1880), 213. Also see Shryock, *Medical Licensing* (n. 22), and Henry Shafer, *The American Medical Profession, 1783–1850* (New York: Columbia University Press, 1936), 53–62, 208–14. The repeal of licensure laws was due not just to Thomsonian agitation but also to a broader public dissatisfaction with the medical profession that stemmed from several sources: see Kaufman (n. 23), 48–51.

24. Thomson, *Narrative* (n. 1), 13, 17–19, 40; Colby (n. 8), 12.

25. Robert Fuller, *Alternative Medicine and American Religious Life* (New York: Oxford University Press, 1989), 19; Thomson, *Narrative* (n. 1), 166; Berman (n. 16), 415; Wilder (n. 23), 460.

26. Berman (n. 16); David Reese, *Humbugs of New York* (New York: Taylor, 1838), 119.

27. F. K. Robertson, *The Book of Health; or, Thomsonian Theory and Practice of Medicine* (Bennington, VT: Cook, 1843), 5.

28. Thomson quoted by Robertson (n. 27), 17.

29. Breeden (n. 13), 160; Catherine Albanese, *Nature Religion in America: From the Algonkian Indians to the New Age* (Chicago: University of Chicago Press, 1990), 130; Berman (n. 16), 407, 417.

30. Colby (n. 8), 12; Samuel Robinson, *A Course of Lectures on Medical Botany* (Boston: Howe, 1834), 10; Thomson, *Narrative* (n. 1), 9.

31. Thomson, *Narrative* (n. 1), 41–2.

32. Thomson, *New Guide* (n. 1), 130–8. For more on Thomson's handling of childbirth, see Chambers (n. 9), 367–89.

33. Thomson, *New Guide* (n. 1), 130–1, 143.

34. Thomson, *New Guide* (n. 1), 131, 134, 145–6.

35. Berman (n. 16), 405.

36. Anonymous, Preface. In: Thomson, *Narrative* (n. 1), 7–8.

37. Thomson, *Narrative* (n. 1), 93.

38. Thomson, *Narrative* (n. 1), 95–106; Thomson, *New Guide* (n. 1), 9.

39. Harris Coulter, *Divided Legacy: A History of the Schism in Medical Thought*, vol. 3, *Science and Ethics in American Medicine, 1800–1914* (Washington, DC: McGrath, 1973), 92–3; Hooker (n. 19), 73, 112; Ticknor (n. 17), 79–83; Mississippi doctor quoted by John Harley Warner, Medical sectarianism, therapeutic conflict, and the shaping of orthodox professional identity in antebellum American medicine. In: W. F. Bynum and Roy Porter, editors, *Medical Fringe and Medical Orthodoxy, 1750–1850* (London: Croom Helm, 1987), 234–60, pp. 239–40.

40. Wesley Herwig, A patient boiled alive (or, why Jehuel Smith, a Thomsonian physician, left East Randolph, Vermont, in a hurry). *VH* (1976) 44:224–7, p. 227.

41. John Uri Lloyd, *Life and Medical Discoveries of Samuel Thomson: Bulletin of the Lloyd Library of Botany, Pharmacy and Materia Medica* (Cincinnati: Lloyd Library, 1909), 67–74; Wilder (n. 23), 475.

42. Lloyd (n. 41), 86–9.

43. Berman (n. 16), 420, 528; Dan King, *Quackery Unmasked, or A Consideration of the Most Prominent Empirical Schemes of the Present Time* (New York: Wood, 1858), 208.

44. John Haller Jr., *Kindly Medicine: Physio-Medicalism in America, 1836–1911* (Kent, OH: Kent State University Press, 1997), 27–35, 112–3.

45. Haller (n. 44), 131, 147–51; Curtis quoted by Alex Berman and Michael Flannery, *America's Botanico-Medical Movements: Vox Populi* (New York: Pharmaceutical Products), 105.

46. John Haller Jr., *Medical Protestants: The Eclectics in American Medicine, 1825–1939* (Carbondale: Southern Illinois University Press, 1994); Haller (n. 44), 19–22; Wilder (n. 23), 512–761.

47. Haller (n. 46); *Medical and Surgical Reporter* quoted by Berman and Flannery (n. 45), 120.

48. Ronald Numbers, The making of an eclectic physician: Joseph M. McElhinney and the Eclectic Medical Institute of Cincinnati. *BHM* (1973) 47:155–66.

49. Ursula Miley and John Pickstone, Medical botany around 1850: American medicine in industrial Britain. In: Roger Cooter, editor, *Studies in the History of Alternative Medicine* (New York: St. Martin's Press, 1988), 139–53; Michael Tierra, The way of herbs. In: Edward Bauman, Armand Brint, Lorin Piper, and Pamela Wright, editors, *The Holistic Health Handbook* (Berkeley, CA: And/Or Press, 1978), 130–6, pp. 131, 135.

CHAPTER 3

1. Worthington Hooker, *Physician and Patient* (New York: Baker and Scribner, 1849), 136; Oliver Wendell Holmes, Review of Homeopathic Domestic Physician. *Atlantic Monthly* (1857–8) 1:250–2, p. 251–2; Dan King, *Quackery Unmasked; or, a Consideration of the Most Prominent Empirical Schemes of the Present Time* (New York: Wood, 1858), 52; Gonzalvo Smythe, *Medical Heresies: Historically Considered* (Philadelphia: Presley Blakiston, 1880), 143; William Leo-Wolf, *Remarks on the Abracadabra of the Nineteenth Century* (New York: Carey, Lea and Blanchard, 1835), 231; Oliver Wendell Holmes, Homeopathy and its kindred delusions. In: *Medical Essays, 1842–1882* (Boston: Houghton, Mifflin, 1899), 1–102, p. 101; David Reese, *Humbugs of New York* (New York: Taylor, 1838), 109.

2. Samuel Hahnemann, *The Lesser Writings of Samuel Hahnemann*, R. E. Dudgeon, translator (New York: Radde, 1852), 410, 417, 426, 512; Harris Coulter, *Divided Legacy: A History of the Schism in Medical Thought*, vol. 2, *Progress and Regress: J. B. Van Helmont to Claude Bernard* (Washington, DC: Weehawken, 1977), 304–19. Also see Thomas Bradford, *The Life and Letters of Dr. Samuel Hahnemann* (Philadelphia: Boericke and Tafel, 1895).

3. Quoted by Coulter (n. 2), 361.

4. Quoted by Coulter (n. 2), 362; Hahnemann, (n. 2), 267

5. Hahnemann (n. 2), 517; Hahnemann, *Organon of the Art of Healing*, 5th American edition, C. Wesselhoeft, translator (Philadelphia: Hahnemann, 1875), 130.

6. Hahnemann, (n. 2), 510, 623, 744; Hahnemann, *Materia Medica Pura*, 4 volumes, Charles Hempel, translator (New York: Radde, 1846), 3:v; Edward Bayard, *Homoeopathia and Nature and Allopathia and Art* (New York: Ludwig, 1858), 3.

7. Coulter (n. 2), 363.

8. Hahnemann, *Materia* (n. 6), 1:vii.

9. Hahnemann, *Organon* (n. 5), 126–7, 130; Hahnemann, *Materia* (n. 6), 1:vii.

10. Hahnemann, *Organon* (n. 5), 127; Constantine Hering quoted by Harris Coulter, *Divided Legacy: A History of the Schism in Medical Thought*, vol. 3, *Science and Ethics in American Medicine, 1800–1914* (Washington, DC: McGrath, 1973), 24.

11. James Dillard and Terra Zipporyn, *Alternative Medicine for Dummies* (New York: IDG Books Worldwide, 1998), 93; Hahnemann, *Materia* (n. 6), 2:iv; Hahnemann, *Organon* (n. 5), 134; Wayne Jonas and Jennifer Jacobs, *Healing With Homeopathy* (New York: Warner, 1996), 27–8.

12. Hahnemann, *Materia* (n. 6), 1: 5, 7, 13, 19, 26, 27, 28, 39, 43, 216; 3:112; 4:14.

13. Hahnemann, *Materia* (n. 6), 1:64, 73, 139, 145, 147; 2:64, 160; 3:66, 179; 4:97.

14. Hahnemann, *Materia* (n. 6), 1:3, 7, 12, 151, 205; 3:185.

15. Hahnemann, *Organon* (n. 5), 137–8; Hahnemann (n. 2), 504, 726–7.

16. Hahnemann (n. 2), 727; Hahnemann, *Organon* (n. 5), iv.

17. Coulter (n. 2), 400–3; Coulter (n. 10), 57.

18. Hahnemann, *Organon* (n. 5), 178; Coulter (n. 2), 402.

19. Coulter (n. 2), 401–2; Hahnemann, (n. 2), 763–4.

20. Hahnemann (n. 2), 728–33; Hahnemann, *Organon* (n. 5), 69.

21. Hahnemann, *Organon* (n. 5), 67, 106.

22. Hahnemann, *Organon* (n. 5), 69; Hahnemann (n. 2), 728–31, 765; Hahnemann, *Materia* (n. 6), 4:vi–vii.

23. Hahnemann, *Organon* (n. 5), 73–5, 101.

24. Hahnemann, *Organon* (n. 5), 74.

25. Julian Winston, *The Faces of Homoeopathy: An Illustrated History of the First 200 Years* (Tawa, New Zealand: Great Auk, 1999), 5; Martin Gumpert, *Hahnemann: The Adventurous Career of a Medical Rebel* (New York: Fischer, 1945), 133–246; Bradford (n. 2), 72–135, 325–420.

26. Martin Kaufman, Homeopathy in America: The rise and fall and persistence of a medical heresy. In: Norman Gevitz, editor, *Other Healers: Unorthodox Medicine in America* (Baltimore: Johns Hopkins University Press, 1988), 99–123; Joseph Kett, *The Formation of the American Medical Profession: The Role of Institutions, 1780–1860* (New Haven, CT: Yale University Press, 1968), 135–7; Thomas Bradford, Homeopathy in New York. In: William King, editor, *History of Homeopathy and Its Institutions in America*, 4 volumes (New York: Lewis, 1905), 1:44–75, pp. 44–5; Bradford, Homeopathy in Pennsylvania. In: King, editor, 1:111–61, pp. 111–3, 142; Calvin Knerr, *Life of Hering* (Philadelphia: Magee, 1940), 197, 214–5, 299–300; W. Bruce Fye, Nitroglycerin: A homeopathic remedy. *Circulation* (1986) 73:21–9. A somewhat less dramatic account of the bushmaster trial is given by Winston (n. 25), 33.

27. Pemberton Dudley, Hahnemann Medical College and Hospital of Philadelphia. In: William King, editor, *History of Homeopathy and Its Institutions in America*, 4 volumes (New York: Lewis, 1905), 2:37–141, pp. 37–42.

28. Naomi Rogers, *An Alternative Path: The Making and Remaking of Hahnemann Medical College and Hospital of Philadelphia* (New Brunswick, NJ: Rutgers University Press); Dudley (n. 27), 42–70; Martin Kaufman, *Homeopathy in America. The Rise and Fall of a Medical Heresy* (Baltimore: Johns Hopkins University Press, 1971), 166.

29. Samuel Hahnemann, *Organon of Homoeopathic Medicine*, 1st American edition (Allentown, PA: Academical Bookstore, 1836); Kaufman (n. 28), 28–9; Coulter (n. 10), 103, 177; J. S. Douglas, *Practical Homoeopathy for the People*, 8th edition (Chicago: Halsey, 1868), v. For accounts of allopaths' conversion to homeopathy, see Walter Johnson, *Homoeopathy: Popular Exposition and Defence of Its Principles and Practice* (London: Simpkin, Marshall, 1852), and John Ellis, *Personal Experience of a Physician* (Philadelphia: Hahnemann, 1892).

30. Coulter (n. 10), 108–9; King (n. 1), 333; Douglas (n. 29), iii; E. E. Marcy, American preface. In: Hahnemann (n. 2), iii–vi, p. iv; Kaufman (n. 28), 29.

31. Knerr (n. 26), 98. For homeopaths' statistical demonstrations of curative supe-riority, see Petrie Hoyle, *Vital Economics* (Philadelphia: Boericke and Tafel, 1902); on the lower cost of their medications, see Albert Bellows, *A Memorial to the Trustees of the Free City Hospital, With Statistics and Facts, Showing the Comparative Merits of Homeopathy and Allopathy, as Shown by Treatment in European Hospitals* (Boston: Clapp, 1863), 23–5. For a refutation of homeopathic claims of better cure rates, see Worthington Hooker, *Homoeopathy: An Examination of Its Doctrines and Evidences* (New York: Scribner, 1851), 107–10.

32. Coulter (n. 10), 114.

33. Hahnemann, *Organon* (n. 5), 67, 149, 158; Coulter (n. 2), 386; Coulter (n. 10), 31.

34. Hannah Creamer, *Delia's Doctors; or, A Glance Behind the Scenes* (New York: Fowlers and Wells, 1852), 55, 69, 78, 93.

35. Hahnemann (n. 2), 719, 744; Hahnemann, *Organon* (n. 5), 178.

36. Constantine Hering, *The Homeopathist, or Domestic Physician*, 2 volumes (Al-lentown, PA: Academical Bookstore, 1835), 2:9.

37. Ronald Numbers, Do-it-yourself the sectarian way. In: Guenter Risse, Ronald Numbers, and Judith Leavitt, editors, *Medicine Without Doctors* (New York: Science His-tory, 1977), 59–61.

38. Hooker (n. 1), 137; Oliver Wendell Holmes, Some more recent views on ho-meopathy. *Atlantic Monthly* (1857) 1:187. Also see Kaufman (n. 28), 101–2.

39. Stephen Mason, *A History of the Sciences*, 2nd edition (New York: Collier, 1962), 296; Mary Jo Nye, *Before Big Science: The Pursuit of Modern Chemistry and Physics, 1800–1940* (New York: Twayne, 1996), 46; Kett (n. 26), 141–54; Robert Fuller, *Alternative Medicine and American Religious Life* (New York: Oxford University Press, 1989), 25–6, 38–58.

40. Oliver Wendell Holmes, The position and prospects of the medical student. In: *Currents and Counter-Currents in Medical Science, With Other Addresses and Essays* (Boston: Ticknor and Fields, 1861), 281–321, p. 318; Alexander Wilder, *History of Medicine* (New Sharon, ME: New England Eclectic Publishing, 1901), 315; P. W. Leland, Empir-icism and its causes. *BMSJ* (1852) 47:292; Holmes, Review (n. 1), 252. See also Hooker (n. 1), 145.

41. Worthington Hooker, *Lessons From the History of Medical Delusions* (New York: Baker and Scribner, 1851), 79–80; Ohio physician quoted by John Harley Warner, Medical sectarianism, therapeutic conflict, and the shaping of orthodox professional iden-tity in antebellum American medicine. In: W. F. Bynum and Roy Porter, editors, *Medical Fringe and Medical Orthodoxy, 1750–1850* (London: Croom Helm, 1987), 234–60, p. 239; C.C.C., Mesmerism. *Lancet* (no. 1, 1842–3): 192; *NYJM* (1847) 9:262; Kaufman (n. 28), 53–62; John Haller Jr. *American Medicine in Transition, 1840–1910* (Urbana: University of Illinois Press, 1981), 256–67; David Cathell, *The Physician Himself and What He Should Add to His Scientific Acquirements*, 4th edition (Baltimore: Cushings and Bailey, 1885), 178, 181. For an example of a defense of the consultation clause, see Jacob Big-elow, Report on homeopathy. In: *Nature in Disease* (New York: Wood, 1855), 104–12, pp. 110–1.

42. Kaufman (n. 28), 63–109; Michael Flannery, Another house divided: Union medical service and sectarians during the Civil War. *JHMAS* (1999) 54:478–510, p. 490.

43. Anonymous, *The Anatomy of a Humbug, of the Genus Germanicus, Species Homoeopathia* (New York: Author, 1837); Coulter (n. 10), 156; Leo-Wolf (n. 1), 230; Elisha Bartlett, *An Essay on the Philosophy of Medical Science* (Philadelphia: Lea and Febinger, 1844), 197; King (n. 1), 58.

44. Hooker (n. 31), ix–x; M. L. Linton, *Medical Science and Common Sense*, 2nd edition (St. Louis: Knapp, 1859), 14 (also quoted by Coulter, [n. 10], 167).

45. Holmes, Homeopathy (n. 1), 59; King (n. 1), 53.

46. Hahnemann, *Materia* (n. 6), 2:5; Hooker (n. 1), 132.

47. Smythe (n. 1), 149; Thomas Blatchford, *Homoeopathy Illustrated* (Albany, NY: Van Benthuysen, 1851), 23–4.

48. Hahnemann (n. 2), 466, 732–3; King (n. 1), 84.

49. Blatchford (n. 47), 71; Holmes, Homeopathy (n. 1), 54; Bartlett (n. 43), 197–8. On allopathic trials, see, for example, Anonymous (n. 43), 22–3.

50. Smythe (n. 1), 149–52; Hooker (n. 1), 125.

51. Holmes, Homeopathy (n. 1), 53; King (n. 1), 32–3; Blatchford (n. 47), 25.

52. P. G. Hanna, Homeopathic soup made from the shadow of a pigeon's wing. *JAIH* (1966) 59:27–9; Hahnemann, *Organon* (n. 5), 69.

53. Susan Cayleff, *Wash and Be Healed: The Water-Cure Movement and Women's Health* (Philadelphia: Temple University Press, 1987), 12; Hooker (n. 1), 123; King (n. 1), 297–8; D. W. Cathell and William Cathell, *Book on the Physician Himself* (Philadelphia: Davis, 1902), 300–1.

54. Holmes, Review (n. 1), 252; Bigelow (n. 41), 107; Leland (n. 40), 292; Cathell (n. 41), 152; Kaufman (n. 28), 30. Nineteenth-century irregulars criticized and competed with one another, not just allopathic medicine; a supporter of Thomson, for example, ridiculed homeopathy as nothing more than nature working: Benjamin Colby, *A Guide to Health* (Nashua, NH: Gill, 1844), 29.

55. King (n. 1), 132–3.

56. Holmes, Review (n. 1), 251; Holmes, Homeopathy (n. 1), xiv. Homeopaths agreed that they were responsible for moderating the severity of allopathic treatments: see, for example, Ellis (n. 29), 18.

57. King (n. 1), 133.

CHAPTER 4

1. Catharine Beecher, *Letters to the People on Health and Happiness* (New York: Harper, 1856), 117–8.

2. Phyllis Hembry, *The English Spa, 1560–1815. A Social History* (London: Athlone Press, 1990); William Addison, *English Spas* (London: Batsford, 1951).

3. Richard Metcalfe, *Life of Vincent Priessnitz, Founder of Hydropathy* (Richmond Hill, England: Metcalfe, 1898).

4. John Forbes, The water-cure. *WCJHR* (1848) 6:33–8, p. 37; M. M. Brashear, Dr. Still and Mark Twain. *JAOA* (1973–4) 73:67–71, p. 71; Joel Shew, *Hand-Book of Hydrop-*

athy (New York: Wiley and Putnam, 1844), 73; Shew, Processes of water cure. *WCJ* (1845–6) 1:17–21, pp. 17–8; Susan Cayleff, *Wash and Be Healed: The Water-Cure Movement and Women's Health* (Philadelphia: Temple University Press, 1987), 38, 40; Benjamin Colby, *A Guide to Health* (Nashua, NH: Gill, 1844), 32–3.

5. Henry Wright, Processes of water cure. *WCJHR* (1849) 7:141–3, p. 141; Charles Scudamore, A medical investigation of the water-cure treatment. In: Roland Houghton, editor, *Bulwer and Forbes on the Water-Treatment* (New York: Fowlers and Wells, 1851), 167–84, p. 177; W. H. McMenemey, The water doctors of Malvern, with special reference to the years 1842 to 1872. *PRSM* (1953) 46:5–12, pp. 7–8; Lawrence Wright, *Clean and Decent: The Fascinating History of the Bathroom and the Water Closet* (New York: Viking Press, 1960), 158–9.

6. L. Wright (n. 5), 158–9; Bostonian quoted by Colby (n. 4), 32; McMenemey (n. 5), 7–8; Wright (n. 5), 142.

7. E. Bulwer Lytton, Confessions of a water patient. In: Roland Houghton, editor, *Bulwer and Forbes on the Water-Treatment* (New York: Fowlers and Wells, 1851), 13–49, p. 30.

8. Joel Shew, *Hydropathy; or The Water-Cure*, 4th edition (New York: Fowlers and Wells, 1851), 141; McMenemey (n. 5), 7; Shew, *Hand-Book* (n. 4), viii; Erasmus Wilson, Two chapters on bathing and the water treatment. In Roland Houghton, editor, *Bulwer and Forbes on the Water-Treatment* (New York: Fowlers and Wells, 1851), 121–65, p. 149. Also see Harry Weiss and Howard Kemble, *The Great American Water-Cure Craze* (Trenton, NJ: Past Times Press, 1967), 7–10.

9. Tennyson quoted by Marshal Legan, Hydropathy in America: A nineteenth-century panacea. *BHM* (1971) 45:267–80, p. 271; American Hydropathic Society. *WCJHR* (1849) 7:185–7; Prospectus of the fourteenth volume. *WCJHR* (1852) 14:16; Russell Trall, Valedictory. *WCJHR* (1851) 12:121–2, p. 122. On hydropathy in Britain, see Richard Metcalfe, *The Rise and Progress of Hydropathy in England and Scotland* (London: Simpkin, Marshall, Hamilton, Kent, 1906); Robin Price, Hydropathy in England, 1840–70. *MH* (1981) 25:269–80; Janet Browne, Spas and sensibilities: Darwin at Malvern. In: Roy Porter, editor, *The Medical History of Spas and Waters: Medical History, Supplement No. 10* (Wellcome Institute for the History of Medicine: London, 1990), 102–13; and Kelvin Rees, Water as a commodity: Hydropathy in Matlock. In: Roger Cooter, editor, *Studies in the History of Alternative Medicine* (New York: St. Martin's Press, 1988), 28–45. For the United States, see Weiss and Kemble (n. 8); Jane Donegan, *"Hydropathic Highway to Health": Women and Water-Cure in Antebellum America* (New York: Greenwood Press, 1986); Cayleff (n. 4); and Frank Mott, *A History of American Magazines*, 2 volumes (New York: Appleton, 1930), 1:441.

10. Cayleff (n. 4), 77–8, 83–90; Glen Haven Water Cure. *WCJHR* (1851) 11:97; A Water Patient, *The Water-Cure in America* (New York: Fowlers and Wells, 1852), 72.

11. Joel Shew, *The Water-Cure Manual* (New York: Fowlers and Wells, 1850), 69. The best source for insight into the diseases treated by American hydropaths, the treatments they employed, the facilities they used, and the prices they charged is A Water Patient (n. 10).

12. A Water Patient (n. 10), 288.

13. A Water Patient (n. 10), 256; Beecher (n. 1), 141–3.

14. Shew, Processes (n. 4), 17; Thomas Nichols, Practice in water-cure. *WCJHR* (1850) 10:18–20, p. 20.

15. Roland Houghton, Observations on hygiene and the water treatment. In: Roland Houghton, editor, *Bulwer and Forbes on the Water-Treatment* (New York: Fowlers and Wells, 1851), 203–58, p. 246; Nathan Bedortha, *Practical Medication; or, The Invalid's Guide* (Albany, NY: Munsell and Rowland, 1860), 61; John Balbirnie, The drinking of water. *WCJ* (1845–6) 1:35–6; James Wilson, Water as a beverage and as a remedy. *WCJ* (1845–6) 1:97–100, p. 100.

16. Joel Shew, Water. *WCJ* (1847) 3:97; Mrs. A. C. Judson, Wash and be healed. *WCJ* (1847) 3:125.

17. W. M. Stephens, Purification. *WCJHR* (1854) 18:122–3, p. 122. Also see Samuel Brown, Physical Puritanism. *Westminster Review* (1852) n.s. 1:405–42; and Virginia Smith, Physical puritanism and sanitary science: Material and immaterial beliefs in popular physiology, 1650–1840. In: William Bynum and Roy Porter, editors, *Medical Fringe and Medical Orthodoxy, 1750–1850* (London: Croom Helm, 1987), 174–97.

18. F. K. Robertson, *The Book of Health; or Thomsonian Theory and Practice of Medicine* (Bennington, VT: Cook, 1843), 12. For discussion of Grahamite health reform, see James Whorton, *Crusaders for Fitness: The History of American Health Reformers* (Princeton, NJ: Princeton University Press, 1982), 38–61; and Stephen Nissenbaum, *Sex, Diet, and Debility in America: Sylvester Graham and Health Reform* (Westport, CT: Greenwood Press, 1980).

19. William Alcott, Preface. *Library of Health and Teacher on the Human Constitution* (1838) 2:3–4.

20. James Whorton, "Tempest in a flesh-pot": The formulation of a physiological rationale for vegetarianism. *JHMAS* (1977) 32:115–39.

21. Sylvester Graham, *Lectures on the Science of Human Life*, 2 volumes (Boston: Marsh, Capen, Lyon, and Webb, 1839), 1: 552; 2:14, 406, 423; David Cambell, Bran bread legislation. *Graham Journal of Health and Longevity* (1839) 3:116–7, p. 116.

22. James Whorton, Christian physiology: William Alcott's prescription for the millennium. *BHM* (1975) 49:466–81; Russell Trall, *The Scientific Basis of Vegetarianism* (Philadelphia: Fowlers and Wells, 1860).

23. Joel Shew, Hydropathy applicable in town and city, as well as country. *WCJ* (1845–6) 1:137–8, p. 137; T. L. Nichols, Address of the American Hydropathic Convention to the people of the United States. *WCJHR* (1850) 10:79–81, p. 81; Russell Trall, Hygeio-therapia. *WCJHR* (1857) 23:37.

24. James Whorton, Russell Trall. In: Martin Kaufman, Stuart Galishoff, and Todd Savitt, editors, *Dictionary of American Medical Biography*, 2 volumes (Westport, CT: Greenwood Press, 1984), 2:751.

25. Cayleff (n. 4), 39.

26. Joel Shew, *Consumption: Its Prevention and Cure by the Water Treatment* (New York: Fowlers and Wells, 1851), 218–9; Ronald Numbers, Health reform on the Delaware. *NJH* (1974) 92:5–12; Weiss and Kemble (n. 8), 85; Bedortha (n. 15), 47–8.

27. Nissenbaum (n. 18), 150–1; Anonymous, Monody. *WCJHR* (1851) 11:129; W. W. Page, Premium crackers. *WCJHR* (1856) 21:110–1; M.P.M., The lay of the Graham cracker. *Journal of Hygeio-Therapy* (1890) 4:59.

28. Edward Bulwer-Lytton, Bulwer on water-cure. *WCJ* (1845) 1:12. For an example of claims for success in treating cholera, see Russell Trall, Eclectics for October. *WCJHR* (1849) 8:113.

29. Russell Trall, *Sexual Physiology*, 28th edition (New York: Fowlers and Wells, 1881), 232, 248.

30. Trall (n. 29), 206. The nineteenth century's confusion over the human menstrual cycle is discussed by James Reed, *From Private Vice to Public Virtue: The Birth Control Movement and American Society Since 1830* (New York: Basic Books, 1978), 13.

31. Trall (n. 29), 257.

32. Trall (n. 29), xi, 201, 244–5.

33. Trall (n. 29), 244–5.

34. Russell Trall, *The Hydropathic Encyclopedia*, 2 volumes (New York: Fowlers and Wells, 1854), 2:393; Trall, Allopathic midwifery. *WCJHR* (1850) 9:121; Mrs. O.C.W., Childbirth—a contrast. *WCJHR* (April 1851) 11:88. See also Donegan (n. 9), 111–29.

35. Joel Shew, *The Hydropathic Family Physician* (New York: Fowlers and Wells, 1856), iii; Shew, Thoughts on domestic water-cure. *WCJHR* (1851) 12:15–6, p. 15. Also see Cayleff (n. 4), 52.

36. Russell Trall, *The New Hydropathic Cook-Book* (New York: Fowlers and Wells, 1854). Trall, Physiological salvation. *WCJHR* (1859) 28:57; Noggs, A business rhyme. *WCJHR* (1850) 9:158; Trall, July matters. *WCJHR* (1850) 10:16; James Jackson, Why shouldst thou die before thy time. *WCJHR* (1856) 21:97–9, p. 98.

37. For discussion of the political climate of antebellum America, see Alice Tyler, *Freedom's Ferment* (New York: Harper, 1962).

38. John Freeze, Reform lyrics. *WCJHR* (1853) 15:108.

39. John Davies, *Phrenology, Fad and Science: A Nineteenth-Century American Crusade* (New Haven, CT: Yale University Press, 1955).

40. Madeleine Stern, *Heads and Headlines: The Phrenological Fowlers* (Norman: University of Oklahoma Press, 1971).

41. Mary Gove Nichols, Woman the physician. *WCJHR* (1851) 12:73–5, p. 74. Also see Cayleff (n. 4), 70–72.

42. Mary Gove Nichols, The new costume. *WCJHR* (1851) 12:30. See also Nichols, A lecture on women's dresses. *WCJHR* (1851) 12:34–6; and A patient of the water-cure. Springfield Bloomer celebration. *WCJHR* (1851) 12:83–4.

43. Mary Williams, The Bloomer and Weber dresses. *WCJHR* (1851) 12:33; Russell Trall, July sentiments. *WCJHR* (1853) 16:13–4; Donegan (n. 9), 136–56, 163–78; Cayleff (n. 4), 18, 126.

44. A patient of the water-cure (n. 42), 84; cartoon in *WCJHR* (1853) 16:120.

45. *WCJHR* (1853) 15: frontispiece; James Jackson, Considerations for common folks. *WCJHR* (1850) 10:97; the cited letters from "Matrimonial Correspondence" are in *WCJHR* (1854) 17:11, 12, 59, 60, 84; *WCJHR* (1855) 19:18, 41, 65, 89, 113; *WCJHR* (1855) 20:42, 65.

46. John Forbes, A review of hydropathy. In: Roland Houghton, editor, *Bulwer and Forbes on the Water-Treatment* (New York: Fowlers and Wells, 1851), 51–119, p. 52; cited by Weiss and Kemble (n. 8), 48.

47. George MacIlwain, *Memoirs of John Abernethy, F.R.S.* (New York: Harper, 1853), 388.

48. Richard Claridge, A letter from Graefenberg. *WCJ* (1846) 2:1–7, pp. 4–5; Russell Trall, *Hydropathic* (n. 34), 1:34; Durham Dunlop, *The Philosophy of the Bath* (London: Kent, 1880), 77; Trall, December doses. *WCJHR* (1850) 10:227–31, pp. 228–9; Scudamore (n. 5), 172; Charles Schieferdecker, Letter from Dr. Schieferdecker. *WCJ* (1845–6) 1:88–90, 89. English hydropath John Smedley claimed that his brother had been killed by aperients given by allopathic doctors to treat constipation and that he himself had taken up the study, then the practice, of hydropathy after a London physician had threatened him with mercury treatment: John Smedley, *Practical Hydropathy*, 14th edition (Blackwood: London, 1872), 5–6.

49. Walter Johnson, *Homoeopathy: Popular Exposition and Defence of Its Principles and Practice* (London: Simpkin, Marshall, 1852), 11.

50. For a much more thorough discussion of the decline of hydropathy, see Cayleff (n. 4), 159–73.

CHAPTER 5

1. Mark Twain, *Christian Science With Notes Containing Corrections to Date* (New York: Harper, 1907), 84–5.

2. Franz Mesmer, *Mémoire sur la Découverte du Magnétisme Animal* (Paris: Didot, 1779), 6, 12–3; Vincent Buranelli, *The Wizard From Vienna* (New York: Coward, McCann and Geogehan, 1975), 34–63; Margaret Goldsmith, *Franz Anton Mesmer: A History of Mesmerism* (Garden City, NY: Doubleday, Doran, 1934), 61–2. Also see Iago Galdston, Mesmer and animal magnetism. *CIBA Symposia* (1948) 9:832–7; Michael Stone, Mesmer and his followers: The beginnings of sympathetic treatment of childhood. *HCQ* (1973) 1: 659–79; and Arnold Ludwig, An historical survey of the early roots of mesmerism. *IJCEH* (1964) 12:205–17.

3. Mesmer (n. 2), 15, 28.

4. Mesmer (n. 2), 74–83; Mesmer, *Memoir of F. A. Mesmer on His Discoveries*, Jerome Eden, translator (Mt. Vernon, NY: Eden, 1957), 55.

5. Mesmer (n. 2), 79.

6. Mesmer (n. 2), 68–70.

7. Charles Hall, On the rise, progress, and mysteries of mesmerism in all ages and countries. *Lancet*, (no. 1, 1845): 149–52, p. 149; Buranelli (n. 2), 109; Franz Mesmer, *Maxims on Animal Magnetism*, Jerome Eden, translator (Mt. Vernon, NY: Eden, 1958), 65–7; Goldsmith (n. 2), 136.

8. Mesmer (n. 7), 76.

9. Robert Darnton, *Mesmerism and the End of the Enlightenment in France* (Cambridge, MA: Harvard University Press, 1968), 40.

10. Benjamin Franklin, *Report of Dr. Benjamin Franklin, and Other Commissioners, Charged by the King of France, With the Examination of the Animal Magnetism* (London: Johnson, 1785); Buranelli (n. 2), 161–7; Darnton (n. 9), 62–4.

11. Alphonse Teste, *A Practical Manual of Animal Magnetism* (Philadelphia: Brown,

Bicking and Guilbert, 1844), 30–1; Hall (n. 7), 149; Buranelli (n. 2), 117; Darnton (n. 9), 54–5.

12. Gilbert Frankau, Introductory monograph. In: Franz Mesmer, *Mesmerism*, V. R. Meyers, translator (London: MacDonald, 1948), 16–7; Goldsmith (n. 2), 166–71; Buranelli (n. 2), 117–20; Théodore Léger, *Animal Magnetism; or, Psychodunamy* (New York: Appleton, 1846), 306–11. For the origins of hypnotism as an outgrowth of mesmerism, see Henri Ellenberger, Mesmer and Puységur: From magnetism to hypnotism. *PR* (1965) 52: 281–97.

13. G. G. Sigmond, Address delivered before the Medico-Botanical Society of London. *Lancet* (no. 1, 1837–8): 769–76, p. 775; George Rosen, Mesmerism and surgery: A strange chapter in the history of anesthesia. *JHMAS* (1946) 1:527–50; Alison Winter, *Mesmerized: Powers of Mind in Victorian Britain* (Chicago: University of Chicago Press, 1998), 165–9, 196–213; Kathy Bocella, Expectant moms look to hypnosis to ease pain. *Tacoma News Tribune* (June 25, 2001), SL1, 4.

14. W.C.O., Animal magnetism. *Lancet* (no. 1, 1837–8): 467–8, p. 467; Correspondence on animal magnetism. *Lancet* (no. 1, 1838–9): 34–5, p. 35; Paul Eve, Mesmerism—a lecture delivered in the Medical College of Georgia (by request of the students), Feb. 18th, 1845. *SMSJ* (1845) 1:167; poem quoted by Rosen (n. 13), 549–50; Mesmerism. *Lancet* (no. 1, 1842–3): 192. For more on Elliotson's plight, see Winter (n. 13), 32–100.

15. Owen Wangensteen and Sarah Wangensteen, *The Rise of Surgery: From Empiric Craft to Scientific Discipline* (Minneapolis: University of Minnesota Press, 1978), 283; Winter (n. 13), 180; American journal quoted by Martin Pernick, *A Calculus of Suffering: Pain, Professionalism, and Anesthesia in Nineteenth-Century America* (New York: Columbia University Press, 1985), 89; Rosen (n. 13), 545–6.

16. Darnton (n. 9), 88–9; Eric Carlson, Charles Poyen brings mesmerism to America. *JHMAS* (1960) 15:121–32; Robert Fuller, *Mesmerism and the American Cure of Souls* (Philadelphia: University of Pennsylvania Press, 1982), 18–20. On the mysterious powers demonstrated by clairvoyants, see Winter (n. 13), 124, 128, 150.

17. George Sandby, *Mesmerism and Its Opponents* (London: Longman, Brown, Green, and Longmans, 1844), v, 4, 200.

18. Sandby (n. 17), 4–5, 178; Edgar Allan Poe, *The Complete Poems and Stories of Edgar Allan Poe*, 2 volumes (New York: Knopf, 1946), 2:663.

19. Thomas Wakley. Animal magnetism. *Lancet* (no. 1, 1838–9): 450–1; Fuller (n. 16), 33–4; Teste (n. 11), 313; J.P.F. Deleuze, *Practical Instruction in Animal Magnetism*, 2d edition (New York: Appleton, 1846), 161.

20. Fuller (n. 16), 20; Carlson (n. 16), 126; Zoroaster, Animal magnetism. *BMSJ* (1838) 17:395–8; Death of Dr. Poyen. *BMSJ* (1844) 31:166–7, p. 167; Mesmerism. *BMSJ* (1843–4) 29:25.

21. Deleuze (n. 19), 43, 67; Léger (n. 12), 15. For details on the procedures used by practitioners to induce a mesmeric trance, see Deleuze (n. 19), 28–41; Teste (n. 11), 119–38; and Charles Hall. On the rise, progress, and mysteries of mesmerism in all ages and countries. *Lancet* (no. 1, 1845): 233–6.

22. Joseph Buchanan, *Neurological System of Anthropology* (Cincinnati: Buchanan,

1854); Laroy Sunderland, *Pathetism* (Boston: White and Potter, 1847). For more discussion of phrenology and magnetism, see T.B.C., Phreno-magnetism. *BMSJ* (1843–4) 29:249–53, 318–21, 437–40.

23. John Bovee Dods, *The Philosophy of Mesmerism and Electrical Psychology* (London: Burns, 1886), iii–v, 5; Lectures on mesmerism. *BMSJ* (1843–4) 29:466.

24. Dods (n. 23), 85.

25. Dods (n. 23), 12–14, 87.

26. Dods (n. 23), 8, 98, 101–3, 189–97.

27. Dods (n. 23), 18, 71, 108–9, 173.

28. Dods (n. 23), 52–9.

29. Dods (n. 23), 122–3, 216. Also see Fuller (n. 16), 85–9.

30. Dods (n. 23), 2; Mesmerism (n. 20); Death (n. 20), 167; Mesmer, Mesmerism. *BMSJ* (1838) 17:125–8, p. 126. On the theatrical performances of mesmerized subjects, see Hall (n. 21).

31. Ralph Major, *Faiths That Healed* (New York: Appleton-Century, 1940), 199–201; Fuller (n. 16), 120; George Quimby, Phineas Parkhurst Quimby. *New England Magazine* (March 1888) 6:267–76, p. 269; Horatio Dresser, editor, *The Quimby Manuscripts* (New Hyde Park, NY: University Books, 1961), 36–8, 43, 45.

32. Dresser (n. 31), 28, 34, 37.

33. Dresser (n. 31), xi–xii, 47–8; Julius Silberger, *Mary Baker Eddy: An Interpretive Biography of the Founder of Christian Science* (Boston: Little, Brown, 1980), 73–4.

34. Dresser (n. 31), 34–5.

35. Dresser (n. 31), 75, 82, 180, 182.

36. Dresser (n. 31), 58, 75, 78, 80.

37. Dresser (n. 31), 83–4.

38. Dresser (n. 31), 117.

39. Dresser (n. 31), 59, 67, 94, 131, 388, 422.

40. Dresser (n. 31), 153, 157; Edwin Dakin, *Mrs. Eddy* (New York: Grosset and Dunlap, 1929), 5–37.

41. Dakin (n. 40), 59, 93, 235; Dresser (n. 31), 433; Georgine Milmine, Mary Baker G. Eddy. *McClure's Magazine* (1907) 29:97–116, pp. 111–2. There are several biographies of Mary Baker Eddy, the most thorough being Robert Peel, *Mary Baker Eddy*, 3 volumes (New York: Holt, Rinehart and Winston, 1966, 1971, 1977); and Gillian Gill, *Mary Baker Eddy* (Reading, MA: Perseus Books, 1998). On the question of plagiarism of Quimby's ideas and writings, see Georgine Milmine, Mary Baker G. Eddy. *McClure's Magazine* (1906–7) 28:506–24; Dresser (n. 31), 19–25, 163; Dakin (n. 40), 44–52; and Gill (n. 41), 139–46.

42. Mary Baker Eddy, *Science and Health With Key to the Scriptures* (Boston: Trustees under the Will of Mary Baker G. Eddy, 1950), 107; Christian Science Publishing Society, *A Century of Christian Science Healing* (Boston: Christian Science Publishing Society, 1966), 3; Dakin (n. 40), 52, 222, 235, 337. For details of Eddy's fall and miraculous recovery, see Georgine Milmine, Mary Baker G. Eddy. *McClure's Magazine* (1906–7) 28: 506–24, pp. 509–13.

43. Dakin (n. 40), 63–4, 90; Twain (n. 1), 29.

44. Eddy (n. 42), 109, 187, 189, 331, 488; Georgine Milmine, Mary Baker G. Eddy. *McClure's Magazine* (1908) 31:179–89, p. 183.

45. Eddy (n. 42), viii, 113, 153, 184, 188, 472, 480.

46. Dakin (n. 40), 73, 120–5, 165, 375–7; Stephen Gottschalk, *The Emergence of Christian Science in American Religious Life* (Berkeley: University of California Press, 1973), x, xviii.

47. Dakin (n. 40), 150, 217, 292, 377, 412; Bryan Wilson, *Sects and Society* (Berkeley: University of California Press, 1961), 149, 198–215; Rennie Schoepflin, Christian Science healing in America. In: Norman Gevitz, editor, *Other Healers: Unorthodox Medicine in America* (Baltimore: Johns Hopkins University Press, 1988), 192–214, pp. 197–9, 204; Twain (n. 1), 102; The "profitess" of Christian Science. *JAMA* (1900) 35:829; Margery Fox. Conflict to coexistence: Christian Science and medicine. *MA* (1984) 8:292–301, p. 296. For detailed figures on the number of Christian Science healers practicing in America from 1901 to 1931, see Louis Reed, *The Healing Cults* (Chicago: University of Chicago Press, 1932), 73.

48. Eddy (n. 42), 610, 632; Milmine (n. 44), 188. For discussion of New Thought, see Horatio Dresser, *A History of the New Thought Movement* (New York: Crowell, 1919), and Charles Braden, *Spirits in Rebellion: The Rise and Development of New Thought* (Dallas: Southern Methodist University Press, 1963). On Eddy's opposition to New Thought, see Gottschalk (n. 46), 109–29. Gottschalk's book is an excellent discussion of late nineteenth-century Protestantism and the popular appeal of Christian Science.

49. Christian Science Publishing Society (n. 42), ix, 18, 24–7, 48–9, 59.

50. Eddy (n. 42), 606, 612–3, 618, 649–50, 679; Dakin (n. 40), 221; Christian Science Publishing Society (n. 42), 36, 237–41; William Simpson. Comparative longevity in a college cohort of Christian Scientists. *JAMA* (1989) 262:1657–8.

51. Edmund Andrews, Christian Science. *JAMA* (1899) 32:578–81, p. 581; Phases of "Christian Science." *JAMA* (1899) 33:297; A test for "Christian Scientists." *JAMA* (1900) 34:759.

52. Christian Science: What it is. *BMJ* (no. 2, 1898): 1515–6; Richard Cabot, One hundred Christian Science cures. *McClure's Magazine* (1908) 31:472–6, pp. 472–4; William Purrington, *Christian Science: An Exposition of Mrs. Eddy's Wonderful Discoveries, Including Its Legal Aspects* (New York: Treat, 1900), 4; William Osler. The faith that heals. *BMJ* (no. 1, 1910): 1470–2, p. 1472; Reed (n. 47), 82. It was not uncommon for allopathic practitioners to give Christian Science credit for demonstrating the power of suggestion and psychotherapy: see, for example, George Dearborn, Medical psychology. *MR* (1909) 75:176–8.

53. Cabot (n. 52), 472–3; Gordon Rice, Pseudomedicine. *JAMA* (1912) 58:360–2, p. 362; Victims of Christian Science. *JAMA* (1900) 34:633–4, p. 633.

54. Three victims of "Christian Science." *JAMA* (1900) 34:117; Death under "Christian Science." *JAMA* (1900), 34:698; Edmund Jacobsen, Christian Science from a medical standpoint. *IMJ* (1922) 42:434–8; An aggressive delusion. *JAMA* (1899) 33:107; Cabot (n. 52), 475; Insanity from Christian Science treatment. *JAMA* (1900) 34:633; Suit against a Christian Scientist. *JAMA* (1900) 34:761.

55. Frederic's case is discussed in The inquest on the late Mr. Harold Frederic. *Lancet* (no. 2, 1898): 1284; Christian Science before the law. *BMJ* (no. 2, 1898): 1508; and

The collapse of the case against the Christian Scientists. *BMJ* (no. 2, 1898): 1916–7; Faith-healing. *BMJ* (no. 2, 1898): 1187; Christian Science legal. *JAMA* (1899) 33:750; "Christian Science" and medical practitioners. *JAMA* (1899) 33:1049; H. L. Mencken, Why the quacks succeed. *IMJ* (1924) 46:240–2, p. 242. For an example of reports of children dying under Christian Science care, see Christian Science foolery. *JAMA* (1899) 33:743. There continue to be instances of deaths of minors under Christian Science care: Gill (n. 41), xv.

56. "Christian Science" and medical practitioners (n. 55); Rice (n. 53), 362; "Christian Science" and death certificates. *JAMA* (1899) 33:1657. See also "Christian Science" and Michigan law. *JAMA* (1899) 33:1498–9.

57. Wilson (n. 47), 195; Dakin (n. 40), 367–9. For more on the legal aspects of Christian Science practice, see Purrington (n. 52); Fox (n. 47); Massachusetts Department of Public Health, Christian Science and community medicine. *NEJM* (1974) 290:401–2; and Nathan Talbot, The position of the Christian Science church. *NEJM* (1983) 309:1641–4.

58. Eddy (n. 42), 101, 178; Milmine (n. 42), 523; Milmine, Mary Baker G. Eddy. *McClure's Magazine* (1907) 29:567–81, pp. 568–9; Silberger (n. 33), 164, 215, 239; Dakin (n. 40), 215, 251, 372; Fuller (n. 16), 38.

59. Editorial announcement. *McClure's Magazine* (1906–7) 28:211–7, p. 217; "Christian Science" Folly. *JAMA* (1899) 33:421.

60. Ambrose Bierce, *The Devil's Dictionary* (Cleveland: World Publishing, 1948), 139; Finley Peter Dunne, *Mr. Dooley's Opinions* (New York: Russell, 1901), 4.

61. Twain (n. 1), 5, 9, 26, 38.

CHAPTER 6

The section-opening poem is from *HHN* (1919) 24:124.

1. Martin Kaufman, *Homeopathy in America: The Rise and Fall of a Medical Heresy* (Baltimore: Johns Hopkins University Press, 1971), 90; Differences between doctors. *Harper's Weekly* (1893) 37:1086.

2. Oliver Wendell Holmes, The position and prospects of the medical student. In: Holmes, *Currents and Counter-Currents in Medical Science, With Other Addresses and Essays* (Boston: Ticknor and Fields, 1861), 281–321, pp. 319–20; D. W. Cathell, Was it wise for the American Medical Association to change its code of ethics? *AM* (1903) 6:618–20, p. 618; Benedict Lust, Editorials. *HHN* (1919) 24:61–2, p. 61. Estimates of the number of alternative practitioners at the turn of the twentieth century are in William Rothstein, *American Physicians in the Nineteenth Century: From Sects to Science* (Baltimore: Johns Hopkins University Press, 1972), 345.

3. Cathell (n. 2), 618, 620; Kaufman (n. 1), 125–40, 153–5; John Haller Jr., *American Medicine in Transition, 1840–1910* (Urbana: University of Illinois Press, 1981), 256–67; Norman Gevitz. The chiropractors and the AMA: Reflections on the history of the consultation clause. *PBM* (1989) 32:281–99, pp. 288–9.

4. Samuel Baker, Physician licensure laws in the United States, 1865–1915. *JHMAS* (1984) 39:173–97; John Duffy, *The Healers: A History of American Medicine* (Urbana: University of Illinois Press, 1979), pp. 291–306; Richard Shryock, *Medical Licensing in America, 1650–1965* (Baltimore: Johns Hopkins University Press, 1967), 51–6.

5. The immorality of "Christian Science." *JAMA* (1899) 33:1299; Christian Science. *JAMA* (1898) 31:1438; Margery Fox, Conflict to coexistence: Christian Science and medicine. *MA* (1984) 8:292–301; Stephen Gottschalk, *The Emergence of Christian Science in American Religious Life* (Berkeley: University of California Press, 1973), 248; Louis Reed, *The Healing Cults* (Chicago: University of Chicago Press, 1932), 83.

6. Henry Wood, Medical slavery through legislation. *Arena* (1893) 8:680–9, pp. 681, 682, 687–8.

7. H. L. Mencken, Why the quacks succeed. *IMJ* (1924), 46:240–2, p. 242.

8. Bernarr Macfadden, The drugless doctors' demand. *Physical Culture* (August 1920), 44:46; Champe Andrews, Medical practice and the law. *Forum* (1901) 31:542–51, p. 547.

9. Andrews (n. 8), 547; E. R. Booth, *History of Osteopathy and Twentieth-Century Medical Practice*, 2d edition (Cincinnati: Jennings and Graham, 1905), 213–4; Alexander Wilder, *History of Medicine* (New Sharon, ME: New England Eclectic Publishing, 1901), 315, 456.

10. A. A. Erz, Medical laws vs. human rights and constitution. *NHH* (1913) 18:438–72, 513–44, 585–97, p. 441, 520; Erz, *The Medical Question: The Truth About Official Medicine and Why We Must Have Medical Freedom* (Butler, NJ: Erz, 1914), xxi, xxviii, 29; Erz, What medicine knows and does not know about rheumatism. *NHH* (1912) 17:563–609, pp. 603–4; Asa Willard, Medicine and politics. *JAOA* (1910–11) 10:155–65, pp. 155, 158; Erz, Friends of medical freedom and voters, attention! *NHH* (1912) 17:707–8.

11. A bill to place Christian Scientists on equal footing with surgeons. *IMJ* (1921) 39:161–2, p. 162; Health Commissioner quoted by J. Stuart Moore, *Chiropractic in America: The History of a Medical Alternative* (Baltimore: Johns Hopkins University Press, 1993), 88.

12. Lyndon Lee, The chiropractic backbone. *Harper's Weekly* (1915) 61:285–8, pp. 287–8; Erz, *Medical* (n. 10), xxiv; R. T. Brown, Why many allopaths are criminals. *HHN* (1920) 25:76–7, p. 77.

13. Chiropractor quoted by Walter Wardwell, *Chiropractic: History and Evolution of a New Profession* (St. Louis: Mosby Year Book, 1992), 106; Booth (n. 9), 213–4; Eugene Christian, Write to your legislators. *Physical Culture* (March 1921) 45:47, 74, p. 74.

14. Paul Wendel, *Standardized Naturopathy* (Brooklyn, NY: Wendel, 1951), 41.

CHAPTER 7

1. Andrew Still, *The Autobiography of Andrew Taylor Still* (Kirksville, MO: Author, 1897), 45, 94–7; E. R. Booth, *History of Osteopathy and Twentieth-Century Medical Practice*, 2d edition (Cincinnati: Jennings and Graham, 1905), 34. Good outlines of Still's life and his development of osteopathy can be found in Booth, 1–70; and Norman Gevitz, *The D.O.'s: Osteopathic Medicine in America* (Baltimore: Johns Hopkins University Press, 1982), 1–47.

2. Still (n. 1), 17, 19–20, 46–7, 65–90.

3. Still, How I came to originate osteopathy. In: George Webster, editor, *Concerning Osteopathy*, 2d edition (Norwood, MA: Plimpton, 1921), 27–37, pp. 30–1; E. Harry Bean,

The Spirit of Osteopathy (New York: Pageant, 1956), 5. Later in life Still claimed to have undertaken a formal course of study at a medical school in Kansas City, but the statement cannot be substantiated: see Still article cited in this note, p. 29. Also see Gevitz (n. 1), 4.

4. Still (n. 1), 98–9, 280, 298.

5. Still (n. 1), 31–2; Still (n. 3), 27–8.

6. Bean (n. 3), 19; Still (n. 3), 32–3.

7. Douglas Graham, *Massage: Manual Treatment Remedial Movements*, 4th edition (Philadelphia: Lippincott, 1913), 1–39; Hartvig Nissen, *Practical Massage and Corrective Exercises With Applied Anatomy*, 5th edition (Philadelphia: Davis, 1929), 18–26; Ellen Gerber, *Innovators and Institutions in Physical Education* (Philadelphia: Lea and Febiger, 1971), 155–62; George Taylor, *An Exposition of the Swedish Movement-Cure* (New York: Fowlers and Wells, 1860); Gevitz (n. 1), 11–5. Also see Elizabeth Lomax, Manipulative therapy: A historical perspective from ancient times to the modern era. In: U.S. Department of Health, Education, and Welfare, *The Research Status of Spinal Manipulative Therapy* (Washington, DC: Government Printing Office, 1975); and Arno Sollmann and Eleonore Blaurock-Busch, Manipulative therapy of the spine: The development of "manual medicine" in Germany and Europe. *CH* (1981) 1:37–41.

8. Robert J. T. Joy, The natural bonesetters with special reference to the Sweet family of Rhode Island. *BHM* (1965) 28:416–41; J. Stuart Moore, *Chiropractic in America: The History of a Medical Alternative* (Baltimore: Johns Hopkins University Press, 1993), 15–8; Roger Cooter, Bones of contention? Orthodox medicine and the mystery of the bone-setter's craft. In: W. F. Bynum and Roy Porter, editors, *Medical Fringe and Medical Orthodoxy, 1750–1850* (London: Croom Helm, 1987), 158–73; Worthington Hooker, *Physician and Patient* (New York: Baker and Scribner, 1849), 146–71; Caleb Ticknor, *A Popular Treatise on Medical Philosophy; or, An Exposition of Quackery and Imposture in Medicine* (New York: Gould and Newman, 1838), 189–93; Alexander Wilder, *History of Medicine* (New Sharon, ME: New England Eclectic Publishing, 1901), 310–11. Natural bonesetting continued in practice in Britain into the twentieth century: see Leonard Minty, *The Legal and Ethical Aspects of Medical Quackery* (London: Heinemann, 1932), 80–95.

9. Still (n. 1), 108, 110–2, 116–7, 330; Bean (n. 3), 19; Booth (n. 1), 26.

10. Booth (n. 1), 28–9, 32; Bean (n. 3), 4–5. Elbert Hubbard described Still as "tall, lanky, homely, angular and chews infinite tobacco": D. D. Palmer, *The Chiropractor's Adjuster: Text-Book of the Science, Art and Philosophy of Chiropractic for Students and Practitioners* (Portland, OR: Portland Printing House, 1910), 715.

11. Still (n. 1), 116, 130–2; Booth (n. 1), 56–7.

12. Still (n. 1), 388; Booth (n. 1), 28, 31, 57; Gevitz (n. 1), 23.

13. Andrew Still, Dr. Still's department. *JO* (1901) 8:68.

14. Still (n. 1), 312, 378; Still (n. 3), 29, 36; Robert Truhlar, *Doctor A. T. Still in the Living* (Cleveland: Truhlar, 1950), 41. The theological basis of osteopathy is discussed by Catherine Albanese, *Nature Religion in America: From the Algonkian Indians to the New Age* (Chicago: University of Chicago Press, 1990), 142–5.

15. Still (n. 1), 223–4.

16. Still (n. 1), 219, 222, 371–2; M. A. Lane, *Dr. A. T. Still: Founder of Osteopathy* (Waukegan, IL: Bunting, 1925), 23–32, 203–5.

17. G. M. Laughlin, What osteopathic lesions are. In: George Webster, *Concerning Osteopathy*, 2d edition (Norwood, MA: Plimpton, 1921), 77–80, p. 77.

18. Truhlar (n. 14), 37, 150.

19. Truhlar (n. 14), 14; Still (n. 1), 219, 310, 417.

20. Still (n. 1), 32.

21. Carl McConnell. Osteopathic diagnosis. *JAOA* (1908–9) 8:108–14; George Webster. Manner of treatment. In: Webster, editor, *Concerning Osteopathy*, 2d edition (Norwood, MA: Plimpton, 1921), 83–89, p. 85, 87–8; Truhlar (n. 14), 22; Donald Thorburn, The case for osteopathy. *American Mercury* (1950) 70:32–42, p. 36. For details on early osteopathic manipulation techniques, supplemented with illustrations, see Charles Murray, *Practice of Osteopathy*, 3d edition (Elgin, IL: Murray, 1912).

22. Bean (n. 3), 16, 20, 31; Booth (n. 1), 33; A. T. Still, Differences between osteopathy and massage. In: George Webster, editor, *Concerning Osteopathy*, 2d edition (Norwood, MA: Plimpton, 1921), 93–4.

23. Truhlar (n. 14), 15, 98, 101; Still (n. 1), 100, 275, 375 (see pp. 212–26 for a sample of Still's visions). Robert Fuller, *Alternative Medicine and American Religious Life* (New York: Oxford University Press, 1989), 81–90, also discusses the religious content of Still's thought.

24. Booth (n. 1), 69–70, 76–9, 81–2; E.R.N. Grigg, Peripatetic pioneer: William Smith, M.D., D.O. (1862–1912). *JHMAS* (1967) 22:169–79; Decision on osteopathy. *JAMA* (1900) 34:86–94, p. 90; Gevitz (n. 1), 19–29, 159.

25. Jenette Bolles, Dr. Still's regard for woman's ability. *JAOA* (1917–8) 17:250–1; Still (n. 1), 117–8, 217–8, 219–20; Roberta Wimer-Ford, Woman and osteopathy. In: George Webster, editor, *Concerning Osteopathy*, 2d edition (Norwood, MA: Plimpton, 1921), 211–3, p. 212. Also see Fannie Carpenter, Dr. Still's character and influence. *JAOA* (1917–8) 17:588–9.

26. Booth (n. 1), 86–94.

27. Booth (n. 1), 67, 74, 271–2; Decision (n. 24), 91; Still (n. 1), 331–2.

28. M. M. Brashear, Dr. Still and Mark Twain. *JAOA* (1973–4) 73:67–71, p. 67; Booth (n. 1), 230, 389–90; Morris Fishbein, *The Medical Follies* (New York: Boni and Liveright, 1925), 67; C. P. McConnell, Dr. McConnell's discussions. *JAOA* (1917–8) 17: 269–75, p. 271; Decision (n. 24), 87; Richard Newton, Is there any good in osteopathy? *AM* (1903) 6:616–7; allopath quoted by Matthew Brennan, Perspectives on chiropractic education in medical literature, 1910–1933. *CH* (1983) 3:25–30, p. 27. Also see John Mitchell, Therapeutics of local massage. In: Solomon Cohen, editor, *A System of Physiologic Therapeutics*, 8 volumes (Philadelphia: Blakiston, 1907), 7:65–80, pp. 79–80.

29. Gevitz (n. 1), 40.

30. Another tragedy of unpreparedness. *JAMA* (1915) 65:2093; Decision (n. 24), 92–4; E. M. Downing, The future of osteopathy or the osteopathy of the future. *JAOA* (1910–1) 10:65–72, p. 69; Gevitz (n. 1), 41; also see The tragedy of unpreparedness in medicine. *JAMA* (1915) 65:2012–3. Osteopaths of course retaliated with their own tales of allopathic malpractice: see, for example, Unpreparedness. *JAOA* (1915–6) 15:246–8. The issue of what constituted the practice of medicine was discussed by Champe Andrews, Medical practice and the law. *Forum* (1901) 31:542–51.

31. E. C. Pickler, Our needs and what we stand for. *JAOA* (1910–1) 10:1–6, p. 2; Andrews (n. 30), 546; Norman Gevitz, Osteopathic medicine: From deviance to difference. In: Gevitz, editor, *Other Healers: Unorthodox Medicine in America* (Baltimore: Johns Hopkins University Press, 1988), 124–56, p. 132; Booth (n. 1), 102–4; Gevitz (n. 1), 26–9.

32. Gevitz (n. 1), 42, 137; Gevitz (n. 31), 134; Downing (n. 30), 68; Booth (n. 1), 106–8, 250–1, 272, 279–80, 285–92 (pp. 95–161 detail the history of all states considering osteopathic licensing laws up to 1905). For more on osteopathic education, see Wilder (n. 8), 776–835.

33. Gevitz (n. 1), 54; George Webster, Scientific proofs of osteopathy. In: Webster, editor, *Concerning Osteopathy*, 2d edition (Norwood, MA: Plimpton, 1921), 99–109, pp. 100–2; Lane (n. 16), 46. For more on early osteopathic research, see J. Deason, A summary of osteopathic research work. In: Webster, editor, 113–8, and Webster, Osteopathic statistics. In: Webster, editor, 167–72.

34. A. G. Hildreth, A few things that deserve our most profound thought. *JAOA* (1910–1) 10:6–12, p. 8; Truhlar (n. 14), 71, 73; Still (n. 1), 312, 353. For discussions of unnecessary surgery in the late nineteenth century, see Ben Barker-Benfield, Sexual surgery in late nineteenth-century America. *IJHS* (1975) 5:279–98; and Ann Dally, *Women Under the Knife: A History of Surgery* (London: Hutchinson Radius, 1991).

35. Truhlar (n. 14), 140; Grigg (n. 24), 176. Also see George Still, Osteopathy and surgery. In: George Webster, editor, *Concerning Osteopathy*, 2d edition (Norwood, MA: Plimpton, 1921), 183–6.

36. F. P. Young, Is conservative surgery compatible with osteopathic practice? *JAOA* (1910–1) 10:232–4; J. I. Dufur, A broader education for osteopathic physicians. *JAOA* (1910–1), 10:77–82, 133–7, p. 134; Still (n. 35), 184–6; Gevitz (n. 1), 62–4. An Osteopathic College of Surgeons was formed in 1917 to promote specialization in surgery among osteopaths: Osteopathic surgeons take notice. *JAOA* (1917–8) 17:108.

37. Young (n. 36), 233–4; Still (n. 1), 50, 226, 286; Booth (n. 1), 348.

38. Still (n. 1), 112, 339; Booth (n. 1), 145, 334. For discussion of drug addiction in the late nineteenth century, see David Musto, *The American Disease: Origins of Narcotic Control*, 2d edition (New York: Oxford University Press, 1987).

39. Truhlar (n. 14), 32, 33, 137; E. E. Tucker, The point of departure between osteopathy and medicine. In: George Webster, editor, *Concerning Osteopathy*, 2d edition (Norwood, MA: Plimpton, 1921), 49–61, p. 59; Lane (n. 16), 48–9.

40. C.M.T. Hulett, Basic difference between osteopathy and drugs. *JAOA* (1915–6) 15:236–9, p. 239; R. E. Hamilton, Osteopathy and the germ theory. In: George Webster, editor, *Concerning Osteopathy*, 2d edition (Norwood, MA: Plimpton, 1921), 197–204; The problem of pain. *JAOA* (1915–6) 15:96; Percy Woodall, What the osteopathic schools should teach. *JAOA* (1915–6) 15:295–7.

41. Lane (n. 16), 55–6, 64, 69, 87; Hulett (n. 40), 239. For a good statement of osteopaths' acceptance of the germ theory, see W. Banks Meacham, Osteopathic consideration of serum therapy. *JAOA* (1908–9) 8:101–8.

42. Harry Dowling, *Fighting Infection: Conquests of the Twentieth Century* (Cambridge, MA: Harvard University Press, 1977).

43. L. von H. Gerdine, Drug teaching and four year course. *JAOA* (1915–6) 15:

315; H. L. Chiles, Emergency remedies in medicine. *JAOA* (1915–6) 15:supplement, 6–11, p. 6; C. W. Young, The medicine question. *JAOA* (1915–6) 15:424–5, p. 424.

44. McConnell (n. 21), 113; C. B. Atzen, Creed vs. science. *JAOA* (1915–6) 15:151–2; S. C. Matthews, Urges the broadest teaching. *JAOA* (1915–6) 15:198–200, p. 199; Young (n. 43), 425.

45. H. M. Vastine, Are we falling from grace. *JAOA* (1915–6) 15:supplement, 1–6, pp. 2–3; The teachings of Dr. Still. *JAOA* (1915–6) 15:93–6, p. 93; Lane (n. 16), 12–7, 40.

46. C.M.T. Hulett, Our professional lesion. *JAOA* (1915–6) 15:465–7; Chiles (n. 43), 8–9; E. C. Pickler, Osteopathy is sufficient. *JAOA* (1915–6) 15:515–7, p. 516; F. E. More, Another former president speaks. *JAOA* (1915–6) 15:634; C. C. Teall, The situation as Dr. Teall sees it. *JAOA* (1915–6) 15:152–3; Vastine (n. 45), 2.

47. Vastine (n. 45), 4; Andrew Taylor Still, An appeal to the thinking osteopaths of the profession. *JAOA* (1915–6) 15:supplement, 52.

48. A. G. Hildreth, Passing of the "old doctor." *JAOA* (1917–8) 17:241–3, p. 243; Funeral of Dr. Still. *JAOA* (1917–8) 17:276–7; What he left us. *JAOA* (1917–8) 17:375–8; Gevitz (n. 1), 74, 81; Fishbein (n. 28), 58–9; Benjamin Israel, Mixers no longer—put on individuality. *HHN* (1922) 27:421–7, p. 423.

49. Grigg (n. 24), 77; Adam Leighton, Leslie's on chiropractic. *JAMA* (1922) 78:299; Calls quackopractic claims "pure bunk." *JAOA* (1920–1) 20:40.

CHAPTER 8

1. P. K. Norman, Chiro bill vetoed. *JAOA* (1912–3) 12:429; Ernest Tucker, As to chiropractors, etc. *JAOA* (1912–3) 12:309–10; Chiropractic—an analogy and a difference. *JAOA* (1912–3) 12:290–3, p. 291; Russell Gibbons, *Chiropractic History: Lost, Strayed or Stolen* (Davenport, IA: Palmer College Student Council, 1976), 4; Morris Fishbein, *The Medical Follies* (New York: Boni and Liveright, 1925), 98.

2. D. D. Palmer, *The Chiropractor's Adjuster: Text-Book of the Science, Art and Philosophy of Chiropractic for Students and Practitioners* (Portland, OR: Portland Printing House, 1910), 502–3, 819–20.

3. Vern Gielow, *Old Dad Chiro: A Biography of D. D. Palmer* (Davenport, IA: Bawden, 1981), 1–41; J. Stuart Moore, *Chiropractic in America: The History of a Medical Alternative* (Baltimore: Johns Hopkins University Press, 1993), 5–14. An additional, and excellent, survey of chiropractic's history is Walter Wardwell, *Chiropractic: History and Evolution of a New Profession* (St. Louis: Mosby Year Book, 1992).

4. Gielow (n. 3), 44, 47, 58.

5. Gielow (n. 3), 131–2; Russell Gibbons, Chiropractic history: Turbulence and triumph. In: *Who's Who in Chiropractic International, 1976–78* (Littleton, CO: Who's Who in Chiropractic International, 1977), 139–48, p. 140; Gibbons, Physician-chiropractors: Medical presence in the evolution of chiropractic. *BHM* (1981) 55:233–45, pp. 237–8.

6. Gielow (n. 3), 56–7, 65, 69–70.

7. Palmer (n. 2), 18.

8. Gielow (n. 3), 79; Palmer (n. 2), 18–9, 101.

9. Palmer (n. 2), 101–5; Gielow (n. 3), 82–3.

10. Palmer (n. 2), 7, 228, 352; see p. 485 for an example of Palmer's distortions of orthodox physiology.

11. Palmer (n. 2), 18–9, 189, 357, 466, 486.

12. Palmer (n. 2), 362, 446, 491–2, 496. The religious content of chiropractic is discussed by Catherine Albanese, *Nature Religion in America: From the Algonkian Indians to the New Age* (Chicago: University of Chicago Press, 1990), 145–9.

13. Palmer (n. 2), 107–8, 124, 128, 504, 674.

14. Palmer (n. 2), 56–7, 78, 98, 101, 296, 782.

15. W. Banks Meacham, Osteopathic consideration of serum therapy. *JAOA* (1908) 8:101–8, p. 101; Palmer (n. 2), 122, 145; Steven Martin, "The only truly scientific method of healing": Chiropractic and American science, 1895–1990. *Isis* (1994) 85:207–27, p. 218; Frank Jett and A. W. Cavins, The chiropractic situation. *JISMA* (1933) 26:169–72, 229–31, p. 230; Confessions of a chiropractor. *JAMA* (1917) 68:732.

16. Palmer (n. 2), 48, 935, 936, 939, 951.

17. Palmer (n. 2), 37–49, 307, 429, 908–9, 914–70; Wardwell (n. 3), 65. For details on early chiropractic adjustment technique, see Joy Loban, *Technic and Practice of Chiropractic*, 3d edition (Pittsburgh: Loban, 1916).

18. Palmer (n. 2), 218, 812, 908; Gielow (n. 3), 81, 91.

19. Palmer (n. 2), 21–2, 380, 496.

20. Palmer (n. 2), 558; Martin (n. 15), 213.

21. Palmer (n. 2), 24, 139–45, 389–93, 399.

22. Gielow (n. 3), 81; Palmer (n. 2), 74.

23. Russell Gibbons, The rise of the chiropractic educational establishment, 1897–1980. In: Fern Lints-Dzaman, editor, *Who's Who in Chiropractic International*, 2d edition (Littleton, CO: Who's Who in Chiropractic International, 1980), 339–51, p. 340; Gibbons, Physician-chiropractors (n. 5), 235; Gielow (n. 3), 43, 91; Palmer (n. 2), 468; Theresa Gromala, Women in chiropractic: Exploring a tradition of equity in healing. *CH* (1983) 3:58–63; Alana Ferguson, "The sweetheart of the PSC"—Mabel Heath Palmer: The early years. *CH* (1984) 4:24–8; Bobby Westbrooks, The troubled legacy of Harvey Lillard: The black experience in chiropractic. *CH* (1982) 2:47–53; Annual Announcement 1921, Palmer School of Chiropractic, Kremers Reference Files, American Institute of the History of Pharmacy, University of Wisconsin, 63 (A) II.

24. Russell Gibbons, Solon Massey Langworthy: Keeper of the flame during the "lost years" of chiropractic. *CH* (1981) 1:15–21, pp. 16–7; R. P. Beideman, Seeking the rational alternative: The National College of Chiropractic from 1906 to 1982. *CH* (1983) 3:17–22, p. 17; Palmer (n. 2), 468; Gielow (n. 3), 32, 97; Wardwell (n. 3), 91; Gibbons (n. 23), 340–4; A. Augustus Dye, *The Evolution of Chiropractic: Its Discovery and Development* (Philadelphia: Author, 1939), 61–77; Matthew Brennan, Perspectives on chiropractic education in medical literature, 1910–1933. *CH* (1983) 3:25–30, p. 27; Lyndon Lee, The chiropractic backbone. *Harper's Weekly* (1915) 61:285–8, p. 285; Chittenden Turner, *The Rise of Chiropractic* (Los Angeles: Powell, 1931), 213. A list of early chiropractic schools is to be found in Joseph Keating, *B. J. of Davenport: The Early Years of Chiropractic* (Davenport, IA: Association for the History of Chiropractic, 1997), 55.

25. Gibbons (n. 1), 7, 13–4; Gibbons, Solon (n. 24), 17–9; Turner (n. 24), 46, 153–64; Hans Baer, A historical overview of British and European chiropractic. *CH* (1984) 4: 10–5.

26. Palmer (n. 2), 99, 778, 854, 894.

27. *Physical Culture* (January 1920) 43:77; Jett and Cavins (n. 15), 171–2; Gibbons, Physician-chiropractors (n. 5), 239; Brennan (n. 24), 28. Chiropractic literature claimed extraordinary cure rates for the full range of diseases, including cancer: see, for example, Turner (n. 24), 46–7, 55, 112.

28. Taking chiropractic seriously. *JAMA* (1921) 76:385.

29. Chiropractor indicted on charge of manslaughter. *JAMA* (1928) 90:38; Patient dies in chiropractor's office. *JAMA* (1928) 90:1633; Neck "twisted"—patient dies. *JAMA* (1928) 90:860; A. G. Hildreth, *The Lengthening Shadow of Dr. Andrew Taylor Still* (Macon, MO: Author, 1938), 44; Palmer (n. 2), 391–2, 809; Moore (n. 3), 18; Arthur Forster, *The White Mark: An Editorial History of Chiropractic* (Chicago: National Publishing, 1921), 140, 144, 149, 151, 156, 159; Stanley Hunter, Chiropractic adequately considered weighed in the balance and found out. *JO* (1909) 16:71–2, p. 72. Also see H. M. Vastine, Are we falling from grace? *JAOA* (1915–6) 15: supplement, 1–6.

30. Palmer (n. 2), 887–8. For examples of chiropractors arrested for practicing osteopathy, see Chiros are worried. *JAOA* (1917–8) 17:401; and Chiropractor convicted. *JAOA* (1915–6) 15:118.

31. Gielow (n. 3), 67, 99–114; Gibbons (n. 1), 10.

32. Arthur Geiger, Chiropractic: Its cause and cure. *ME* (August 1942) 19:41–3, 72–8, p. 42; R. P. Beideman, Seeking the rational alternative: The National College of Chiropractic from 1906 to 1982. *CH* (1983) 3:17–22, p. 17; Gibbons, The rise (n. 23), 342; Walter Wardwell, The cutting edge of chiropractic recognition: Prosecution and legislation in Massachusetts. *CH* (1982) 2:55–65, pp. 55–6; Moore (n. 3), 73.

33. Wardwell (n. 32), 56, 60; Palmer (n. 2), 60.

34. Moore (n. 3), 73–4; Bucks County boisterous chiropractors jailed, *JAMA* (1928) 91:506; Practicing chiropody from the county jail, *IMJ* (1923) 44:83–4.

35. Wardwell (n. 32), 61; Moore (n. 3), 74.

36. Turner (n. 24), 126, 173; Moore (n. 3), 75–7; Gibbons (n. 1), 10; Keating (n. 24), 127–33.

37. W. H. Rafferty, *Health and Love a la Chiropractic* (no city, no publisher, no date, no pagination), Kremers Reference Files, American Institute of the History of Pharmacy, University of Wisconsin, 63 (A) II.

38. Rafferty (n. 37).

39. Rafferty (n. 37).

40. Moore (n. 3), 89–92; Norman Gevitz, "A coarse sieve": Basic science boards and medical licensure in the United States. *JHMAS* (1988) 43:36–63, p. 39; Palmer (n. 2), 789; Brennan (n. 24), 28; H. L. Mencken, *Prejudices: Sixth Series* (New York: Octagon, 1977), 224. Also see Miscellany I. *CH* (1982) 2:13, and Turner (n. 24), 95–120; in pp. 300–73, Turner provides a compendium of state laws regulating chiropractic as of 1931. By 1950 eleven states allowed chiropractors to deliver babies, but during the second half of the century all but one repealed the provision: Russell Gibbons, Forgotten perameters [sic] of general practice: The chiropractic obstetrician. *CH* (1982) 2:27–33.

41. Gibbons, Physician-chiropractors (n. 5), 237; Gibbons (n. 1), 9; Paul Smallie, *Chiropractic History* (Stockton, CA: World-Wide Books, 1992), 7; Dye (n. 24), 117, 123–4, 157–72; Palmer (n. 2), 286, 307, 884; Melvin Rosenthal, The structural approach to chiropractic: From Willard Carver to present practice. *CH* (1981) 1:25–9.

42. Beideman (n. 32), 18; Gibbons, Physician-chiropractors (n. 5), 238. Also see Forster (n. 29) for similar statements regarding the scientific simplicity of D. D. Palmer's version of chiropractic: "How much better it would have been to have originally admitted that . . . subluxations of the vertebrae are not the only cause of disease" (44).

43. Turner (n. 24), 273; Palmer (n. 2), 79, 146, 256, 695, 713, 883; advertisement in *Physical Culture* (September 1920) 44:79; Gibbons, Physician-chiropractors (n. 5), 240.

44. Forster (n. 29), 70–5, 130; Palmer (n. 2), 146; W. J. Gassett, The au-to-chiropractor. *Naturopath* (1924) 29:726. For discussion of the range of mixer therapies, see James Ransom, The origins of chiropractic physiological therapeutics: Howard, Forester and Schulze. *CH* (1984) 4:46–52; Dye (n. 24), 113–53; and Moore (n. 3), 42–57.

45. Wardwell (n. 32), 60; Turner (n. 24), 48, 208–11; Albanese (n. 12), 147–8; Martin (n. 15), 219; Moore (n. 3), 41.

46. Keating (n. 24), 7–10.

47. Keating (n. 24), 15–6; Palmer (n. 2), 508, 616, 629, 752. Events surrounding the passing of the Palmer School from father to son are somewhat confused: see Keating (n. 24), 26, 44; Gielow (n. 3), 96–8; Dye (n. 24), 15–20.

48. Palmer (n. 2), 5, 506, 626; Dye (n. 24), 22, 47–57; Gielow (n. 3), 123–8; Kathleen Crisp, Chiropractic lyceums: The colorful origins of chiropractic continuing education. *CH* (1984) 4:16–22, p. 18. A detailed rendering of the conflict between the Palmers *père* and *fils* can be found in Keating (n. 24), 85–103.

49. Arthur Seyse, Chiropractic from the inside. *NYSJM* (1924) 24:550–2, p. 551 (Brennan [n. 24] quotes another allopath who called B. J. "as egotistic as a Chinese God" [29]); Geiger (n. 32), 63.

50. Keating (n. 24), 53, 158; Turner (n. 24), 36–7; Annual (n. 23), 2, 13, 17, 18, 22, 39; Brennan (n. 24), 27.

51. Annual (n. 23), 19, 31–2, 35; Keating (n. 24), 159; Chiropractic candor. *JAMA* (1920) 75:1276.

52. Herbert Shelton, Chiropractic popularity. *HHN* (1922) 27:476–80, p. 476; Schools of chiropractic and of naturopathy in the United States. *JAMA* (1928) 90:1733–8, p. 1736; Forster (n. 29), 177; Steven Martin, Chiropractic and the social context of medical technology, 1895–1925. *TC* (1993) 34:808–34, p. 819; Theresa Gromala, Broadsides, epigrams, and testimonials: The evolution of chiropractic advertising. *CH* (1984) 4:40–5; George Dock, A visit to a chiropractic school. *JAMA* (1922) 78:60–3, p. 60; Turner (n. 24), 229–30. B. J. Palmer's emphasis on advertising is discussed in Keating (n. 24), 139–52.

53. Wardwell (n. 32), 57; Crisp (n. 48), 17; Moore (n. 3), 58; Keating (n. 24), 229–32.

54. Palmer (n. 2), 315; Martin (n. 52); Moore (n. 3), 58–62.

55. Martin (n. 52), 828; Moore (n. 3), 59–60; Crisp (n. 48), 20; Keating (n. 24), 169, 201–6. Fees for using the neurocalometer were gradually decreased, eventually falling so low as $150 initial payment plus $5 monthly rental: Wardwell (n. 3), 80.

56. Keating (n. 24), 204; Moore (n. 3), 59–62; Gibbons, The rise (n. 23), 346–7.

57. Martin (n. 52), 811; Turner (n. 24), 289, 292–3; Dye (n. 24), 273–94.

CHAPTER 9

1. Sebastian Kneipp, *My Water-Cure*, 36th edition (Kempten, Germany: Koesel, 1896), 1–3; Friedhelm Kirchfeld and Wade Boyle, *Nature Doctors. Pioneers in Naturopathic Medicine* (Portland, OR: Medicina Biologica, 1994), 75, 93; Harry Weiss and Howard Kemble. *The Great American Water-Cure Craze* (Trenton, NJ: Past Times Press, 1967), 100–8. Kneipp drew upon a long tradition of "nature cure" in Germany: see Thomas Maretzki and Eduard Seidler, Biomedicine and naturopathic healing in West Germany: A historical and ethnomedical view of a stormy relationship. *CMP* (1985) 9:383–421.

2. Kneipp (n. 1), 15, 63–6, 121–93.

3. Kneipp (n. 1), 9, 15, 22–33; Kirchfeld and Boyle (n. 1), 77.

4. Edward Purinton, Where to find health. *NHH* (1914) 19:275–86, p. 279; Benedict Lust, The growth of Woerishofen. *B. Lust's Gesundheits-Kalender* (1899) 1:77–8; Kirchfeld and Boyle (n. 1), 83, 90, 93; Kneipp (n. 1), xviii.

5. Benedict Lust, The American Naturopathic Association. *NHH* (1942) 47:198–200, p. 198; Kirchfeld and Boyle (n. 1), 185; Benedict Lust, History of the naturopathic movement. *HHN* (1921) 26:479–80; Jesse Gehman, The birth—crucifixion—and rise of naturopathy. *NP* (1946) 50:506, 526, p. 526.

6. Benedict Lust, Kneippism in America. *B. Lust's Gesundheits-Kalender* (1899) 1: 73–5; James Faulkner, Speaking of naturopaths. *NHH* (1934) 33:102–3, p. 102; Paul Wendel, *Standardized Naturopathy* (Brooklyn, NY: Wendel, 1951), 18; Kirchfeld and Boyle (n. 1), 91, 187–90, 202 (this volume is the best English-language survey of the German nature cure tradition); Lust, History (n. 5), 479; Proclamation. *NP* (1927) 32:473–7, p. 473. The only work purporting to be a history of naturopathy in America is George Cody, History of naturopathic medicine. In: Joseph Pizzorno and Michael Murray, editors, *Textbook of Natural Medicine*, 2d edition, 2 volumes (New York: Churchill Livingstone, 1999), 1: 17–40.

7. Kirchfeld and Boyle (n. 1), 200; Henry Lindlahr, *Nature Cure*, 12th edition (Chicago: Nature Cure Publishing, 1919), 12.

8. Lindlahr (n. 7), 1; *NHH* (1913) 18:766; Benedict Lust, Dr. Lust speaking. *NHH* (1934) 33:259–60, p. 259; Lust, Dr. Lust speaking. *NP* (1945) 49:290, 296, 301, 318, p. 318; Lust, Our lord's kindness in the healing herbs. *Naturopath* (1925), 30:111–7; Lust, Dr. Lust speaking. *NP* (1944) 48:202, 212, 224, p. 212.

9. Wendel (n. 6), 26–7; Benedict Lust, Health incarnate. *NHH* (1903), 4:164–7, p. 165.

10. Naturopathic legislation series. *NHH* (1914) 19:143–50, 183–7, 217–58, p. 145; Lust, Naturopathy vs. nature cure. *NHH* (1902) 3:262–3; advertisement for American School of Naturopathy, *HHN* (1921) 26:576.

11. Benedict Lust, Editorial drift. *NHH* (1902) 3:168–71, pp. 170–1; Edward Purinton, Naturopathic creed-crystals. *NHH* (1902) 3:no page; advertisement for American School of Naturopathy, *NHH* (1902) 3:no page.

12. Henry Lindlahr, How I became acquainted with naturopathic cure. In: Benedict Lust, editor, *Universal Naturopathic Encyclopedia Directory and Buyers' Guide Year Book of Drugless Therapy for 1918–19* (Butler, NJ: Lust, 1918), 33–50, p. 33; Lust, The organization and establishment of the "American Yungborn." *NHH* (1913), 18:no page.

13. Per Nelson, Naturopathy versus medicine. *HHN* (1920) 25:78–82, p. 80; Edward Purinton, Efficiency in drugless healing. In: Benedict Lust, editor, *Universal Naturopathic Encyclopedia Directory and Buyers' Guide Year Book of Drugless Therapy for 1918–19* (Butler, NJ: Lust, 1918), 65–165, p. 88; James Clauson, The dawn of a new era. *NHH* (1910) 15:513–7, p. 516; Lust, A happy new year! 1907. *NHH* (1907) 8:1–4, p. 2; Wendel (n. 6), 153.

14. Benedict Lust, Personal advice to our readers. *NHH* (1907) 8:39; Lust, Naturopathy in Southern California. *NHH* (1907) 8:40–1; Henry Lindlahr, *Philosophy of Natural Therapeutics*, 3d edition (Chicago: Lindlahr, 1921), viii; Lust, A happy (n. 13), 3.

15. Lust, A happy (n. 13), 4; Lust, Naturopathic news. *HHN* (1922) 27:88–9, p. 88; *NHH* (1912) 17:421; Kirchfeld and Boyle (n. 1), 80.

16. Lust, A happy (n. 13), 4; A New York Physician, How a doctor was disillusioned. *NHH* (1902) 3:251–4, p. 252; Kirchfeld and Boyle (n. 1), 116; Purinton (n. 4), 279; T.C.M., The nature cure at Butler. *NHH* (1904) 5:151.

17. J. Austin Shaw, J. Austin Shaw explains Yungborn nature cure. *NHH* (1911) 16:145–55, pp. 149–53; advertisement in Benedict Lust, editor, *Universal Naturopathic Encyclopedia Directory and Buyers' Guide Year Book of Drugless Therapy for 1918–19* (Butler, NJ: Lust, 1918), 1207; Purinton (n. 4), 281, 284.

18. Advertisement for Yungborn. *HHN* (1916), 21:no page; Shaw (n. 17), 148; Edward Purinton, Where to find health. *NHH* (1915) 20: i–xxviii, pp. xvii.

19. Joe Riley, Benedict Lust. *NHH* (1921) 26:525.

20. Benedict Lust, Art versus nature in the process of healing. *KWCM* (1900), 1: 120; William Havard, The naturopath's creed. *HHN* (1919) 24:268; Byron Stillman, Back to nature. *NHH* (1905) 6:151.

21. Benedict Lust, Editorial drift. *NHH* (1902) 3:296–9, p. 298.

22. D. D. Palmer, *The Chiropractor's Adjuster: Text-Book of the Science, Art and Philosophy of Chiropractic for Students and Practitioners* (Portland, OR: Portland Printing House, 1910), 286; Phrenological section. *NHH* (1912) 17:615–8, p. 617; Astroscopy department. *HHN* (1917) 22:188–9; J. Haskel Kritzer, *Textbook of Iridiagnosis* (Chicago: Kritzer, 1921); Henry Lindlahr, *Iridiagnosis and Other Diagnostic Methods* (Chicago: Lindlahr, 1922). For a recent discussion of iridiagnosis, see Armand Brint, Iridology. In: Edward Bauman, Armand Brint, Lorin Piper, and Pamela Wright, editors, *The Holistic Health Handbook* (Berkeley, CA: And/Or Press, 1978), 155–63.

23. *NHH* (1904) 5:no page; William Moat, Rectal manipulation. *HHN* (1916) 21: 502–4, p. 502; Arnold Ehret, My mucusless diet and naturopathy. *HHN* (1919) 24:233–5; An Ehretist "derailed." *Naturopath* (1923) 28:12; Apyrotropher section. *NHH* (1912) 17: 819–26; Dr. Lust enjoys an apyrotropher dinner. *NHH* (1913) 18:418–22, p. 421; advertisement for "raw food" in *NHH* (1906) 7:no page; Typhoid Mary. *NHH* (1915) 20:650. See Eugene Christian, *Why Die?* (New York: Christian, 1928) for more on the theory of apyrotrophy.

24. Advertisement for the Parker Vibratory Electric Bath Blanket. *NP* (1928) 33:90; ad for the Toxo-Absorbent Pack. NHH (November 1906), 7:28; ad for the Golden Sunlight Radiator. *NHH* (April 1907), 8:18; ad for the Burdick Infra-Red Generator. *Naturopath* (1923) 28:201; ad for Vi-Rex. *Physical Culture* (Feb 1920) 43:1; ad for X-Ray. *NHH* (August 1905), 6:no page.

25. Benedict Lust, *The Fountain of Youth* (New York: Macfadden, 1923), 91–6, 100–2, 116–8.

26. Lust (n. 25), 104–10, 118–9.

27. Benedict Lust, Editorial drift. *NHH* (1902), 3:82–7, p. 84.

28. A. A. Erz, *The Medical Question: The Truth About Official Medicine and Why We Must Have Medical Freedom* (Butler, NJ: Erz, 1914), xxix–xxx; Benedict Lust, True method of healing. *NHH* (1902) 3:72–3, p. 72; Purinton (n. 4), 282.

29. Benedict Lust, Your great life work. *Naturopath* (1923) 28:5–10, p. 7; Lust (n. 17), 10–1; Louis Reed, *The Healing Cults* (Chicago: University of Chicago Press, 1932), 62, 66; advertisement for Lindlahr College of Natural Therapeutics. *HHN* (1920) 25:257; Schools of chiropractic and of naturopathy in the United States. *JAMA* (1928) 90:1733–8, p. 1735.

30. Benedict Lust, Dr. Lust reports. *NHH* (1934) 33:36–7, p. 36; William Hunt, *Body Love: The Amazing Career of Bernarr Macfadden* (Bowling Green, OH: Bowling Green State University Popular Press, 1989), 66–7; Morris Fishbein, *The Medical Follies* (New York: Boni and Liveright, 1925), 179; Bernarr Macfadden, A physical outrage. *Physical Culture* (1921) 45:44; Benedict Lust, Naturopathic news. *HHN* (1922) 27:293–5, p. 294; Lust, History (n. 5), 480. For more on Macfadden, see James Whorton, *Crusaders for Fitness: The History of American Health Reformers* (Princeton, NJ: Princeton University Press, 1982), 296–303.

31. William Bradshaw, "Yungborn," Tangerine, Fla., the Home of Health. *HHN* (1918) 23:884–90, p. 887; advertisment for Lindlahr, *Physical Culture* (March 1921) 45:119; Wendel (n. 6), 133; Lust, Your (n. 29), 8; Fishbein (n. 30), 52; Schools (n. 29), 1734; Reed (n. 29), 67.

32. Benedict Lust, Who will give the first million to promote naturopathy? *HHN* (1920) 25:61–2; R. L. Alsaker, Do germs cause disease? *Physical Culture* (February 1920) 43:46, 87, 89–90, p. 89; Nelson (n. 13), 78–80.

33. Nelson (n. 13), 80, 82.

34. Martin Kaufman, The American anti-vaccinationists and their arguments. *BHM* (1967) 41:463–78 (homeopath quoted on p. 473); Judith Leavitt, *The Healthiest City: Milwaukee and the Politics of Health Reform* (Princeton, NJ: Princeton University Press, 1982), 76–121.

35. The sinfulness of inoculation. *WCJHR* (1849) 7:12. Also see Evils of vaccination. *WCJ* (1845–6) 1:125.

36. Kaufman (n. 34), 471.

37. Vern Gielow, *Old Dad Chiro: A Biography of D. D. Palmer* (Davenport, IA: Bawden, 1981), 48; W. Banks Meacham, Osteopathic consideration of serum therapy. *JAOA* (1908–9) 8:101–8: p. 102; L. H. Anderson, Natural healing. *NHH* (1902), 3:149–53, p. 153; Erz (n. 28), 255; Benedict Lust, What I stand for. *Naturopath* (1927) 32:217–20, p. 218.

38. Benedict Lust, Naturopathic news. *HHN* (1922) 27:32; A. A. Erz, What medicine knows and does not know about rheumatism. *NHH* (1912) 17:563–609, p. 597; Lust, How vaccine virus is made. *NHH* (1912) 17:614; Anti-Vaccination League of America. *NHH* (1910) 15:549–50.

39. A. A. Erz, Official medicine—as it is—and what it is not. *NHH* (1914) 19:573–604, p. 602; Benedict Lust, The principles and program of the nature cure system. In: Lust, editor, *Universal Naturopathic Encyclopedia Directory and Buyers' Guide Year Book of Drugless Therapy for 1918–19* (Butler, NJ: Lust, 1918), 13–25, p. 17; Lust, How (n. 38); Edmund Vance-Cooke, A serum-comic tragedy. *NHH* (1911) 16:314.

40. Albert Leffingwell, *The Vivisection Question*, 2d edition (Chicago: Vivisection Reform Society, 1907), 52; Henry Salt, *Animals' Rights Considered in Relation to Social Progress* (New York: Macmillan, 1894), 81. For the history of opposition to animal experimentation, see James Whorton, Animal research: Historical aspects. In: Warren Reich, editor, *Encyclopedia of Bioethics*, revised edition, 5 volumes (New York: Simon and Schuster Macmillan, 1995), 1: 143–7; Richard French, *Antivivisection and Medical Science in Victorian Society* (Princeton, NJ: Princeton University Press, 1975); James Turner, *Reckoning With the Beast: Animals, Pain, and Humanity in the Victorian Mind* (Baltimore: Johns Hopkins University Press, 1980); Susan Lederer, The controversy over animal experimentation in America, 1880–1914. In: Nicolaas Rupke, editor, *Vivisection in Historical Perspective* (London: Croom Helm, 1987), 236–58.

41. Vern Gielow, Daniel David Palmer: Rediscovering the frontier years, 1845–1887. *CH* (1981) 1:11–13, p. 13; Gielow (n. 37), 62; Erz (n. 39), 602; Regular allopathic drug doctors. *HHN* (1921) 26:138.

42. Quoted by James Burrow, *Organized Medicine in the Progressive Era: The Move Toward Monopoly* (Baltimore: Johns Hopkins University Press, 1977), 52 (the campaign for a national health department is discussed on pp. 100–2); A. A. Erz, Medical laws vs. human rights and constitution. *NHH* (1913) 18:438–72, 513–44, 585–97, p. 459.

43. J. T. Robinson, The National Bureau of Health. *NHH* (1910) 15:555–6; Robinson, The origin and workings of the medical trust. *NHH* (1912) 17:528–30; Erz (n. 38), 604; Erz (n. 42), 449; Charles Zurmuhlen, The fight for medical freedom against the allopathic trust. *NHH* (1912) 17:609; Robert Baker, Fighting the doctor-drug trust. *NHH* (1912) 17:513–5.

44. Erz (n. 38), 600.

45. Erz (n. 38), 600; Kirchfeld and Boyle (n. 1), 188; Benedict Lust, Medical liberty versus unconstitutional health laws. *NHH* (1934) 33:296–8. For an eloquent example of naturopaths' appeals for licensing protection, see Naturopathic (n. 10).

46. Lust, History (n. 5); Lust (n. 45), 297; Paid prayer curing declared illegal. *New York Times* (July 11, 1914), 4.

47. Lust (n. 45), 298; Lust, History (n. 5), 480; *NHH* (1912) 17:610.

48. J. W. Bush, The arrest and persecution of Benedict Lust. *NHH* (1912) 17:462; Lust, Naturopathic news. *NHH* (1912) 17:742–5, p. 743; Lust, History (n. 5), 480; Lust (n. 45), 297; Lust, Intolerance of official medicine. *HHN* (1919) 24:438–40, p. 439.

49. A. A. Erz, Friends of medical freedom and voters, attention! *NHH* (1912) 17:707–8; Erz (n. 28); Wendel (n. 6), 35; advertisement for American Naturopathic Association. *HHN* (1918) 23:603; James Whorton, Drugless healing in the 1920s: The thera-

peutic cult of sanipractic. *PH* (1986) 28:14–25; State of Washington. *Naturopath* (1925) 30:147–52; Treatment à la carte. *NM* (1919) 18:70–1; Kirchfeld and Boyle (n. 1), 210. For a compendium of naturopathic legislation as of the mid-1930s, see Naturopathic laws of various states. *NHH* (1934) 33:79–82, 117–21, 144–8, 181–4.

50. Advertisement. *HHN* (1920) 25:300; Our declaration of independence. *HHN* (1920) 25:219–20. Also see Platform adopted by Constitutional Liberty League. *HHN* (1920) 25:221–3.

51. Per Nelson, Why all-drugless methods? In: Benedict Lust, editor, *Universal Naturopathic Encyclopedia Directory and Buyers' Guide Year Book of Drugless Therapy for 1918–19* (Butler, NJ: Lust, 1918), 63–4. p. 63; Louis Kuhne, *Neo-Naturopathy: The New Science of Healing* (Butler, NJ: Lust, 1918); Drugless practitioners in convention. *NHH* (1912) 17:709–10; Constitution of the National Association of Drugless Practitioners. *NHH* (1912) 17:710–2, p. 710; Benedict Lust, Editorials. *HHN* (1920) 25:269; Lust, Naturopathic news. *HHN* (1922) 27:32; advertisement for American School of Naturopathy, *HHN* (1921) 26:576; Ernest Napolitano, The struggle for accreditation in chiropractic: A unique history of educational bootstrapping. *CH* (1981) 1:23–4; cartoon in *Naturopath* (1923) 28:196.

52. Benedict Lust, Naturopathic news. *HHN* (1922) 27:88–9, p. 89; Lust, Dr. Lust speaking. *NHH* (1935) 40:2–3, 9, p. 3.

53. Benedict Lust, Naturopathic news. *HHN* (1922) 27:191–2, p. 192; Lust, Editorials (n. 51); Lust, Editorials. *HHN* (1920) 25:283; Lust, Naturopathic news. *HHN* (1922) 27: 293–5. Many other naturopaths became disgusted with chiropractic by the 1920s and predicted its imminent demise: see, for examples, Herbert Shelton, Chiropractic popularity. *HHN* (1922) 27:476–80; and Benjamin Israel, Chiropractic supremacy. *HHN* (1923) 28: 213–6; Wendel (n. 6), 37.

54. Lust, Editorials (n. 51); Lust, Editorials. *HHN* (1920) 25:283.

55. Benedict Lust, Dr. Lust speaking. *NP* (1944) 48:362, 377; Jesse Gehman, To honor the father of naturopathy. *NP* (1947) 51:19, 53; Benedict Lust Permanent Memorial Association, *The Light of Naturopathy* (Butler, NJ: Benedict Lust Permanent Memorial Association, 1947); Wendel (n. 6), 40; Lust, Dr. Wendel fights medical gestapo. *NP* (1945) 49:453.

CHAPTER 10

The section-opening quotation is from Frederick Stenn, Thoughts of a dying physician. *FM* (1980) 3:718–9, p. 719.

1. Louis Reed, *The Healing Cults* (Chicago: University of Chicago Press, 1932), 2–3.

2. John Haller Jr., *Kindly Medicine: Physio-Medicalism in America, 1836–1911* (Kent, OH: Kent State University Press, 1997), 147; Haller, *Medical Protestants. The Eclectics in American Medicine, 1825–1939* (Carbondale: Southern Illinois University Press, 1994), 246; Martin Kaufman, Homeopathy in America: The rise and fall and persistence of a medical heresy. In: Norman Gevitz, editor, *Other Healers: Unorthodox Medicine in America* (Baltimore: Johns Hopkins University Press, 1988), 99–123, pp. 112–3; Morris Fishbein, *The Medical Follies* (New York: Boni and Liveright, 1925), 46.

3. Joseph Sullivan, Osteopathic technique—the hope of the D.O. for individuality.

JAOA (1910–11) 10:317–24, p. 317; speaker quoted by Annie Riley Hale, *These Cults* (New York: National Health Foundation, 1926), 19; Edward Beardsley, Why the public consult the pseudo medical cults. *JMSNJ* (1924) 21:275–81, p. 275; California the battle ground for the legal recognition of various cults. *IMJ* (1923) 44:389–90, p. 389.

4. Fishbein (n. 2), 61–2; Irvin Arthur, The medical profession and the people. *JISMA* (1923) 16:369–70, p. 369; Selwyn Collins, Frequency and volume of doctors' calls among males and females in 9,000 families, based on nationwide periodic canvasses, 1928–31. *PHR* (1940) 55:1977–2020, p. 1988; Beardsley (n. 3), 277; Buda Keller, The laity's idea of the physician. *IMJ* (1923) 44:13–20, p. 14; David Eisenberg, Ronald Kessler, Cindy Foster, Frances Norlock, David Calkins, and Thomas Delbanco, Unconventional medicine in the United States. *NEJM* (1993) 328:246–52.

5. Osteopathy. Special report of the Judicial Council to the AMA House of Delegates. *JAMA* (1961) 177:774–6, p. 774; Arthur Geiger, Chiropractic: Its cause and cure. *ME* (February 1942), 19:56–9, 96–102, p. 56.

6. Edward Purinton, Efficiency in drugless healing. In: Benedict Lust, editor, *Universal Naturopathic Encyclopedia Directory and Buyers' Guide Year Book of Drugless Therapy for 1918–19* (Butler, NJ: Lust, 1918), 65–165, pp. 103–4.

7. Benedict Lust, The science of nature-cure. *NHH* (1908) 9:1–3, p. 2; Lust, Nature cure methods or allopathy. *Naturopath* (1927) 32:213–6, p. 214; A. A. Erz, Medical laws vs. human rights and constitution. *NHH* (1913) 18:438–72, p. 451; Henry Lindlahr, How I became acquainted with nature cure. *HHN* (1918) 23:21–29, p. 27.

8. Charles Zurmuhlen, The true cause of vaccination. *NHH* (1912) 17:725–6, p. 725; chiropractor quoted by Steven Martin, "The only truly scientific method of healing": Chiropractic and American science, 1895–1990. *Isis* (1994) 85:207–27, p. 213; L. H. Anderson, Natural healing. *NHH* (1902) 3:149–53, p. 153.

9. Benedict Lust, The principles and program of the nature cure system. In: Lust, editor, *Universal Naturopathic Encyclopedia Directory and Buyers' Guide Year Book of Drugless Therapy for 1918–19* (Butler, NJ: Lust, 1918), 13–25, p. 25; Arthur Forster, *The White Mark: An Editorial History of Chiropractic* (Chicago: National Publishing Association, 1921), 254–5, 301–2; R. L. Alsaker, Do germs cause disease? *Physical Culture* (February 1920) 43:46, 87, 89–90, p. 87; Norman Gevitz, *The D.O.'s: Osteopathic Medicine in America* (Baltimore: Johns Hopkins University Press, 1982), 72. Homeopaths also claimed superior cure rates against influenza: Julian Winston, *The Faces of Homoeopathy: An Illustrated History* (Tawa, New Zealand: Great Auk, 1999), 236–8.

10. Carl Frischkorn, Naturopaths now control cancer. *Naturopath* (1925) 30:258–9; Abraham Flexner, *Medical Education in the United States and Canada* (New York: Carnegie Foundation for the Advancement of Teaching, 1910), 28, 216, 233, 319. For a detailed examination of the Flexnerian revolution, see Kenneth Ludmerer, *Learning to Heal: The Development of American Medical Education* (New York: Basic Books, 1985).

11. Flexner (n. 10), 156–66, 253.

12. Fishbein (n. 2), 61; The menace of chiropractic. *JAMA* (1923) 80:715–6; Schools of chiropractic and of naturopathy in the United States. *JAMA* (1928) 90:1733–8, p. 1737; George Dock, A visit to a chiropractic school. *JAMA* (1922) 78:60–3, p. 61; Thomas Duhigg, Where chiropractors are made. *JAMA* (1915) 65:2228–9; Arthur Seyse, Chiro-

practic from the inside. *NYSJM* (1924) 24:550–2, p. 550; Frank Jett and A. W. Cavins, The chiropractic situation. *JISMA* (1933) 26:169–72, 229–31, pp. 172, 230. To be sure, by the 1920s chiropractic students had more cadavers to use for anatomical study, but the rigor of their dissection work was questionable: see Schools of chiropractic (this note, above), 1737. For a survey of the history of allopathic opposition to chiropractic, see Susan Smith-Cunnien, *A Profession of One's Own: Organized Medicine's Opposition to Chiropractic* (Lanham, MD: University Press of America, 1998). Also see Gordon Rice, Pseudomedicine. *JAMA* (1912) 58:360–2; A. W. Meyer, "Chiropractic Fountain Head": An inside view. *CWM* (1925) 23:610–3; and J. Stuart Moore, *Chiropractic in America: The History of a Medical Alternative* (Baltimore: Johns Hopkins University Press, 1993), 108–15.

13. Jett and Cavins (n. 12), 229; Steven Martin, Chiropractic and the social context of medical technology, 1895–1925. *TC* (1993) 34:808–34, p. 815; Fishbein (n. 2), 63; Flexner (n. 10), 19; H. L. Mencken, *Prejudices: Sixth Series* (New York: Octagon, 1977), 218, 222. Also see Chittenden Turner, *The Rise of Chiropractic* (Los Angeles: Powell, 1931), 37.

14. Reed (n. 1), 66–9; Fishbein (n. 2), 135; advertisement in *Physical Culture* (January 1920) 43:113; *HM* (February 1926), 21; James Whorton, Drugless healing in the 1920s: The therapeutic cult of sanipractic. *PH* (1986) 28:14–25, pp. 21–3.

15. Suppression of diploma mill. *NM* (1925) 24:145; Schools (n. 12), 1734, 1738; Herbert Shelton, Medical propaganda—a reply. *Naturopath* (1924) 29:124–8, p. 124; Correction. *JAMA* (1928) 91:654.

16. Ford Wilson, History of class of '22, Universal Sanipractic College. *DA* (January 1923) 4:4–5; Purinton (n. 6), 90; Seyse (n. 12), 550.

17. Benedict Lust, Editorial drift. *NHH* (1902) 3:168–71, p. 168; Lust, Naturopathy vs. nature cure. *NHH* (1902) 3:262–3, p. 262; Paul Wendel, *Standardized Naturopathy* (Brooklyn, NY: Wendel, 1951), 41; Herbert Shelton, The Procrustean bedstead. *NP* (1927) 32:477; Purinton (n. 6), 102; Purinton, Where to find health. *NHH* (1914) 14:275–86, p. 284.

18. Norman Gevitz, "A coarse sieve": Basic science boards and medical licensure in the United States. *JHMAS* (1988) 43:36–63; Public Health League. *MS* (1921) 29:40; Channing Frothingham, Osteopathy, chiropractic, and the profession of medicine. *Atlantic Monthly* (1922) 130:75–81, p. 81.

19. Results of basic science examinations. *NM* (1928) 27:206; Gevitz (n. 18), 47–8; B. J. admits chiropractic is doomed. *JAMA* (1928) 90:864. Chiropractors questioned "if it [the basic science act] is administered fairly and honestly": the quotation is from A. Augustus Dye, *The Evolution of Chiropractic: Its Discovery and Development* (Philadelphia: Author, 1939), 231.

20. Gevitz (n. 18), 61–3.

21. Gevitz (n. 9), 75–87, 107–10.

22. Erwin Blackstone, The A.M.A. and the osteopaths: A study of the power of organized medicine. *Antitrust Bulletin* (1977) 22:405–40, pp. 408–9.

23. Lyndon Lee, The chiropractic backbone. *Harper's Weekly* (1915), 61:285–8; Russell Gibbons, The rise of the chiropractic educational establishment, 1897–1980. In: Fern Lints-Dzaman, editor, *Who's Who in Chiropractic International*, 2d edition (Littleton, CO: Who's Who in Chiropractic International, 1980), 339–51, pp. 348–9; Turner (n. 13), 194;

Chiropractors: Healers or quacks? *PM* (April 1976) 79:45–56, pp. 46, 49. Also see Ernest Napolitano, The struggle for accreditation in chiropractic: A unique history of educational bootstrapping. *CH* (1981) 1:23–4; Moore (n. 12), 112–5; and Paul Smallie, *Chiropractic History* (Stockton, CA: World-Wide Books, 1992), pp. 31–45.

24. Shelton (n. 15), 124–5, 128; A. A. Erz, *The Medical Question: The Truth About Official Medicine and Why We Must Have Medical Freedom* (Butler, NJ: Erz, 1914), xxi.

25. Wendel (n. 17), 30, 135–6; Herbert Shelton, What have we, nature cure or a bag of tricks? *HHN* (1921) 26:283–7, p. 283; Shelton, Naturopaths, forward! *Naturopath* (1923) 28:635–7, p. 636.

26. Benedict Lust, Dr. Lust speaking. *NHH* (1942) 47:258; Lust, The American Naturopathic Association. *NHH* (1942) 47:198–200, pp. 199–200; Friedhelm Kirchfeld and Wade Boyle, *Nature Doctors: Pioneers in Naturopathic Medicine* (Portland, OR: Medicina Biologica, 1994), 203, 207–8; Wendel (n. 17), i.

27. Arthur Schramm, editor, *Year Book of the International Society of Naturopathic Physicians* (Los Angeles: International Society of Naturopathic Physicians, 1948), 7–65, 86–7; *A Study of the Healing Arts With Particular Emphasis Upon Naturopathy: A Report to the Utah Legislative Council by the Legislative Council Staff*, November 1958, Bastyr University Library, pp. 6, 14, 71.

28. Osteopathy (n. 5), 774; Blackstone (n. 22), 412–4.

29. Blackstone (n. 22), 417–8; Nelson Crawford, Consult with D.O.'s? We've done it for years, *ME* (March 12, 1962) 39:236–50, p. 239; Osteopathy (n. 5), 775; Jean Pascoe, Green light for osteopaths. *ME* (July 31, 1961) 38:97–115, pp. 97, 105.

30. Osteopathy (n. 5), 775.

31. Victory! *JAOA* (1974) 73:713–4, p. 713; Gevitz (n. 9), 99–102, 114–6; Blackstone (n. 22), 418–9.

32. George Northrup, Sixty-five pieces of silver. *JAOA* (1961–2) 61:555–6, p. 555; Northrup, A matter of degrees. *JAOA* (1961–2) 61:999; A blessing in disguise. *JAOA* (1961–2) 61:559; Northrup, Voices in the night. *JAOA* (1962–3) 62:778–80, p. 780; Northrup, A new m.d. *JAOA* (1962–3) 62:4–5; Northrup, A new year—a new era. *JAOA* (1962–3) 62:278–9, p. 279; Irvin Korr, Osteopathy and medical evolution. *JAOA* (1961–2) 61:515–26, p. 521. It appears that 321 osteopaths in California declined the invitation to become MDs: Editorial comment. *JAOA* (1962–3) 62:686–7.

33. Carl McConnell, Individuality. *JAOA* (1910–1) 10:367–8, p. 368; E. C. Pickler, Our needs and what we stand for. *JAOA* (1910–1) 10:1–6, p. 5.

34. Wayne Pollock, The present relationship of osteopathy and scientific medicine. *WMJ* (1962) 9:337–9, p. 339; AOA-AMA Relationships. No. 3. White Paper prepared by the American Osteopathic Association Department of Public Relations, August 1970, 3–4; AOA-AMA Relationships. No. 2. White Paper prepared by the American Osteopathic Association Department of Public Relations, March 1968, 4; Blackstone (n. 22), 411; Northrup, Sixty-five (n. 32), 556.

35. Professional briefs. *ME* (August 27, 1962) 39:111; Northrup, A New (n. 32); AOA-AMA Relationships. No. 2 (n. 34), 1–2; Blackstone (n. 22), 420–1.

36. Victory! (n. 31), 713; California: Reprise. *JAOA* (1974) 73:792; George Northrup. An affirmative 'no.' *JAOA* (1961–2) 61:997–9, p. 998; Victory and visions. *JAOA* (1974)

73:792–3, p. 793; Jean Crum, The saga of osteopathy in California. *WJM* (1975) 122:87–90.

37. Gevitz (n. 9), 124, 134–6.

38. Gevitz (n. 9), 124; Benedict Lust, Editorial. *HHN* (1918) 23:523–4, p. 524; Bob Jones, *The difference a D.O. makes: Osteopathic medicine in the Twentieth Century* (Oklahoma City: Times-Journal Publishing, 1978), 34–5. For a sample of osteopathic protest at being excluded from the military medical corps, see Our appeal to Washington. *JAOA* (1917–8) 17:319–22.

39. W. J. Cohen, *Independent Practitioners Under Medicare* (Washington, DC: Department of Health, Education, and Welfare, 1969), 142, 197; Norman Gevitz, The chiropractors and the AMA: Reflections on the history of the consultation clause. *PBM* (1989) 32:281–99: p. 290; Walter Wardwell, *Chiropractic: History and Evolution of a New Profession* (St. Louis: Mosby Year Book, 1992), 37; Edward Bauman, Armand Brint, Lorin Piper, and Pamela Wright, editors, *The Holistic Health Handbook* (Berkeley, CA: And/Or Press, 1978). Also see Barrie Cassisleth, Is osteopathic medicine "alternative"? *JAMA* (1999) 281: 1893.

40. Korr (n. 32), 521, 525; Korr, The function of the osteopathic profession: A matter for decision. *JAOA* (1959–60) 59:77–90, p. 89.

41. Osteopathic medicine: Philosophy vs. manipulative therapy. *JAOA* (1973–4) 73: 604–5; Korr (n. 32), 524.

42. Carl McConnell, The making of an osteopath. *JAOA* (1915–6) 15:493–9, pp. 493, 496; Korr (n. 32), 520, 525; George Northrup, A strategy for service. *JAOA* (1961–2) 61: 474; Crawford (n. 29), 244. On the history of psychosomatic medicine, see Erwin Ackerknecht, The history of psychosomatic medicine. *PAM* (1982) 12:17–24; and Z. J. Lipowski, Psychosomatic medicine: Past and present. *CJP* (1986) 31:2–13.

43. George Northrup, The story of the clock, *JAOA* (1963–4) 63:216–7, is a representative discussion of ecological medicine.

44. True Eveleth, Osteopathy today. *JAOA* (1962–3) 62:249–52, p. 252.

45. Victory! (n. 31), 714.

CHAPTER 11

1. Ivan Illich, *Medical Nemesis: The Expropriation of Health* (New York: Pantheon, 1976), 4, 35; Paul Starr, *The Social Transformation of American Medicine* (New York: Basic Books, 1982), 381; Thomas McKeown, *The Role of Medicine: Dream, Mirage, or Nemesis?* (London: Nuffield Provincial Hospitals Trust, 1976); Rick Carlson, *The End of Medicine* (New York: Wiley, 1975); Marcia Millman, *The Unkindest Cut: Life in the Backrooms of Medicine* (New York: Morrow, 1977). For an outline of the emergence of holistic medicine, see Howard Berliner and J. Warren Salmon, The holistic alternative to scientific medicine: History and analysis. *IJHS* (1980) 10:133–47.

2. Norman Cousins, The holistic health explosion. *Saturday Review* (March 31, 1979) 6:17–20; quoted by Kristine Alster, *The Holistic Health Movement* (Tuscaloosa: University of Alabama Press, 1989), 1.

3. Robert Brandon, Holism in philosophy of biology. In: Douglas Stalker and Clark Glymour, editors, *Examining Holistic Medicine* (Buffalo: Prometheus Books, 1985), 127–

36, p. 129. Smuts introduced the word "holism" in his *Holism and Evolution* (New York: Macmillan, 1926). For discussion of medical holism in the earlier twentieth century, see Christopher Lawrence and George Weisz, editors, *Greater Than the Parts: Holism in Biomedicine, 1920–1950* (New York: Oxford University Press, 1998).

4. Quoted by John Burnham, American medicine's golden age: What happened to it? *Science* (1982) 215:1474–9, p. 1475; Robert Moser, *Diseases of Medical Progress* (Springfield, IL: Charles Thomas, 1959), 8; In England now. *Lancet* (no. 2, 1956): 1155. For fuller discussion of overprescribing of wonder drugs, see James Whorton, "Antibiotic abandon": The resurgence of therapeutic rationalism. In: John Parascandola, editor, *The History of Antibiotics. A Symposium* (Madison, WI: American Institute of the History of Pharmacy, 1980), 125–36.

5. Illich (n. 1), 1, 4; Editors of Consumer Reports, Chiropractors: Healers or quacks? *DMJ* (1977) 49:277–300, p. 294; Robert Moser, editor, *Diseases of Medical Progress*, 2d edition (Springfield, IL: Thomas, 1964), xi; Moser, *Diseases of Medical Progress* (Springfield, IL: Thomas, 1959); Moser, editor, *Diseases of Medical Progress*, 3d edition (Springfield, IL: Thomas, 1969), 819. Also see Brian Inglis, *The Case for Unorthodox Medicine* (New York: Putnam, 1965), 15–64; and Knight Steel, Paul Gertman, Caroline Crescenzi, and Jennifer Anderson, Iatrogenic illness on a general medical service at a university hospital. *NEJM* (1981) 304:638–42.

6. Harry Dowling, A new generation. *AMCT* (1956) 3:25–6, p. 26.

7. Carlson (n. 1), 34.

8. Buda Keller, The laity's idea of the physician. *IMJ* (1923) 44:13–20, p. 15; Charles Rosenberg, Holism in twentieth-century medicine. In: Christopher Lawrence and George Weisz, editors, *Greater Than the Parts: Holism in Biomedicine, 1920–1950* (New York: Oxford University Press, 1998), 335–55; Frederick Stenn, Thoughts of a dying physician. *FM* (1980) 3:718–9, p. 718.

9. John Millis, *The Graduate Education of Physicians* (Chicago: American Medical Association, 1966), 34; Walter Alvarez, Constitutional inadequacy. *JAMA* (1942) 119:780–3, pp. 780–1; Kerr White, Health care arrangements in the United States: A.D. 1972, *MMFQ* (October 1972), 50:17–40, pp. 20–1. For detailed discussion of the growth of specialization in American medicine in the twentieth century, see Rosemary Stevens, *American Medicine and the Public Interest* (New Haven, CT: Yale University Press, 1971).

10. Burnham (n. 4); Carlson (n. 1), 24, 29. Illich (n. 1) stresses medical impotence as well, and for McKeown (n. 1) that is the major theme of the book.

11. Stanley Gross, Holistic perspective on professional licensure. *JHM* (1981) 3:38–45, p. 38. For discussion of the counterculture and medicine, see Alster (n. 2), 136–55; and June Lowenberg, *Caring and Responsibility: The Crossroads Between Holistic Practice and Traditional Medicine* (Philadelphia: University of Pennsylvania Press, 1989), 53–80.

12. Edward Bauman, Armand Brint, Lorin Piper, and Pamela Wright, editors, *The Holistic Health Handbook* (Berkeley, CA: And/Or Press, 1978), dedication page; Norman Cousins, *Anatomy of an Illness as Perceived by the Patient* (New York: Norton, 1979), 48; Edward Purinton, *The Laugh Cure*, advertised in Benedict Lust, editor, *Universal Naturopathic Encyclopedia Directory and Buyers' Guide Year Book of Drugless Therapy for 1918–19* (Butler, NJ: Lust, 1918), 1233; Herbert Shelton, Phobiotherapy. *Naturopath* (1926) 31:184–7; Sheldon Solomon, Laughing all the way to the bank. *AIM* (1991), 404. For a particularly

good succinct statement of holistic philosophy, see James Gordon, Holistic medicine: Toward a new medical model. *JCP* (1981) 42:114–9.

13. McKeown (n. 1), 9–10; Keller (n. 8), 16; Morris Fishbein, *The Medical Follies* (New York: Boni and Liveright, 1925), 56; Cousins (n. 12), 48.

14. Arnold Relman, Holistic medicine. *NEJM* (1979) 300:312–3, p. 313. For a critical survey of holistic medicine, see Douglas Stalker and Clark Glymour, *Examining Holistic Medicine* (Buffalo, NY: Prometheus, 1985).

15. George Dearborn, Medical psychology. *MR* (1909) 75:176–8; Abraham Flexner, *Medical Education in the United States and Canada* (New York: Carnegie Foundation for the Advancement of Teaching, 1910), 26; Irvin Arthur, The medical profession and the people. *JISMA* (1923) 16:369–70.

16. Ernest Dichter, Do your patients really like you? *NYSJM* (1954) 54:222–6; Herrman Blumgart, Caring for the patient. *NEJM* (1964) 270:449–56, p. 449.

17. George Engel, The need for a new medical model: A challenge for biomedicine. *Science* (1977) 196:129–36, pp. 129–30. Also see Engel, The clinical application of the biopsychosocial model. *AJP* (1980) 137:535–44.

18. Ad Hoc Committee on Education for Family Practice, *Meeting the Challenge of Family Practice* (Chicago: American Medical Association, 1966), 4; E. Richard Brown, *Rockefeller Medicine Men: Medicine and Capitalism in America* (Berkeley: University of California Press, 1979), 215. For a general discussion of the move toward specialization, see Frank Campion, *The AMA and Health Policy Since 1940* (Chicago: Chicago Review Press, 1984), 31–7.

19. Millis (n. 9), 33, 52; Ad Hoc Committee (n. 18), 7. For an extensive examination of the challenges confronting physicians in the mid-1960s, see Richard Magraw, *Ferment in Medicine: A Study of the Essence of Medical Practice and of Its New Dilemmas* (Philadelphia: Saunders, 1966).

20. James Bryan, *The Role of the Family Physician in America's Developing Medical Care Program* (St. Louis: Green, 1968), 4, 6, 19.

21. John Schwab, Psychosomatic medicine: Its past and present. *Psychosomatics* (1985) 26:583–93; Z. J. Lipowski, Psychosomatic medicine: Past and present. Part I. Historical background. *CJP* (1986) 31:2–7; Lipowski, Psychosomatic medicine: Past and present. Part II. Current state. *CJP* (1986) 31:8–13; Lipowski, Psychosomatic medicine in the seventies: An overview. *AJP* (1977) 134:233–44; Erwin Ackerknecht, The history of psychosomatic medicine. *PAM* (1982) 12:17–24.

22. Lipowski, Psychosomatic medicine in the seventies (n. 21), 235–42; Schwab (n. 21), 591–3; Janice Kiecolt-Glaser and Ronald Glaser, Psychoneuroimmunology: Past, present, and future. *HP* (1989) 8:677–82. Awareness of the relation of stress to health was fostered particularly by Herbert Benson's *The Relaxation Response* (New York: Morrow, 1975). For early discussion of biofeedback, see Neal Miller and Barry Dworkin, Effects of learning on visceral functions—biofeedback. *NEJM* (1977) 296:1274–8.

23. Lipowski, Psychosomatic medicine in the seventies (n. 21), 233; Lipowski, Psychosomatic medicine: Past and present. Part II. (n. 21), 12; Bryan (n. 20), 20.

24. Herbert Otto and James Knight, Wholistic healing: Basic principles and concepts. In: Otto and Knight, editors. *Dimensions in Holistic Healing* (Chicago: Nelson-Hall, 1979), 3–27, pp. 19–25; *JHM* (spring/summer 1980) 2:2; *JHM* (1981) 3:2.

25. James Gordon, Holistic health centers in the United States. In: J. Warren Salmon, editor, *Alternative Medicines: Popular and Policy Perspectives* (New York: Tavistock, 1984), 229–51.

26. James Reston, Now, about my operation in Peking. *New York Times* (July 26, 1971), 1, 6. For a condensed account of the episode, see Gary Kaplan, A brief history of acupuncture's journey to the West, *JACM* (1997), 3:S5-S10.

27. E. Grey Dimond, Acupuncture anesthesia: Western medicine and Chinese traditional medicine. *JAMA* (1971) 218:1558–63; Ian Capperauld, Acupuncture anesthesia and medicine in China today. *SGO* (1972) 135:440–5.

28. Dimond (n. 27), 1561, 1563; Walter Tkach, "I have seen acupuncture work," says Nixon's doctor. *Today's Health* (July 1972) 50:50–6, p. 51.

29. Tkach (n. 28), 51–2, 54, 56. Tkach acknowledged that his comment "I have seen the past, and it works" originated with Samuel Rosen, one of the physicians in the previous American delegation. British physicians confirmed American observations: see P. E. Brown, Use of acupuncture in major surgery. *Lancet* (no. 2, 1972): 1328–30.

30. Felix Mann, *Acupuncture: The Ancient Chinese Art of Healing* (New York: Random House, 1962); Nguyen van Nghi, Guido Fisch, and John Kao, An introduction to classical acupuncture. *AJCM* (1973) 1:75–83. The definition of qi as vital energy is an oversimplification of the concept in Chinese thought, where it carries a much broader and more subtle set of meanings: see Stephen Birch and Robert Felt, *Understanding Acupuncture* (New York: Harcourt Brace, 1999), 105, 148–50.

31. Ilza Veith, Acupuncture in traditional Chinese medicine—an historical review. *CM* (1973) 118:70–9, p. 73. Also see Veith, *The Yellow Emperor's Classic of Internal Medicine* (Berkeley: University of California Press, 1966); Joseph Needham and Lu Gwei-Djen, Chinese medicine. In: F.N.L. Poynter, editor, *Medicine and Culture* (London: Wellcome Institute of the History of Medicine, 1969), 255–84; Birch and Felt (n. 30), 14–5. For comprehensive treatment of the history of Chinese medicine in general, see Paul Unschuld, *Medicine in China: A History of Ideas* (Berkeley: University of California Press, 1985); and Lu Gwei-Djen and Joseph Needham, *Celestial Lancets: A History and Rationale of Acupuncture and Moxa* (Cambridge: Cambridge University Press, 1980).

32. Veith, Acupuncture (n. 31), 76–7; Veith, Acupuncture: Ancient enigma to east and west. *AJP* (1972) 129:333–6. For discussion of the evolution of acupuncture over time in China and changes imposed by other cultures to which it was exported, see Birch and Felt (n. 30), 3–60.

33. Robert Carrubba and John Bowers, The Western world's first detailed treatise on acupuncture: Willem Ten Rhijne's *De Acupunctura. JHMAS* (1974) 29:371–98; Willem Ten Rhijne, *Dissertatio de Arthritide* (London: Chiswell, 1683), 186.

34. John Elliotson, Acupuncture. In: John Forbes, Alexander Tweedie, and John Conolly, editors, *The Cyclopaedia of Practical Medicine*, 4 volumes (Philadelphia: Lea and Blanchard, 1847), 1: 54–7, pp. 55–6; John Haller Jr., Acupuncture in nineteenth-century Western medicine. *NYSJM* (1973) 73:1213–21, pp. 1215, 1217; Jacques Quen, Acupuncture and Western medicine. *BHM* (1975) 49:196–205, pp. 198–201. Also see Quen, Case studies in nineteenth-century scientific rejection: Mesmerism, Perkinism, and acupuncture. *JHBS* (1975) 11:149–56; and When acupuncture came to Britain. *BMJ* (no. 4, 1973) 687–8.

35. Bache's experiments were reported in Cases illustrative of the remedial effects

of acupuncturation. *NAMSJ* (1826) 1:311–21; the article has been reproduced, with commentary, by James Cassedy, Early uses of acupuncture in the United States, with an addendum (1826) by Franklin Bache, M.D. *BNYAM* (1974) 50:892–906. The surgical text cited is Samuel Gross, *A System of Surgery: Pathological, Diagnostic, Therapeutic and Operative*, 2 volumes (Philadelphia: Blanchard and Lea, 1859), 1: 575–6 (also quoted by Cassedy, 896).

36. Cassedy (n. 35), 896–8, 902–3.

37. Cassedy (n. 35), 902; Mr. Wansbrough, Acupuncturation. *Lancet* (1826) 10:846–8 (the case of Mr. W. is also reported by Haller [n. 34], 1216); Elliotson (n. 34), 55.

38. Wansbrough (n. 37), 848.

39. Charles [sic] Baunscheidt, *Baunscheidtism; or, A New Method of Cure*, Theophilus Clewell, translator, 8th edition (Cleveland: Linden, 1865), 36. Baunscheidtism is also discussed in Haller (n. 34), 1218–20.

40. Baunscheidt (n. 39), 27, 34, 76.

41. Baunscheidt (n. 39), 43, 161.

42. Baunscheidt (n. 39), 46–64, 79. On Victorians' dread of being buried alive, see Alison Winter, *Mesmerized: Powers of Mind in Victorian Britain* (Chicago: University of Chicago Press, 1998), 171.

43. Baunscheidt (n. 39), 226 (testimonials from American patients are published on pp. 219–30); Georg Kirchner, *Baunscheidt—Die Akupunktur des Westens: Gesund Durch Hautreizbehandlung* (Genf: Ariston Verlag, 1976).

44. William Osler, *The Principles and Practice of Medicine* (New York: Appleton, 1894), 282, 820; Harvey Cushing, *The Life of Sir William Osler* (London: Oxford University Press, 1940), 177.

45. Pang Man and Calvin Chen, Mechanism of acupunctural anesthesia. *DNS* (1972) 33:730–5, pp. 730–1; Unschuld (n. 31), 251; Capperauld (n. 27), 441. For more detailed discussion of the revival of traditional medicine in twentieth-century China, see Ralph Crozier's excellent monograph *Traditional Medicine in Modern China* (Cambridge, MA: Harvard University Press, 1968); and Unschuld (n. 31), 229–62.

46. Tkach (n. 28), 51; Capperauld (n. 27), 444–5; Man and Chen (n. 45), 731; Veith, Acupuncture: Ancient enigma (n. 32), 335.

47. J. Elizabeth Jeffress, Acupuncture: Witchcraft or wizardry? *JAMWA* (1972) 27: 519–21; David Goldstein, The cult of acupuncture. *WIMJ* (October 1972) 71:14–7, pp. 15, 17.

48. Ronald Malt and Frank McDowell, Cable from Cathay. *NEJM* (1973) 288:1353–4, p. 1353; William Kroger, Letters to the editor. *MWN* (August 4, 1972) 13:12; Kroger, Hypnotism and acupuncture. *JAMA* (1972) 220:1012–3, p. 1012.

49. Goldstein (n. 47), 17; E. Grey Dimond, More than herbs and acupuncture. *Saturday Review* (December 18, 1971) 54:17–9, 71, p. 19; Needham and Gwei-Djen (n. 31), 281; Theodore Rowan, letter, *WIMJ* (December 1972) 71:14.

50. Barbara Culliton, Acupuncture: Fertile ground for faddists and serious NIH research. *Science* (1972) 177:592–4, p. 592; Jane Lee, Needle power. *CM* (August 1972) 117:74–5; Jeffress (n. 47), 519–20.

51. Jeffress (n. 47), 520; Needling the profession. *JMSNJ* (1973) 70:2263–4, p. 263; Agnes Fagan, Everyone is talking about acupuncture. *CAH* (February 1973) 50:57–8, p. 57;

Culliton (n. 50), 592; "Vast number of human pin-cushions" feared from acupuncture fad. *DS* (May 1972), 48:13; Dimond (n. 49), 19; Joseph Davis and Lillian Yin, Acupuncture: Past and present. *FDA Consumer* (May 1973), 7:17–23, p. 23. Also see Acupuncture therapy may hit spot, but is it legal? *MWN* (August 4, 1972) 13:15–17; Don Mills, Acupuncture—a measured view. *JAOA* (1973–4), 73:22–3; and Birch and Felt (n. 30), 68.

52. Needling (n. 51); Acupuncture and the acuchiropractors. *JAMA* (1973) 223:682–3, p. 682.

53. Acupuncture therapy (n. 51), 15–17; Robert Wild, Acupuncture—a current legal analysis. *AJCM* (1973) 1:123–33.

54. Acupuncture. *JAMA* (1973) 226:354; G.G.L., The two-armed bandit. *JAMA* (1973) 225:297.

55. Birch and Felt (n. 30), 62–5, 78.

56. Vast (n. 51); Acupuncture: The plot thickens. *SAMJ* (1973) 47:1387. Also see Nicholas Greene, This is no humbug—or is it? *JA* (1972) 36:101–2.

57. Culliton (n. 50); Wei-Chi Liu, Acupuncture anesthesia: A case report. *JAMA* (1972) 221:87–8; Wild (n. 53), 125; Acupuncture anaesthesia. *Lancet* (no. 2, 1973): 849–50, p. 849.

58. Alfred Peng, Yoshiaki Omura, Huan Cheng, and Louis Blancato, Acupuncture for relief of chronic pain and surgical analgesia. *AS* (1974) 40:50–3; Teruo Matsumoto, Bruce Levy, and Victor Ambruso, Clinical evaluation of acupuncture. *AS* (1974) 40:400–5; Henry Nemerof, Acupuncture in the service of osteopathic medicine: A pathway to comprehensive patient management. *JAOA* (1972–3) 72:346–51, p. 347.

59. Wei-Chi Liu (n. 57), 88; Ronald Melzack and Patrick Wall, Pain mechanisms: A new theory. *Science* (1965) 150:971–9; Man and Chen (n. 45); Nemerof (n. 58), 347. For a review of theories of acupuncture's effects on pain, see Birch and Felt (n. 30), 154–69. On the research basis of acupuncture, see Lyn Freeman and G. Frank Lawlis, *Mosby's Complementary and Alternative Medicine: A Research-Based Approach* (St. Louis: Mosby, 2001), 311–44.

CHAPTER 12

1. Acupuncture works. *Time* (November 17, 1997), 150:84; NIH Consensus Development Panel on Acupuncture, Acupuncture. *JAMA* (1998) 280:1518–24, p. 1522.

2. Edzard Ernst, Karl-Ludwig Resch, and Adrian White, Complementary medicine: What physicians think of it: a meta-analysis. *AIM* (1995) 155:2405–8.

3. Elisha Bartlett, *An Essay on the Philosophy of Medical Science* (Philadelphia: Lea and Blanchard, 1844), 201.

4. William Rothstein, *American Physicians in the Nineteenth Century: From Sects to Science* (Baltimore: Johns Hopkins University Press, 1972), 235, 345; William Holcombe, *The Truth About Homeopathy* (Philadelphia: Boericke and Tafel, 1894), 11–12; Martin Kaufman, *Homeopathy in America: The Rise and Fall of a Medical Heresy* (Baltimore: Johns Hopkins University Press, 1971), 166–73, 183; Kaufman, Homeopathy in America: The rise and fall and persistence of a medical heresy. In: Norman Gevitz, editor, *Other Healers: Unorthodox Medicine in America* (Baltimore: Johns Hopkins University Press, 1988), 99–123, pp. 110–5; Dana Ullman, *Homeopathy: Medicine for the Twenty-first Century* (Berkeley,

CA: North Atlantic Books, 1988), 47; Wayne Jonas and Jennifer Jacobs, *Healing With Homeopathy: The Complete Guide* (New York: Warner, 1996), 39–41.

5. The Connecticut society president is quoted by Julian Winston, *The Faces of Homoeopathy: An Illustrated History of the First 200 Years* (Tawa, New Zealand: Great Auk, 1999), 287; William Wesner, President's address, Bedford Springs convention. *JAIH* (1958) 51:55; Roger Schmidt, Presidential message. *JAIH* (1959) 52:117–8, p. 117; Kaufman, *Homeopathy* (n. 4), 183.

6. Ullman (n. 4), 50; Kaufman, Homeopathy (n. 4), 117, 121–3; Christina Chambreau and C. Edgar Sheaffer, Homeopathic care for the whole animal. Program for National Center for Homeopathy, 1997 Annual Meeting and Conference.

7. Jonas and Jacobs (n. 4), 98; Frederic Schmid, The president's welcoming address. *JAIH* (1979) 72:197–9, p. 198. For advertisements for homeopathic medicine kits, see *Discover Homeopathy*, mail-order brochure from Homeopathic Educational Services, Berkeley, California.

8. William Gutman, Presidential address. *JAIH* (1965) 58:266–8, p. 268; Gutman, A word from the president. *JAIH* (1965) 58:2; Kaufman, Homeopathy (n. 4), 116–7; Winston (n. 5), 370–2. For information on current homeopathic education in the United States, see Ullman (n. 4), 2466–7.

9. Ullman (n. 4), xxiii; Elizabeth Hubbard, The meaning of homeopathy. *JAIH* (1965) 58:46–9; Margery Blackie, *The Patient, not the Cure: The Challenge of Homeopathy* (Santa Barbara, CA: Woodbridge, 1978).

10. Ullman (n. 4), 224; Robert Avina and Lawrence Schneiderman, Why patients choose homeopathy. *WJM* (1978) 128:366–9.

11. Jonas and Jacobs (n. 4), 94–5; British editorial. *JAIH* (1958) 51:80–1, p. 81.

12. Jos Kleijnen, Paul Knipschild, and Gerben ter Riet, Clinical trials of homoeopathy. *BMJ* (1991) 302:316–23, p. 316. Also see Edzard Ernst and Ted Kaptchuk, Homeopathy revisited. *AIM* (1996) 156:2162–4; and Ullman (n. 4), 55–69. For comprehensive discussion of recent theories of homeopathic drug action, see Paolo Bellavite and Andrea Signorini, *Homeopathy: A Frontier in Medical Science*, Anthony Steele, translator (Berkeley, CA: North Atlantic Books, 1995).

13. Klaus Linde, Nicola Clausius, Gilbert Ramirez, Dieter Melchart, Florian Eitel, Larry Hedges, and Wayne Jonas, Are the clinical effects of homoeopathy placebo effects? A meta-analysis of placebo-controlled trials. *Lancet* (1997) 350:834–43, p. 839 (also see, in that same issue of *Lancet*, Jan Vandenbroucke, Homoeopathy trials: Going nowhere, p. 824, and M.J.S. Langman, Homoeopathy trials: Reason for good ones but are they warranted? p. 825); Winston (n. 5), 455; physician quoted in See me, feel me, touch me, heal me. *Life* (September 1996), 121:34–50, p. 42; Wallace Sampson, Homeopathy does not work. *AT* (1995) 1:48–52, p. 49. The article on childhood diarrhea was Jennifer Jacobs, L. Margarita Jimenez, Stephen Gloyd, James Gale, and Dean Crothers, Treatment of acute childhood diarrhea with homeopathic medicine: A randomized clinical trial in Nicaragua. *Paediatrics* (1994) 93:719–25. Another, and controversial, example of orthodox disbelief in homeopathy is the flap that developed over the publication in *Nature* in 1988 of an article documenting activity of antibodies in homeopathic dilution: see John Maddox, James Randi, and Walter Stewart, "High-dilution" experiments a delusion. *Nature* (1988)

334:287–90; Jacques Benveniste, Dr. Benveniste replies. *Nature* (1988) 334:291; and Carol Bayley, Homeopathy. *JMP* (1993) 18:129–45.

14. Jonas and Jacobs (n. 4), 88–9; Workshop on Alternative Medicine, *Alternative Medicine: Expanding Medical Horizons* (Washington, DC: Government Printing Office, 1992), 45, 134–8. Also see Jeffrey Migdow, An introduction to homeopathic medicine and the utilization of bioenergetics for healing. *JHM* (1982) 4:137–45; Keith Sehnert, Convergence, energy and optimal health. *JHM* (1985) 7:178–93; and William Tiller, Rationale for an energy medicine. In: Herbert Otto and James Knight, editors, *Dimensions in Wholistic Healing: New Frontiers in the Treatment of the Whole Person* (Chicago: Nelson-Hall, 1979), 165–79.

15. Dolores Krieger, Therapeutic touch: Two decades of research, teaching and clinical practice. *Imprint* (no. 3, 1990) 37:83–8, p. 83; Ronni Sandroff, A skeptic's guide to therapeutic touch. *RN* (January 1980) 43:25–30, 82–3, p. 26; Maxine Karpen, Dolores Krieger, Ph.D., R.N. *ACT* (1994–5) 1:142–6.

16. Dolores Krieger, Therapeutic touch. *NT* (1976) 72:572–4. On the similarity of mesmerism to therapeutic touch, see Alison Winter, *Mesmerized: Powers of Mind in Victorian Britain* (Chicago: University of Chicago Press, 1998), 64–5, 139–40.

17. Krieger (n. 15), 83; Krieger (n. 16); Sandroff (n. 15), 26–7; Linda Rosa, Emily Rosa, Larry Sarner, and Stephen Barrett, A close look at therapeutic touch. *JAMA* (1998) 279:1005–10, p. 1005. Also see Krieger, *The Therapeutic Touch: How to Use Your Hands to Help or Heal* (New York: Prentice-Hall, 1986).

18. Krieger (n. 15), 83; Joe Maxwell, Nursing's new age? *Christianity Today* (no. 2, 1996), 40:96–8, p. 96; Therapeutic touch fails a rare scientific test. *Skeptical Inquirer* (May-June 1998) 22:6.

19. Florence Nightingale, *Notes on Nursing* (New York: Dover, 1969), 133; Finley Peter Dunne, *Mr. Dooley's Opinions* (New York: Russell, 1901), 9. On holism in nursing, see Susan Williams, Holistic nursing. In: Douglas Stalker and Clark Glymour, editors, *Examining Holistic Medicine* (Buffalo, NY: Prometheus, 1985), 49–63.

20. John Bovee Dods, *The Philosophy of Mesmerism and Electrical Psychology* (London: Burns, 1886), 162–3; Horatio Dresser, editor, *The Quimby Manuscripts* (New Hyde Park, NY: University Books, 1961), 179.

21. O. Carl Simonton, Stephanie Matthews-Simonton, and James Creighton, *Getting Well Again* (Los Angeles: Tarcher, 1978), 6–10; Bernie Siegel, *Love, Medicine and Miracles* (New York: Harper and Row, 1986).

22. Nathan Talbot, The position of the Christian Science church. *NEJM* (1983) 309:1641–4; Randolph Byrd, Positive therapeutic effects of intercessory prayer in a coronary care unit population. *SMJ* (1988) 81:826–9.

23. David Van Blema, A test of the healing power of prayer. *Time* (October 12, 1998) 152:72–3; Harold Koenig, *The Healing Power of Faith* (New York: Simon and Schuster, 1999); Jeffrey Levin, David Larson, and Christina Puchalski, Religion and spirituality in medicine: Research and education. *JAMA* (1997) 278:792–3; Richard Sloan, Emilia Bagiella, Larry VandeCreek, Margot Hover, Carlo Casalone, Trudi Hirsch, Yusuf Hasan, Ralph Kreger, and Peter Poulos, Should physicians prescribe religious activities? *NEJM* (2000) 342:1913–6, p. 1913; Faith is good for your health. Brochure from the

National Institute for Healthcare Research, no date; Mike Mitka, Getting religion seen as help in getting well. *JAMA* (1998) 280:1896–7; Charles Marwick, Should physicians prescribe prayer for health? Spiritual aspects of well-being considered. *JAMA* (1995) 273: 1561–2; physician quoted by Sharon Driedger, Prayer power. *Maclean's* (1995) 108:42. For discussion of the full range of experiments utilizing prayer to effect physical change, see Larry Dossey, *Reinventing Medicine: Beyond Mind-Body to a New Era of Healing* (San Francisco: HarperCollins, 1999). For criticism of studies linking health to religious commitment, see R. P. Sloan, E. Bagiella, and T. Powell, Religion, spirituality, and medicine. *Lancet* (1999) 353:664–7.

24. Dossey (n. 23), 8, 19, 53.

25. Dossey (n. 23), 8 (the statement dismissing the healing power of prayer as "crap" is taken from my notes of a lecture by Dossey at the University of Washington, December 5, 1995; in his text, p. 34, the sentence used is "This is the sort of thing I would not believe, even if it were true"); Siegel (n. 21), vi; Edward Friedlander, Dream your cancer away. In: Douglas Stalker and Clark Glymour, editors, *Examining Holistic Medicine* (Buffalo, NY: Prometheus, 1985), 273–85; Philip Clark and Mary Jo Clark, Therapeutic touch: Is there a scientific basis for the practice? *NR* (1984) 33:37–41, p. 40; Robert Park, The danger of voodoo science. *New York Times* (July 9, 1995), A15; Park, Buying snake oil with tax dollars. *New York Times* (January 3, 1996), A11.

26. Rosa et al. (n. 17).

27. Michael Lemonick, Emily's little experiment. *Time* (April 13, 1998) 151:67; Thomas Ball and Dean Alexander, Catching up with eighteenth-century science in the evaluation of therapeutic touch. *Skeptical Inquirer* (July-August 1998) 22:31–4. The validity of Emily's experiment has been challenged by Daniel Eskinazi and David Muehsam, Is the scientific publishing of complementary and alternative medicine objective? *JACM* (1999) 5:587–94. Recent positive trials of therapeutic touch include Joan Turner, Ann Clark, Dorothy Gauthier, and Monica Williams, The effect of therapeutic touch on pain and anxiety in burn patients. *JAN* (1998) 28:10–20; and Andrea Gordon, Joel Merenstein, Frank D'Amico, and David Hudgens, The effect of therapeutic touch on patients with osteoarthritis of the knee. *JFP* (1998) 47:271–7. For discussion of clinical trials of therapeutic touch, see Vern Bullough and Bonnie Bullough, Therapeutic touch: Why do nurses believe? *Skeptical Inquirer* (1993) 17:69–74; and Clark and Clark (n. 25).

28. Empathology handbill placed under windshield wiper, 1997; Harold Vanderpool, The holistic hodgepodge: A critical analysis of holistic medicine and health in America today. *JFP* (1984) 19:773–81; Michael Specter, The outlaw doctor. *New Yorker* (February 5, 2001), 48–61. p. 52.

29. Lyn Freeman and G. Frank Lawlis, *Mosby's Complementary and Alternative Medicine: A Research-Based Approach* (St. Louis: Mosby, 2001), 225–59; David Gelman, Illusions that heal. *Newsweek* (November 17, 1986), 108:74–6; American Medical Association, *Digest of Official Actions, 1959–1968* (Chicago: American Medical Association, 1971), 335; Stephen Rushmore, The bill to register chiropractors. *NEJM* (1932) 206:614–5, p. 615; What is chiropractic? *NEJM* (1932) 206:298–9, p. 299; Jean Pascoe, Chiropractic is cracking up! *ME* (Aug. 18, 1961) 38:181–93, p. 181.

30. Norman Gevitz, The chiropractors and the AMA: Reflections on the history of the consultation clause. *PBM* (1989) 32:281–99, pp. 292–3; AMAgrams. *JAMA* (1966) 197:

9; AMAgrams. *JAMA* (1969) 209:1600; How the new ethics code affects you. *ME* (October, 1949) 27:54–8, p. 56. The book supplied by the AMA was Ralph Smith, *At Your Own Risk: The Case Against Chiropractic* (New York: Trident, 1969).

31. Wilbur Cohen, *Independent Practitioners Under Medicare* (Washington, DC: Department of Health, Education, and Welfare, 1968), 197; AMAgrams. *JAMA* (1971) 216: 586; A call to arms. *JAMA* (1971) 217:959; Walter Wardwell, *Chiropractic: History and Evolution of a New Profession* (St. Louis: Mosby Year Book, 1992), 166; Editors of Consumer Reports, Chiropractors: Healers or quacks? *DMJ* (1977) 49:277–300, p. 299; William Jarvis, Chiropractic: A challenge for health education. *Journal of School Health* (1974) 44: 210–4. On the passage of Medicare and Medicaid, and the role of the AMA in deliberations over the legislation, see Frank Campion, *The AMA and Health Policy Since 1940* (Chicago: Chicago Review Press, 1984), 253–83.

32. Jarvis (n. 31), 213; Ray Casterline, Unscientific cultism: "Dangerous to your health." *JAMA* (1972) 220:1009–10 p. 1009; J. Stuart Moore, *Chiropractic in America: The History of a Medical Alternative* (Baltimore: Johns Hopkins University Press, 1993), 130.

33. Susan Getzendanner, Permanent injunction order against AMA. *JAMA* (1988) 259:81–2; Wardwell (n. 31), 11, 168–78; Moore (n. 32), 131–7.

34. Gevitz (n. 30), 294–6.

35. Requirements for admission to schools of chiropractic. *JAMA* (1964) 190:763–4; American Medical Association (n. 29), 335; Cohen (n. 31), 197; Susan Smith-Cunnien, *A Profession of One's Own: Organized Medicine's Opposition to Chiropractic* (Lanham, MD: University Press of America, 1998), 20.

36. Russell Gibbons, The rise of the chiropractic educational establishment, 1897–1980. In: Fern Lints-Dzaman, editor, *Who's Who in Chiropractic International*, 2d edition (Littleton, CO: Who's Who in Chiropractic International, 1980), 339–51, p. 350; Editors (n. 31), 46; Robert Fuller, *Alternative Medicine and American Religious Life* (New York: Oxford University Press, 1989), 71–81; B. D. Inglis, *Chiropractic in New Zealand* (Wellington, New Zealand: Government Printer, 1979), 1–2; D. A. Chapman-Smith, The New Zealand Commission of Inquiry: Its significance in chiropractic history. *CH* (1983) 3:32–40. For a survey of the research basis for chiropractic, see Freeman and Lawlis (n. 29), 286–310. On the efficacy of chiropractic for treating back pain, see T. W. Meade, Sandra Dyer, Wendy Browne, Joy Townsend, and A. O. Frank, Low back pain of mechanical origin: Randomised comparison of chiropractic and hospital outpatient treatment. *BMJ* (1990) 300:1431–7. On the continuing straight-mixer conflict, see Wardwell (n. 31), 131–4, 195–205; John Coulehan, Adjustment, the hands and healing. *CMP* (1985) 9:353–82, p. 361; and Smith-Cunnien (n. 35), 18.

37. Editors (n. 31), 277, 290; Wardwell (n. 31), 194.

38. Editors (n. 31); Dan Cherkin, Frederick MacCornack, and Alfred Berg, Family physicians' views of chiropractors: Hostile or hospitable? *AJPH* (1989) 79:636–7; Brian Berman, B. Krishna Singh, Lixing Lao, Betsy Singh, Kevin Ferentz, and Susan Hartnoll, Physicians' attitudes toward complementary or alternative medicine: A regional survey. *JABFP* (1995) 8:361–6; Wardwell (n. 31), 245–6; Inglis (n. 36), 2–5.

39. Paul Wendel, *Standardized Naturopathy* (Brooklyn, NY: Wendel, 1951), 37, 57.

40. Friedhelm Kirchfeld and Wade Boyle, *Nature Doctors: Pioneers in Naturopathic Medicine* (Portland, OR: Medicina Biologica, 1994), 203–4, 310; Hans Baer, The potential

rejuvenation of American naturopathy as a consequence of the holistic health movement. *MA* (1991–2) 13:369–83, pp. 373–4; Cohen (n. 31), 140; Julius Roth, *Health Purifiers and Their Enemies* (New York: Prodist, 1977), 121.

41. Cohen (n. 31), 142; Kirchfeld and Boyle (n. 40), 204–6.

42. Kirchfeld and Boyle (n. 40), 306, 311; Joseph Pizzorno and Pamela Snider, Naturopathic medicine. In: Marc Micozzi, editor, *Fundamentals of Complementary and Alternative Medicine* (New York: Churchill Livingstone, 2001), 159–92, p. 171; Baer (n. 40), 375; *Bastyr 22*, brochure published by Bastyr University, 2000.

43. Pizzorno and Snider (n. 42), 171; *Bastyr 22* (n. 42); *Bastyr University Catalog 2000/2001* (Bothel, WA: Bastyr University, 2000); *University Data Book*, 1998 (Bastyr University Library).

44. Joseph Pizzorno, State of the college. *JNM* (winter 1985) 3:111–4; Joseph Pizzorno and Michael Murray, *Textbook of Natural Medicine*, 2d edition, 2 volumes (New York: Churchill Livingstone, 1999); Jared Zeff and Pamela Snider, *Report to the American Association of Naturopathic Physicians From the Select Committee on the Definition of Naturopathic Medicine*, September 1988 (Bastyr University Library), 17.

45. Pizzorno and Snider (n. 42), 179–81, 188; American Associaton of Naturopathic Physicians, *Position Paper and Organizational Documents*, 1995 (Bastyr University Library); Jared Zeff, The process of healing: A unifying theory of naturopathic medicine. *JNM* (no. 1, 1997) 7:122–5, p. 124. For comprehensive discussion of modern naturopathic diagnosis and therapy, see Pizzorno and Murray (n. 44).

46. Benedict Lust, Why federal and state naturopathic laws should be enacted. *NHH* (1942) 47:252; Pizzorno and Snider (n. 42), 184; Rob Cagen, Dealing openly and honestly with standards issues. *JNM* (1990) 1:74–5; personal communication from several naturopathic physicians.

47. Pizzorno and Murray (n. 44), 1: 797–805, 943–6.

48. Charles Vincent and Adrian Furnham, *Complementary Medicine: A Research Perspective* (New York: Wiley, 1997), 155; Office of Technology Assessment, *Assessing the Safety and Efficacy of Medical Technology* (Washington, DC: U.S. Congress, 1978), 7, 42–4; Richard Smith, Where is the wisdom . . . ? *BMJ* (1991) 303:798–9, p. 798; Thomas Preston, Marketing an operation. *Atlantic Monthly* (December 1984) 254:32–40; Paul Wolpe, The holistic heresy: Strategies of ideological challenge in the medical profession. *SSM* (1990) 31:913–23, p. 921.

49. Obstacles to research in alternative medicine are discussed by Vincent and Furnham (n. 48), 153–74; Arthur Margolin, S. Kelly Avants, and Herbert Kleber, Investigating alternative medicine therapies in randomized controlled trials. *JAMA* (1998) 280:1626–8; and Mahesh Patel, Evaluation of alternative medicine. *SSM* (1987) 24:169–75. Also see: Anne Coulter, Alternative and Complementary Therapies presents an objective response to a recent *New York Times* series that disparages alternative medicine. *ACT* (1996) 2: 253–8; Foundation for Integrated Medicine, *Integrated Healthcare: A Way Forward for the Next Five Years?* (no city: Foundation for Integrated Medicine, 1997), 10; and Pizzorno and Snider (n. 42), 188.

50. Joseph Pizzorno, Natural medicine approach to the treatment of cystitis. *ACT* (1994) 1:32–4; Pizzorno and Snider (n. 42), 188; Vincent and Furnham (n. 48), 166; Eliot Marshall, The politics of alternative medicine. *Science* (1994) 265:2000–2, p. 2000.

51. James Harvey Young, The development of the Office of Alternative Medicine in the National Institutes of Health, 1991–1996. *BHM* (1998) 72:279–98, pp. 279–82, 290; Paul Trachtman, NIH looks at the implausible and the inexplicable. *Smithsonian* (1994) 25:110–23, p. 121; Walter Wardwell, Limited and marginal practitioners. In: Howard Freeman, Sol Levine, and Leo Reeder, editors, *Handbook of Medical Sociology*, 3d edition (Englewood Cliffs, NJ: Prentice-Hall, 1979), 230–50, p. 241.

52. Young (n. 51), 280–1; Baynan McDowell, The National Institutes of Health Office of Alternative Medicine. *ACT* (1994–5) 1:17–25; Charles Marwick, Advisory group insists on "alternative" voice. *JAMA* (1994) 272:1239–40.

53. Young (n. 51), 290, 293; McDowell (n. 52), 19–21; Robert Park and Ursula Goodenough, Buying snake oil with tax dollars. *New York Times* (January 3, 1996), A11; Lisa Stiffler, On science's frontier—or fringe? *Seattle Post-Intelligencer* (May 10, 2001), A1, A5.

54. Alterations are ahead at the OAM. *JAMA* (1998) 280:1553; McDowell (n. 52), 17.

CONCLUSION

1. Tom Delbanco, Leeches, spiders, and astrology: Predilections and predictions. *JAMA* (1998) 280:1560–2, p. 1560; Wayne Jonas, Alternative medicine—learning from the past, examining the present, advancing to the future. *JAMA* (1998) 280:1616–7, p. 1617.

2. See me, feel me, touch me, heal me. *Life* (September 1996), 121:34–50, p. 40. For discussion of possible futures for alternative medicine, see Institute for Alternative Futures, *The Future of Complementary and Alternative Approaches (CAAs) in U.S. Health Care* (Des Moines, IA: NCMIC Insurance Company, 1998).

3. Michael Sergeant, Medical school courses in alternative medicine. *JAMA* (1999) 281:609–10; Eliot Marshall, The politics of alternative medicine. *Science* (1994) 265:2000–2; Kathleen Finn, Seattle first to open natural medicine public health clinic. *Delicious!* (November 1995), 12–3; Timothy Egan, Seattle officials seeking to establish a subsidized natural medicine clinic. *New York Times* (January 3, 1996), A6; David Holzman, Seattle's new alternative medicine clinic. *ACT* (1996) 3:176–8; Cindy Breed, The King County Natural Medicine Clinic—a preliminary report. *JNM* (1997) 7:90. On the role of cost in the appeal of alternative medicine, see Adrian White, Do complementary therapies offer value for money? In: Edzard Ernst, editor, *Complementary Medicine: An Objective Appraisal* (Oxford: Butterworth-Heinemann, 1996), 89–105; and Foundation for Integrated Medicine, *Integrated Healthcare. A Way Forward for the Next Five Years?* (no city: Foundation for Integrated Medicine, 1997).

4. Mike Maharry, Insurance companies study their alternatives. *Tacoma News Tribune* (January 1, 1996), A1; Eileen Stretch and Nancy Faass, The evolution of integrative medicine in Washington State. In: Nancy Faass, editor, *Integrating Complementary Medicine Into Health Systems* (Gaithersburg, MD: Aspen, 2001), 32–5; John Weeks, Major trends in the integration of complementary and alternative medicine. In: Faass, editor, 4–11, p. 6.

5. Washington State Hospital Association, "Mainstreaming Alternative Medicine" (November 6, 1995), Tukwila, Washington; Kristin White, The Richard and Hinda Rosenthal Center for Alternative/Complementary Medicine. *ACT* (1994–5) 1:158–64; Major

metropolitan hospital establishes alternative medicine department. *ACT* (1998) 4:224; The White House Commission on Complementary and Alternative Medicine Policy. In: Nancy Faass, editor, *Integrating Complementary Medicine Into Health Systems* (Gaithersburg, MD: Aspen, 2001), 167; Jacqueline Wootton, The White House Commission on Complementary and Alternative Medicine Policy: Meeting on the access to, and delivery of, complementary and alternative medical services. *JACM* (2001) 7:109–10.

6. The University of Arizona Program in Integrative Medicine, 1996 announcement; Andrew Weil, The body's healing systems. *ACT* (1994–5) 1:305–10; Richard Horton, Andrew Weil: Working towards an integrated medicine. *Lancet* (1997) 350:1374. On the content and philosophy of Weil's program, see Tracy Gaudet, Integrative medicine: The evolution of a new approach to medicine and to medical education. *IM* (1998) 1:67–73.

7. Brian Berman, B. Krishna Singh, Lixing Lao, Betsy Singh, Kevin Ferentz, and Susan Hartnoll, Physicians' attitudes toward complementary or alternative medicine: A regional survey. *JABFP* (1995) 8:361–6, p. 363; Jeffrey Borkan, Jon Neher, Ofra Anson, and Bret Smoker, Referrals for alternative therapies. *JFP* (1994) 39:545–50; Mary Burg, Shae Kosch, Allen Neims, and Eleanor Stoller, Personal use of alternative medicine therapies by health science center faculty. *JAMA* (1998) 280:1563; James quoted by Annie Riley Hale, *These Cults* (New York: National Health Foundation, 1926), 34.

8. Richard Claridge, A letter from Graefenberg. *WCJ* (1846) 2:1–7, pp. 4–5; Russell Trall, Results of hydropathy. *WCJHR* (1849) 8:21–3, p. 22; Edythe Ashmore, A toast to Dr. Still. *JAOA* (1910–11) 10:632–3; Benedict Lust, Naturopathic news. *Naturopath* (1925) 30:363–80, p. 366; Lust, Editorial drift. *NHH* (1902) 3:376–8, p. 377.

9. D. W. Cathell, Was it wise for the American Medical Association to change its code of ethics? *AM* (1903) 6:618–20, p. 619; John Forbes, A review of hydropathy. In: Roland Houghton, editor, *Bulwer and Forbes on the Water-Treatment* (New York: Fowlers and Wells, 1851), 51–119, p. 54.

10. Anonymous, *The Anatomy of a Humbug, of the Genus Germanicus, Species Homoeopathia* (New York: Author, 1837), 7; John Nichols, Medical sectarianism. *JAMA* (1913) 60:331–7, p. 333; See (n. 2), 46.

11. William Leo-Wolf, *Remarks on the Abracadabra of the Nineteenth Century* (New York: Carey, Lea and Blanchard, 1835), 260; Thomas Blatchford, *Homoeopathy Illustrated* (Albany, NY: Van Benthuysen, 1851), 76.

12. John Astin, Why patients use alternative medicine. *JAMA* (1998) 279:1548–53; Adrian Furnham, Why do people choose and use complementary therapies? In: Edzard Ernst, editor, *Complementary Medicine: An Objective Appraisal* (Oxford: Butterworth-Heinemann, 1996), 71–88, p. 73; Robert Avina and Lawrence Schneiderman, Why patients choose homeopathy. *WJM* (1978) 128:366–9.

13. Stretch and Faass (n. 4), 35.

14. Karen Rappaport, *Directory of Schools for Alternative and Complementary Health Care* (Phoenix, AZ: Oryx, 1998). The most extensive discussion of the practical problems to be solved in bringing about medical integration is Nancy Faass, editor, *Integrating Complementary Medicine Into Health Systems* (Gaithersburg, MD: Aspen, 2001). Also see Joanna Murray and Simon Shepherd, Alternative or additional medicine? A new dilemma for the doctor. *JRCGP* (1988) 38:511–4.

15. Abraham Flexner, *Medical Education in the United States and Canada* (New York: Carnegie Foundation for the Advancement of Teaching, 1910), 157; Phil Fontanarosa and George Lundberg, Alternative medicine meets science. *JAMA* (1998) 280:1618–9, p. 1618; Mark Tonelli and Timothy Callahan, Why alternative medicine cannot be evidence-based. *ACM* (2001) 76:1213–9.

16. Robert Anderson, On doctors and bonesetters in the sixteenth and seventeenth centuries. *CH* (1983) 3:11–5, p. 15; Joseph Pizzorno and Pamela Snider, Naturopathic medicine. In: Marc Micozzi, editor, *Fundamentals of Complementary and Alternative Medicine* (New York: Churchill Livingstone, 2001), 159–92, p. 189.

17. John Bastyr. *JNM* (1991) 2:40; Jared Zeff and Pamela Snider, *Report to the American Association of Naturopathic Physicians From the Select Committee on the Definition of Naturopathic Medicine*, September 1988 (Bastyr University Library); Pizzorno and Snider (n. 16), 173.

18. Hippocrates, *Hippocrates*, W.H.S. Jones, translator, 4 volumes (Cambridge, MA: Harvard University Press, 1948), 1: 165; Jason Lazarou, Bruce Pomeranz, and Paul Corey, Incidence of adverse drug reactions in hospitalized patients. *JAMA* (1998) 279:1200–5; David Bates, Drugs and adverse drug reactions. How worried should we be? *JAMA* (1998) 279:1216–7, p. 1217.

19. Paul Wendel, *Standardized Naturopathy* (Brooklyn, NY: Wendel, 1951), 59 (also see Stanley Lief, The germ fallacy. *NP* [1946] 50:551; and N. H. Blachman, The germ theory. *NP* [1946] 50:527); Patrick Bufi quoted in Zeff and Snider (n. 17), 79; physio-medical resolution quoted by John Haller Jr., *Kindly Medicine: Physio-Medicalism in America, 1836–1911* (Kent, OH: Kent State University Press, 1997), 114. For the concept of "terrain" in medicine, see Ilana Löwy, "The terrain is all": Metchnikoff's heritage at the Pasteur Institute, from Besredka's "antivirus" to Bardach's "orthobiotic serum." In: Christopher Lawrence and George Weisz, editors, *Greater Than the Parts: Holism in Biomedicine, 1920–1950* (New York: Oxford University Press, 1998), 257–82.

20. Frederick Kao, China, Chinese medicine, and the Chinese medical system. *AJCM* (1973) 1:1–59, pp. 3–4; Tom Monte, *World Medicine: The East-West Guide to Healing Your Body* (New York: Putnam, 1993); Gerard Bodeker, Global context. In: Marc Micozzi, editor, *Fundamentals of Complementary and Alternative Medicine* (New York: Churchill Livingstone, 2001), 72–83, p. 72.

21. Thomas Shepherd, From the president. In: *Bastyr University Catalog 2000/2001* (Bothel, WA: Bastyr University, 2000), 3; Paul Hoaken, Alternative medicine. *NEJM* (1984) 310:1196; René Dubos, Introduction. In: Norman Cousins, *Anatomy of an Illness as Perceived by the Patient* (New York: Norton, 1979), 11–23, p. 23.

22. Weeks (n. 4), 11.

23. Walter Johnson, *Homoeopathy: Popular Exposition and Defence of Its Principles and Practice* (London: Simpkin, Marshall, 1852), viii; John Bovee Dods, *The Philosophy of Mesmerism and Electrical Psychology* (London: Burns, 1886), 173.

24. Edward Purinton, Efficiency in drugless healing. In: Benedict Lust, editor, *Universal Naturopathic Encyclopedia Directory and Buyers' Guide Year Book of Drugless Therapy for 1918–19* (Butler, NJ: Lust, 1918), 65–165, p. 165.

Index